T0348397

2013
YEAR BOOK OF
NEONATAL AND
PERINATAL MEDICINE®

The 2013 Year Book Series

Year Book of Critical Care Medicine®: Drs Dries, Zanotti-Cavazzoni, Latenser, Martinez, Rincon, and Zwank

Year Book of Emergency Medicine®: Drs Hamilton, Bruno, Handly, Minczak, Quintana, and Ramoska

Year Book of Endocrinology®: Drs Schott, Apovian, Clarke, Eugster, Meikle, Oetgen, Ovalle, Schteingart, and Toth

Year Book of Hand and Upper Limb Surgery®: Drs Yao, Adams, Isaacs, and Rizzo

Year Book of Medicine®: Drs Barker, Garrick, Gersh, Khardori, LeRoith, Panush, Talley, and Thigpen

Year Book of Neonatal and Perinatal Medicine®: Drs Fanaroff, Benitz, Donn, Neu, Papile, and Van Marter

Year Book of Neurology and Neurosurgery®: Drs Klimo, Minagar, Gandhi, Liu, Panagariya, Rezania, Riel-Romero, Riesenburger, Robottom, Schwendimann, Shafazand, and Yang

Year Book of Obstetrics, Gynecology, and Women's Health®: Drs Dungan and Shulman

Year Book of Oncology®: Drs Arceci, Bauer, Chiorean, Gordon, Lawton, Murphy, Thigpen, and Tsao

Year Book of Ophthalmology®: Drs Rapuano, Cohen, Flanders, Hammersmith, Milman, Myers, Nagra, Nelson, Penne, Pyfer, Sergott, Shields, Talekar, and Vander

Year Book of Orthopedics®: Drs Morrey, Huddleston, Rose, Swiontkowski, and Trigg

Year Book of Otolaryngology-Head and Neck Surgery®: Drs Sindwani, Balough, Franco, Gapany, and Mitchell

Year Book of Pathology and Laboratory Medicine®: Drs Raab and Bissell

Year Book of Pediatrics®: Dr Stockman

Year Book of Plastic and Aesthetic Surgery™: Drs Miller, Boehmler, Gosman, Gutowski, Ruberg, Salisbury, and Smith

Year Book of Psychiatry and Applied Mental Health®: Drs Talbott, Ballenger, Buckley, Frances, Krupnick, and Mack

Year Book of Pulmonary Disease®: Drs Barker, Jones, Maurer, Spradley, Tanoue, and Willsie

Year Book of Sports Medicine®: Drs Shephard, Cantu, Feldman, Galea, Jankowski, Janssen, Lebrun, and Nieman

2013

The Year Book of
NEONATAL AND
PERINATAL
MEDICINE®

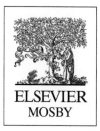

ELSEVIER
MOSBY

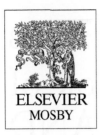

ELSEVIER
MOSBY

Vice President, Global Medical Reference: Mary Gatsch
Editor: Kerry Holland
Production Supervisor, Electronic Year Books: Donna M. Skelton
Electronic Article Manager: Mike Rainey
Illustrations and Permissions Coordinator: Dawn Vohsen

Printed and bound by CPI Group (UK) Ltd, Croydon, CR0 4YY

Transferred to digital print 2012

Editorial Office:
Elsevier
Suite 1800
1600 John F. Kennedy Blvd.
Philadelphia, PA 19106-3399

International Standard Serial Number: 8756-5005
International Standard Book Number: 978-1-4557-7278-0

Editorial Board

Contributing Editors

David H. Adamkin, MD
Professor of Pediatrics; Director of Division of Neonatology; Director of Nutritional Research; Rounsavall Chair of Neonatal Medicine; Co-Director of Neonatal Fellowship, University of Louisville, Louisville, Kentucky

Vishnu Priya Akula, MD
Neonatology Fellow, Stanford University, Palo Alto, California

Mohammad Attar, MD
Associate Professor, Department of Pediatrics and Infectious Disease, University of Michigan, Ann Arbor, Michigan

Heather H. Burris, MD, MPH
Instructor in Pediatrics, Division of Newborn Medicine, Boston Children's Hospital; Attending Neonatologist, Department of Neonatology, Beth Israel Deaconess Medical Center, Boston, Massachusetts

Helen Christou, MD
Assistant Professor of Pediatrics, Harvard Medical School; Associate Director, Harvard Perinatal-Neonatal Fellowship Program; Brigham and Women's Hospital and Boston Children's Hospital, Boston, Massachusetts

Karl Coe Desch, MD
Assistant Professor, Department of Pediatrics and Communicable Diseases, Division of Neonatal-Perinatal Medicine, University of Michigan, C.S. Mott Children's Hospital, Ann Arbor, Michigan

Judy A. Estroff, MD
Chief, Fetal-Neonatal Imaging, Department of Radiology, Advanced Fetal Care Center, Boston Children's Hospital; Associate Professor of Radiology, Harvard Medical School, Boston, Massachusetts

Jonathan M. Fanaroff, MD, JD
Associate Professor of Pediatrics, Case Western Reserve University School of Medicine; Director, Rainbow Center for Pediatric Ethics; Co-Director, Neonatal Intensive Care Unit, Rainbow Babies & Children's Hospital, Cleveland, Ohio

Sandra Fucile, OTR, PhD
Division of Neonatology, Department of Pediatrics, University of Florida College of Medicine, Gainesville, Florida

A. Greenough, MD
Professor of Neonatology and Clinical Respiratory Physiology, Division of Asthma, Allergy and Lung Biology, MRC-Centre for Allergic Mechanisms in Asthma, King's College London, London, United Kingdom

Thor Willy Ruud Hansen, MD, PhD, MHA, FAAP
FAAP Professor, Department of Neonatology, Women's & Children's Division; Director of Clinical Ethics; Director of Pediatric Education; Associate Director of Academic Pediatrics, Faculty of Medicine, University of Oslo, Oslo, Norway

Jonathan Hellmann, MBBCh, FCP(SA), FRCPC, MHSc
Professor of Paediatrics, University of Toronto; Staff Neonatologist, The Hospital for Sick Children, Toronto, Ontario, Canada

Naomi Laventhal, MD, MA
Assistant Professor, Department of Pediatrics and Communicable Diseases, Division of Neonatal-Perinatal Medicine, University of Michigan, C.S. Mott Children's Hospital, Ann Arbor, Michigan

M. Jeffrey Maisels MD, DSc
Chair Emeritus and Professor; Director, Academic Affairs, Department of Pediatrics, Oakland University William Beaumont School of Medicine, Royal Oak, Michigan

Camilia R. Martin, MD, MS
Assistant Professor of Pediatrics, Harvard Medical School; Associate Director, NICU, Department of Neonatology; Director for Cross-Disciplinary Research Partnerships, Division of Translational Research Beth Israel Deaconess Medical Center, Boston, Massachusetts

Richard J. Martin, MD
Drusinsky-Fanaroff Chair in Neonatology, Rainbow Babies & Children's Hospital; Professor of Pediatrics, Case Western Reserve University, Cleveland, Ohio

Matthew F. Niedner, MD
Assistant Professor of Pediatrics & Communicable Diseases, Pediatric Critical Care Medicine & Pediatric Palliative Care Service, University of Michigan Medical Center, C.S. Mott Children's Hospital, Ann Arbor, Michigan

Ola Didrik Saugstad, MD, PhD, FRCPE
Professor of Pediatrics; Director, Department of Pediatric Research, Oslo University Hospital, University of Oslo, Oslo, Norway

Sadath Sayeed, MD
Assistant Professor of Global Health and Social Medicine and Pediatrics, Harvard Medical School, Division of Newborn Medicine, Boston Children's Hospital, Boston, Massachusetts

Nidhi Agrawal Shah, MD
Clinical Fellow, Department of Neonatology, Stanford University, Lucille Packard Children's Hospital, Palo Alto, California

Seetha Shankaran, MD
Professor of Pediatrics, Wayne State University School of Medicine; Director, Neonatal-Perinatal Medicine, Children's Hospital of Michigan and Hutzel Women's Hospital, Detroit Michigan

Faye S. Silverstein, MD
Professor, Pediatrics and Neurology, University of Michigan, Ann Arbor, Michigan

Martha Sola-Visner, MD
Attending Neonatologist, Boston Children's Hospital; Assistant Professor of Pediatrics, Harvard Medical School, Boston, Massachusetts

Sohini Stone, MD, MBA
Stanford University, Department of Neonatal and Developmental Medicine, Palo Alto, California

Win Tin, FRCPCH
Consultant Neonatologist, The James Cook University Hospital, Middlesbrough, United Kingdom

Table of Contents

Journals Represented

Journals represented in this YEAR BOOK are listed below.
Acta Obstetricia et Gynecologica Scandinavica
Acta Paediatrica
American Journal of Cardiology
American Journal of Clinical Nutrition
American Journal of Obstetrics and Gynecology
American Journal of Perinatology
American Journal of Physiology, Gastrointestinal and Liver Physiology
Anaesthesia and Intensive Care
Annals of Neurology
Archives of Disease in Childhood Fetal and Neonatal Edition
Archives of Pediatrics & Adolescent Medicine
British Journal of Obstetrics and Gynaecology
British Journal of Ophthalmology
British Journal of Surgery
British Medical Journal
Canadian Medical Association Journal
Childs Nervous System
Clinical Endocrinology
Dermatologic Therapy
Disease Models & Mechanisms
European Respiratory Journal
Gastroenterology
Genome Biology
Human Reproduction
Intensive Care Medicine
International Journal of Cardiology
Journal of Child Psychology and Psychiatry
Journal of Clinical Endocrinology & Metabolism
Journal of Clinical Psychiatry
Journal of Medical Ethics
Journal of Neurosurgery Pediatrics
Journal of Parenteral and Enteral Nutrition
Journal of Pediatric Gastroenterology and Nutrition
Journal of Pediatric Surgery
Journal of Pediatrics
Journal of Perinatology
Journal of Surgical Research
Journal of the American Medical Association
Journal of the American Medical Association Pediatrics
Journal of the American Medical Association Otolaryngology, Head & Neck Surgery
Journal of Urology
Journal of Women's Health (Larchmt)
Lancet
Medical Care
Nephrology Dialysis Transplantation
New England Journal of Medicine
Nutrition in Clinical Practice

Obstetrics & Gynecology
Pediatric Cardiology
Pediatric Emergency Care
Pediatric Infectious Disease Journal
Pediatric Physical Therapy
Pediatric Radiology
Pediatric Research
Pediatrics
Placenta
Prenatal Diagnosis
Proceedings of the National Academy of Sciences of the United States of America
Public Library of Science One
Respiratory Care
Thrombosis Research
Ultrasound in Obstetrics & Gynecology

STANDARD ABBREVIATIONS

The following terms are abbreviated in this edition: acquired immunodeficiency syndrome (AIDS), cardiopulmonary resuscitation (CPR), central nervous system (CNS), cerebrospinal fluid (CSF), computed tomography (CT), deoxyribonucleic acid (DNA), electrocardiography (ECG), health maintenance organization (HMO), human immunodeficiency virus (HIV), intensive care unit (ICU), intramuscular (IM), intravenous (IV), magnetic resonance (MR) imaging (MRI), ribonucleic acid (RNA), and ultrasound (US).

NOTE

The YEAR BOOK OF NEONATAL AND PERINATAL MEDICINE® is a literature survey service providing abstracts of articles published in the professional literature. Every effort is made to assure the accuracy of the information presented in these pages. Neither the editors nor the publisher of the YEAR BOOK OF NEONATAL AND PERINATAL MEDICINE® can be responsible for errors in the original materials. The editors' comments are their own opinions. Mention of specific products within this publication does not constitute endorsement.

To facilitate the use of the YEAR BOOK OF NEONATAL AND PERINATAL MEDICINE® as a reference tool, all illustrations and tables included in this publication are now identified as they appear in the original article. This change is meant to help the reader recognize that any illustration or table appearing in the YEAR BOOK OF NEONATAL AND PERINATAL MEDICINE® may be only one of many in the original article. For this reason, figure and table numbers will often appear to be out of sequence within the YEAR BOOK OF NEONATAL AND PERINATAL MEDICINE®.

Introduction

This is the 27th edition of the YEAR BOOK OF NEONATAL AND PERINATAL MEDICINE, and it is loaded with a variety of manuscripts and critical comments reflecting the issues foremost on practitioners' problem lists. Whereas once again there has been no sea change or wow publication in the past 12 months, we, the editors, have included a wealth of information that focuses on key topics ranging from fetal diagnosis and therapy to a comprehensive section on perinatal ethics. Recent research has highlighted the variation in attitudes to end-of-life decision making and important influences on this that cross different continents and cultures. Accurate information on outcomes for infants born at the edges of viability is critical to informing management decisions. The importance a single day makes at this time period is documented by the difference in outcomes between the first and second half of the 23rd week of gestation. Whenever available, we have selected appropriately powered, randomized, controlled trials and have also included a smattering of meta-analyses and Cochrane reviews. There is an abundance of information on short-term survival and long-term neurodevelopmental outcome of term and preterm infants with due attention to the longer term outcomes of newer therapies, such as hypothermia for neuroprotection. This issue has extensive coverage on hyperbilirubinemia, including the economic impact of universal screening, value of phototherapy, benefits of transcutaneous measurements, and the prevalence of kernicterus. The gastrointestinal tract and nutrition section dominates the 2013 YEAR BOOK. There is detailed coverage of the benefits of human milk, the growing importance of the gut microbiome, the value of probiotics and, of course, various considerations in the diagnosis, prevention, management, and long-term outcome of necrotizing enterocolitis.

We all strive to provide palatable perspective and insight into the thorny, persistent problems in neonatal perinatal medicine. Our goal is not only to present the current state of the art, but also to pose questions that will stimulate further research to fill the gaps that continue to exist. We are forever grateful to our colleagues who lent their expertise to the process in order to enhance the quality of the book. We thank Kerry Holland, our editor, for her continued assistance and for helping us to complete our task on time. In the electronic era, it is vital that commentaries are completed each quarter rather than with a flurry of activity at the end of the cycle. Kerry has helped considerably in accomplishing this task. We thank the Elsevier team for their professionalism and support in producing this book.

"It is not the strongest of the species that survives, nor the most intelligent that survives. It is the one that is the most adaptable to change."

—Charles Darwin

Avroy A. Fanaroff, MD

1 The Fetus

4D ultrasound evaluation of fetal facial expressions during the latter stages of the second trimester

Kanenishi K, Hanaoka U, Noguchi J, et al (Kagawa Univ School of Medicine, Miki, Japan; Kagawa Prefectural College of Health Sciences, Takamatsu, Japan; et al)

Int J Gynecol Obstet 121:257-260, 2013

Objective.—To assess the frequency of fetal facial expressions at 25–27 weeks of gestation using 4D ultrasound.

Methods.—Twenty-four normal fetuses were examined using 4D ultrasound. The face of each fetus was recorded continuously for 15 minutes. The frequencies of tongue expulsion, yawning, sucking, mouthing, blinking, scowling, and smiling were assessed and compared with those observed at 28–34 weeks of gestation in a previous study.

Results.—Mouthing was the most common facial expression at 25–27 weeks of gestation; the frequency of mouthing was significantly higher than that of the other 6 facial expressions ($P < 0.05$). Yawning was significantly more frequent than the other facial expressions, apart from mouthing ($P < 0.05$). The frequencies of yawning, smiling, tongue expulsion, sucking, and blinking differed significantly between 25–27 and 28–34 weeks ($P < 0.05$).

Conclusion.—The results indicate that facial expressions can be used as an indicator of normal fetal neurologic development from the second to the third trimester. 4D ultrasound may be a valuable tool for assessing fetal neurobehavioral development during gestation (Fig 2).

▶ Fetal behavior is defined as any fetal action seen by the mother or fetus diagnosed by objective methods, such as cardiotocography or ultrasound scan. Observations made with 4-dimensional (4D) ultrasound scan suggest that fetal behavior reflects development and maturation of the central nervous system, and abnormal fetal behavior patterns make possible the early recognition of fetal brain impairment. More data are accumulating on these 4D assessments, and the normal patterns are being defined.

Kurjak et al,[1,2] prime movers in this field, have detected variations in facial expression frequency in the second and third trimesters. The frequencies of all of the examined facial expressions peaked during the latter stages of the second trimester, except for that of isolated eye blinking, which increased at the start of week 24. This has been further defined in the study abstracted above, with evidence of maturation of the brain in the third trimester (Fig 2). The fetuses

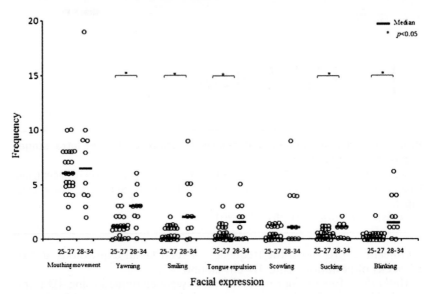

FIGURE 2.—Comparison of the frequency of each fetal facial expression between 25–27 and 28–34 weeks of gestation. Data regarding frequencies of fetal facial expressions at 28–34 weeks were obtained from a previous study. (Reprinted from International Journal of Gynecology and Obstetrics. Kanenishi K, Hanaoka U, Noguchi J, et al. 4D ultrasound evaluation of fetal facial expressions during the latter stages of the second trimester. *Int J Gynecol Obstet.* 2013;121:257-260, Copyright 2013, with permission from Elsevier.)

are even smiling. What they are smiling about is, of course, still a mystery. In the study by Yigiter and Kavak,[3] the frequencies of yawning, sucking, swallowing, smiling, mouthing, and tongue expulsion were highest at 24 to 32 weeks, whereas grimacing peaked at 28 to 36 weeks and eye blinking peaked after week 32.

It is fascinating to start discovering fetal behavior and the cues that we might be able to read indicating abnormal brain development. Remember that these studies are only done for an intense 15 to 20 minutes, and the interpretation of the 4D images are subjective. Studies validating the interobserver variability and reliability of fetal facial expressions are needed. However, we are finally validating Prechtl's suggestion[4] that we would be able to study fetal behavior.

A. A. Fanaroff, MBBCh, FRCPE

References

1. Kurjak A, Andonotopo W, Hafner T, et al. Normal standards for fetal neurobehavioral developments—longitudinal quantification by four-dimensional sonography. *J Perinat Med.* 2006;34:56-65.
2. Kurjak A, Abo-Yaqoub S, Stanojevic M, et al. The potential of 4D sonography in the assessment of fetal neurobehavior—multicentric study in high-risk pregnancies. *J Perinat Med.* 2010;38:77-82.
3. Yigiter AB, Kavak ZN. Normal standards of fetal behavior assessed by four-dimensional sonography. *J Matern Fetal Neonatal Med.* 2006;19:707-721.
4. Prechtl HF. State of the art of a new functional assessment of the young nervous system. An early predictor of cerebral palsy. *Early Hum Dev.* 1997;50:1-11.

Microcystic congenital pulmonary airway malformation with hydrops fetalis: steroids vs open fetal resection

Loh KC, Jelin E, Hirose S, et al (Univ of California at San Francisco)
J Pediatr Surg 47:36-39, 2012

Background/Purpose.—Congenital pulmonary airway malformations (CPAM) are rare lesions often diagnosed during routine prenatal ultrasound. The presence of hydrops fetalis is an indicator of poor prognosis. Here we present a retrospective review of fetuses undergoing either open fetal surgery or steroids for predominantly microcystic CPAM with hydrops fetalis.

Method.—A retrospective review of patients undergoing open fetal surgery or steroids for CPAM at our institution was performed. The primary outcome was survival.

Results.—A retrospective review of all patients referred to our institution with the diagnosis of CPAM was performed. Fetuses with predominantly microcystic CPAM and the presence of hydrops fetalis treated with steroid or surgery were included. Thirteen patients were treated with steroids, and 11 patients underwent open fetal surgery. In the steroid group 12 (92%) of 13 fetuses survived to delivery versus 9 (82%) of 11 in the open fetal surgery group. Only 5 (56%) of 9 of the patients in the open fetal surgery group survived to neonatal discharge compared to 10 (83%) of 12 in the steroid group.

Conclusions.—In the present retrospective study, improved survival was seen in fetuses with hydrops fetalis and predominantly microcystic CPAM treated with steroids when compared with open fetal surgery. Steroids should be considered for first-line therapy in these cases.

▶ The authors retrospectively describe their experience with the rare, but life-threatening fetal condition of hydrops occurring secondary to very large fetal lung masses in 24 fetuses, 13 of whom were given glucocorticoids in an attempt to reverse the hydrops, and 11 of whom underwent open fetal surgery to resect the causative lesion. This article discusses neonatal outcomes in terms of survival until birth and also discharge home from the hospital.

This article is important because, before attempts at intervention, either pharmacologically or surgically, a hydropic fetus with a lung mass was nearly certain to die in utero. Those who had open fetal surgery often delivered early and did not survive the neonatal period because of the combination of immature lungs and reduced residual lung tissue, leaving very little functioning lung to support life.

Nomenclature has changed significantly in the past several years, and there is now some degree of consensus to term all fetal lung masses as congenital pulmonary airway malformations. This change reflects our fairly recent understanding that the previously separated entities of congenital cystic adenomatoid malformation, sequestration (intralobar and extralobar), and bronchogenic cyst are pathologically part of a spectrum of airway and lung malformations. Those that appear completely or predominately solid in nature and echogenic, or brighter, on sonography are termed "microcystic." This appearance is more often associated with an increased risk for fetal hydrops when the lesion reaches a certain proportional, large size in relation to fetal gestational age.

Before this article, there were small reports of cases or series in which administration of steroids to the pregnant patient reversed or ameliorated fetal hydrops, leading to increased survival, both in utero and after birth. For a condition that even in the most experienced hands most often resulted in fetal death, the option to administer steroids offers great hope.

J. Estroff, MD

The risks of selective serotonin reuptake inhibitor use in infertile women: a review of the impact on fertility, pregnancy, neonatal health and beyond

Domar AD, Moragianni VA, Ryley DA, et al (Harvard Med School, Waltham, MA; et al)
Hum Reprod 1-12, 2012

Study Question.—What is the current literature on the safety and efficacy of selective serotonin reuptake inhibitor (SSRI) use in infertile women?

Summary Answer.—There is little evidence that infertile women benefit from taking an SSRI, therefore they should be counseled appropriately about the risks and be advised to consider alternate safer treatments to treat depressive symptoms.

What is Known Already.—SSRI use is associated with possible reduced infertility treatment efficacy as well as higher rates of pregnancy loss, preterm birth, pregnancy complications, neonatal issues and long-term neurobehavioral abnormalities in offspring.

Study Design, Size, Duration.—Review of existing literature.

Participants/Materials, Setting, Methods.—We conducted a review of all published studies that evaluate females with depressive symptoms who are taking antidepressant medications and who are experiencing infertility.

Main Results and the Role of Chance.—Antidepressant use during pregnancy is associated with increased risks of miscarriage, birth defects, preterm birth, newborn behavioral syndrome, persistent pulmonary hypertension of the newborn and possible longer term neurobehavioral effects. There is no evidence of improved pregnancy outcomes with antidepressant use. There is some evidence that psychotherapy, including cognitive-behavioral therapy as well as physical exercise, is associated with significant decreases in depressive symptoms in the general population; research indicates that some forms of counseling are effective in treating depressive symptoms in infertile women.

Limitations, Reasons for Caution.—Our findings are limited by the availability of published studies in the field, which are often retrospective and of small size.

Wider Implications of the Findings.—Practitioners who care for infertility patients should have a thorough understanding of the published literature so that they can adequately counsel their patients.

▶ This is a review article by a group of maternal fetal medicine specialists, aiming to examine the available evidence for the use of selective serotonin reuptake inhibitors (SSRIs) in women undergoing infertility treatment and during pregnancy. Because no randomized, controlled studies have been conducted, a review article is as close to a meta-analysis as we will probably get and, given the widespread use of SSRIs, it is worth evaluating the important issues it raises. It is estimated that up to 13.7% of pregnant women have taken SSRIs during pregnancy. Most commonly prescribed antidepressants are classified as Pregnancy Category C, which implies that they can be taken if the perceived benefits outweigh the risks. A notable exception is paroxetine (Pregnancy Category D because of the association with congenital heart disease). This review article highlights the risks associated with SSRI use but also questions the efficacy of SSRI treatment in cases of mild-to-moderate depression. Citing well-conducted individual studies and meta-analyses, the authors make a well-supported argument that the risk-benefit ratio is likely unfavorable and urge health care providers either to consider alternatives to SSRIs, or, if unable to avoid them, to at least inform patients of the well-described risks associated with their use. These risks include reduced efficacy of infertility treatments, increased risk of preeclampsia, and pregnancy loss. For infants exposed to SSRIs in utero, the risks include low birth weight, respiratory distress, persistent pulmonary hypertension of the newborn, birth defects, newborn behavioral syndrome, and long-term neurobehavioral abnormalities, including autism.

H. Christou, MD

Can we select fetuses with intra-abdominal calcification for delivery in neonatal surgical centres?
Zerhouni S, Mayer C, Skarsgard ED (Univ of British Columbia, Vancouver, Canada)
J Pediatr Surg 48:946-950, 2013

Background.—Prenatal ultrasound (US) diagnosis of fetal intra-abdominal calcification (iAC) is frequently caused by an in utero perforation causing meconium peritonitis. Our ability to predict which fetuses will require postnatal surgery is limited. The aim of our study is to correlate iAC and associated US findings with postnatal outcome.

Methods.—A single centre retrospective review of all cases of fetal iAC diagnosed between 2004 and 2010 was performed. Maternal demographics, fetal US findings, and outcomes (need for surgery and mortality) were collected. Descriptive and comparative statistical analyses were performed.

Results.—Twenty-three cases of iAC were identified. There were no cases of fetal demise or postnatal deaths. Three liveborns (13%) required abdominal surgery at a median of 2 days (0—3) for intestinal atresia. US findings of iAC and dilated bowel with ($p = 0.008$) or without ($p = 0.005$) polyhydramnios predicted a need for postnatal surgery as did the combination of iAC, polyhydramnios, and ascites ($p = 0.008$). Conversely, iAC alone or associated with oligohydramnios, polyhydramnios, ascites, or growth restriction did not predict need for postnatal surgery.

Conclusion.—The majority of fetuses with iAC on prenatal US do not require surgery. Associated US findings (bowel dilation) can be used to select fetuses for delivery in neonatal surgical centres.

▶ Intra-abdominal calcifications (iAC) and other echogenic masses are relatively common findings during fetal sonography. Many are associated with no additional risk for the fetus or neonate. They may arise from the liver, gallbladder, spleen, kidneys, adrenal glands, gastrointestinal tract, or peritoneal cavity. The initial consideration when calcifications are visualized within the fetal abdomen is whether they are scattered in the abdomen and/or associated with a mass, or if they are in the liver.

The prenatal diagnosis of fetal iAC can be easily made with prenatal ultrasound scan (US). Whereas the initial thoughts may turn to cystic fibrosis with meconium ileus and intrauterine perforation, the differential diagnosis of iAC is quite broad. Conditions to be taken into consideration include congenital infection, tumors such as neuroblastoma or Wilms tumor, hemangiomata, gall stones, hepatic calcification, and aneuploidy. Other US features, such as a karyotype and gene array and infectious screening including polymerase chain reaction, usually permit exclusion of cases in which the calcification is caused by something other than meconium peritonitis (MP). Assuming this exclusion, the finding of iAC is most likely caused by fetal intestinal perforation resulting in a sterile chemical inflammatory response. This report, the largest series to date, was undertaken to identify those infants with iAC that need to deliver at the surgical center. Prior reports of the outcome of prenatally diagnosed MP had used variable diagnostic criteria and were initially associated with limited technical US capability.

Kamata et al reported 20 cases of MP collected over a 17-year period, all of which required surgery.[1] However, among this group, only 5 (25%) had iAC reported on prenatal US, with the rest having ascites or pseudocyst as the predominant sonographic findings. A similar observation was made, in the largest published series to date, of 38 patients with a prenatal diagnosis of MP, of whom 31 required postnatal surgery; yet, only 8 fetuses (21%) were reported to have iAC.[2] In reviewing their indications for early surgery and, therefore, the candidates for delivery at the perinatal center if iAC is present, Zerhouni identified those fetuses with iAC together with fetal bowel dilation (and possibly ascites and polyhydramnios). Fetuses with iAC as a solitary finding were, in their experience, unlikely to require surgical intervention.

An allied condition to intra-abdominal calcification is the condition of hyperechoic colon. Amat et al[3] noted that the presence of a hyperechoic colon at routine US before 36 weeks of gestation should prompt screening for cystinuria at birth, whereas later observation (> 36 weeks) of this finding does not appear to be related to any disease.

A. A. Fanaroff, MBBCh, FRCPE

References

1. Kamata S, Nose K, Ishikawa S, et al. Meconium peritonitis in utero. *Pediatr Surg Int.* 2000;16:377-379.
2. Nam SH, Kim SC, Kim DY, et al. Experience with meconium peritonitis. *J Pediatr Surg.* 2007;42:1822-1825.
3. Amat S, Czerkiewicz I, Benoist J-F, Eurin D, Fontanges M, Muller F. Isolated hyperechoic fetal colon before 36 weeks' gestation reveals cystinuria. *Ultrasound Obstet Gynecol.* 2011;38:543-547.

Use of magnetic resonance imaging in prenatal prognosis of the fetus with isolated left congenital diaphragmatic hernia
Victoria T, Bebbington MW, Danzer E, et al (The Children's Hosp of Philadelphia, PA)
Prenat Diagn 32:715-723, 2012

Objectives.—To investigate the prognostic value of magnetic resonance-calculated fetal lung volumes (FLV) in fetuses with isolated left congenital diaphragmatic hernia (L-CDH) who receive standardized prenatal and postnatal care at a single institution.

Materials and Methods.—A retrospective review was undertaken to identify fetuses with isolated L-CDH between 2001 and 2010.

Results.—Eighty-five cases of isolated L-CDH were identified. The overall survival was 65% (55/85). Survival was 45% if there was 'liver up' (23/51) and 94% if there was 'liver down' (32/34). Univariate statistical analysis showed that 'liver up' ($p = 0.001$), lung-to-head ratio (LHR) at diagnosis ($p = 0.009$), observed/expected (O/E) LHR ($p = 0.01$), total FLV ($p = 0.03$), right LV ($p = 0.04$), magnetic resonance imaging (MRI) observed versus expected (O/E) FLV ($p = 0.002$), intrathoracic versus intra-abdominal stomach ($p = 0.002$), percentage of herniated liver ($p = 0.004$), and postnatal extracorporeal membrane oxygenation use ($p = 0.001$) are predictive of postnatal survival. Multivariate analysis of only prenatal factors showed that the most important determinants of postnatal outcome are percentage of herniated liver, presence of liver up, and MRI O/E FLV.

Conclusion.—Herniated intrathoracic liver expressed as 'liver up' or as percent herniated liver and MRI measurement of FLV expressed as a O/E ratio are strong prenatal indicators of postnatal survival.

▶ Though relatively rare, congenital diaphragmatic hernia remains one of the most life-threatening fetal malformations, especially when the liver is up in the chest and residual lung becomes hypoplastic as a result. With the widespread use of fetal sonography and magnetic resonance imaging (MRI), many diaphragmatic hernias are identified in utero. Though it makes intuitive sense that when more abdominal organs are herniated into the chest, less lung will be available to oxygenate the newborn, it has been difficult for fetal centers to predict which fetuses will survive and which will not, despite the availability of and willingness to offer all manner of heroic measures. These heroic measures have included: open surgical in utero repair, fetal tracheal occlusion (either by placing a clip across the trachea or a balloon within the lumen) with the goal of forcing the lungs to grow, delivering the fetus by the EXIT procedure (ex utero intrapartum treatment, in which the fetus is partially delivered but the umbilical cord is not cut, leaving the fetus/infant on placental circulation), and ECMO (extracorporeal membrane oxygenation, a form of heart-lung bypass). These heroic procedures involve maternal and fetal risk and are not offered unless the prediction of pulmonary hypoplasia is likely.

Attempts to estimate fetal lung volumes have been frustrating and difficult to reproduce from center to center. Though many centers have published articles on this topic, this paper from a high-volume fetal center meticulously evaluates the current major approaches to predicting fetal outcome, including the fetal sonographic measure of lung—head ratio (LHR) and the MRI determined: observed to expected (O/E) LHR, total fetal lung volume, intrathoracic vs intra-abdominal stomach, and the percentage of herniated liver. Necessity of postnatal ECMO use is also evaluated as a predictor of outcome. Results in this work validate the previous concepts that MRI-derived fetal lung volumes are helpful and adds the new information that the presence of an intrathoracic stomach worsens prognosis, as does the percent of intrathoracic liver.

J. Estroff, MD

Prenatal diagnosis and outcome of fetal posterior fossa fluid collections
Gandolfi Colleoni G, Contro E, Carletti A, et al (Univ of Bologna, Italy; et al)
Ultrasound Obstet Gynecol 39:625-631, 2012

Objective.—To evaluate the accuracy of fetal imaging in differentiating between diagnoses involving posterior fossa fluid collections and to investigate the postnatal outcome of affected infants.

Methods.—This was a retrospective study of fetuses with posterior fossa fluid collections, carried out between 2001 and 2010 in two referral centers for prenatal diagnosis. All fetuses underwent multiplanar neurosonography. Parents were also offered fetal magnetic resonance imaging (MRI) and karyotyping. Prenatal diagnosis was compared with autopsy or postnatal MRI findings and detailed follow-up was attempted by consultation of medical records and interview with parents and pediatricians.

Results.—During the study period, 105 fetuses were examined, at a mean gestational age of 24 (range, 17—28) weeks. Sonographic diagnoses (Blake's pouch cyst, $n = 32$; megacisterna magna, $n = 27$; Dandy—Walker malformation, $n = 26$; vermian hypoplasia, $n = 17$; cerebellar hypoplasia, $n = 2$; arachnoid cyst, $n = 1$) were accurate in 88% of the 65 cases in which confirmation was possible. MRI proved more informative than ultrasound in only 1/51 cases. Anatomic anomalies and/or chromosomal aberrations were found in 43% of cases. Blake's pouch cysts and megacisterna magna underwent spontaneous resolution in utero in one third of cases and over 90% of survivors without associated anomalies had normal developmental outcome at 1—5 years. Isolated Dandy—Walker malformation and vermian hypoplasia were associated with normal developmental outcome in only 50% of cases.

Conclusion.—Prenatal neurosonography and MRI are similarly accurate in the categorization of posterior fossa fluid collections from mid gestation. Blake's pouch cyst and megacisterna magna are risk factors for associated anomalies but when isolated have an excellent prognosis, with a high probability of intrauterine resolution and normal intellectual development in almost all cases. Conversely, Dandy—Walker malformation and vermian hypoplasia, even when they appear isolated antenatally, are associated with an abnormal outcome in half of cases.

▶ Fluid collections in the fetal posterior fossa encompass a wide spectrum of entities ranging from normal variants to severe anomalies. In this retrospective, observational report, the authors evaluated the diagnostic accuracy of fetal neurosonography and magnetic resonance imaging in 106 fetuses with posterior fossa fluid collections and assessed the outcomes of affected infants.

The most common diagnosis was Blake's pouch cyst (32%), followed by megacisterna magna (26%). Intrauterine regression of the abnormal posterior fossa findings was documented in 27% of the fetuses. Chromosomal aberrations and genetic syndromes were noted in 6% of the fetuses and an additional 23% were noted to have cerebral abnormalities alone. Termination of the pregnancy occurred in 18% of the cases, the majority of which had a fetus identified with Dandy-Walker malformation. Of the 65 cases in which there was confirmation of the diagnosis either postnatally or at autopsy, there was harmonization in 88%. There was 1 false-positive diagnosis and discordance in the diagnosis for 7 additional fetuses. Additional evaluation with fetal magnetic resonance was completed for 51 cases and there was only 1 case in which the diagnosis differed from that ascertained with neurosonography. Because neurological development was not evaluated in a uniform manner, but rather abstracted from medical charts and interviews with parents and primary care providers, the reliability of the follow-up data is uncertain. Nevertheless, the most relevant result of the study is the demonstration that fetal ultrasonography is as accurate as fetal magnetic resonance in the diagnosis and categorization of posterior fossa fluid collections in the fetus.

L. A. Papile, MD

In Utero Closure of Myelomeningocele Does Not Improve Lower Urinary Tract Function
Lee NG, Gomez P, Uberoi V, et al (Children's Hosp Boston, MA; et al)
J Urol 188:1567-1571, 2012

Purpose.—Recent data comparing prenatal to postnatal closure of myelomeningocele showed a decreased need for ventriculoperitoneal shunting and improved lower extremity motor outcomes in patients who underwent closure prenatally. A total of 11 children whose spinal defect was closed in utero were followed at our spina bifida center. We hypothesized that in utero repair of myelomeningocele improves lower urinary tract function compared to postnatal repair.

Materials and Methods.—Eleven patients who underwent in utero repair were matched to 22 control patients who underwent postnatal repair according to age, gender and level of spinal defect. Urological outcomes were retrospectively reviewed including urodynamic study data, need for clean intermittent catheterization, use of anticholinergic agents and prophylactic antibiotics, and surgical history. The need for ventriculoperitoneal shunting or spinal cord untethering surgery was also reviewed.

Results.—Mean followup was 7.2 years for patients who underwent in utero repair and 7.3 years for those who underwent postnatal repair. Mean patient age at compared urodynamic studies was 5.9 years for in utero repair and 6.0 years for postnatal repair. The in utero repair group was comprised of 5 lumbar and 6 sacral level defects with equal matching (1:2) in the postnatal repair cohort. There were no differences between the groups in terms of need for clean intermittent catheterization, incontinence between catheterizations or anticholinergic/antibiotic use. Urodynamic parameters including bladder capacity, detrusor pressure at capacity, detrusor overactivity and the presence of detrusor sphincter dyssynergia were not significantly different between the groups. There was no difference in the rate of ventriculoperitoneal shunting ($p = 0.14$) or untethering surgery ($p = 0.99$).

Conclusions.—While in utero closure of myelomeningocele has been shown to decrease rates of ventriculoperitoneal shunting and improve motor function, it is not associated with any significant improvement in lower urinary tract function compared to repair after birth.

▶ Publication of the Management of Myelomeningocele Study (MOMS Trial) results in 2011 represents a landmark in the history of fetal therapies, providing the first demonstration that intrauterine fetal surgery could substantially improve postnatal outcomes.[1] In that trial, prenatal repair of open myelomeningocele reduced the prevalence of hindbrain herniation and the need for placement of cerebrospinal fluid shunts by 12 months of age and led to better mental development and motor function, including higher rates of independent ambulation at 30 months of age. However, prenatal surgery was associated with increased rates of preterm delivery and uterine dehiscence at delivery. Other case-control and retrospective case series reports have described similar encouraging results, tempered by concerns about increased rates of fetal death, premature birth, chorioamnionitis, premature rupture of membranes, oligohydramnios, and respiratory distress syndrome requiring assisted ventilation. Whether early benefits are sustained through later childhood and the extent to which they offset maternal and neonatal complications remain uncertain, however. This case-control analysis begins to provide information for at least one aspect of this multifaceted condition. These investigators found no differences in urodynamic testing performed at 6 years of age as well as equal rates of surgery to correct spinal cord tethering. Like infants treated with postnatal closure, most infants treated with prenatal surgery required intermittent bladder catheterization, anticholinergic agents, and a bowel regimen, indicating that prenatal surgery does not fully salvage bowel and bladder function. Although the sample size was modest, these results do not appear to simply reflect a lack of statistical power. These observations are of general importance for 3 reasons: (1) we must await longer-term follow-up of MOMS trial subjects regarding outcomes, including ventriculoperitoneal shunting, orthopedic and gross motor function, and neurodevelopmental/cognitive performance; (2) vigilant management of affected infants is still necessary after in utero myelomeningocele repair; and (3) counseling of women considering prenatal interventions must still be circumspect, reflecting ongoing uncertainty about the optimal approach to management of these pregnancies. For the moment, this treatment should be offered at a limited number of sites to ensure comprehensive capture of long-term outcomes and to maximize the opportunity for technical refinements, such as migration from open to endoscopic surgical methods.

W. E. Benitz, MD

Reference

1. Adzick NS, Thom EA, Spong CY, et al. A randomized trial of prenatal versus postnatal repair of myelomeningocele. *N Engl J Med.* 2011;364:993-1004.

Outcome of infants presenting with echogenic bowel in the second trimester of pregnancy

Buiter HD, Holswilder-Olde Scholtenhuis MA, Bouman K, et al (Univ of Groningen, The Netherlands)
Arch Dis Child Fetal Neonatal Ed 98:F256-F259, 2013

Objective.—Fetal echogenic bowel (FEB) is a soft marker found on second trimester sonography. Our main aim was to determine the outcome of infants who presented with FEB and secondarily to identify additional sonographic findings that might have clinical relevance for the prognosis.

Design.—We reviewed all pregnancies in which the diagnosis FEB was made in our Fetal Medicine Unit during 2009-2010 (N=121). We divided all cases into five groups according to additional sonographic findings. Group 1 consisted of cases of isolated FEB, group 2 of FEB associated with dilated bowels, group 3 of FEB with one or two other soft markers, group 4 of FEB with major congenital anomalies or three or more other soft markers, and group 5 consisted of FEB with isolated intrauterine growth restriction (IUGR).

Results.—Of 121 cases, five were lost to follow-up. Of the remaining 116 cases, 48 (41.4%) were assigned to group 1, 15 (12.9%) to group 2, 15 (12.9%) to group 3, 27 (23.2%) to group 4, and 11 (9.5%) to group 5. The outcome for group 1 was uneventful. In group 2 and 3, two anomalies, anorectal malformation and cystic fibrosis, were detected postnatally (6.7%). In group 4, mortality and morbidity were high (78% resp. 22%). Group 5 also had high mortality (82%) and major morbidity (18%).

Conclusions.—If FEB occurs in isolation, it is a benign condition carrying a favourable prognosis. If multiple additional anomalies or early IUGR are observed, the prognosis tends to be less favourable to extremely poor.

▶ Progressive improvements in fetal imaging offer the benefit of far greater knowledge of structural fetal abnormalities, enabling optimal preparation of caregivers and parents for each newborn's anticipated medical or surgical issues. The relative paucity of outcome studies in this new era of advance fetal imaging has created new uncertainty regarding optimal pregnancy and perinatal management. This is especially relevant for some conditions such as echogenic bowel (EB), the focus of a study by Buiter et al. Outcomes of 121 fetuses identified by prenatal ultrasonographic imaging as having EB were retrospectively reviewed. Most fetuses with isolated EB did well, regardless of the presence or absence of bowel dilation. Of the 48 fetuses in the group with isolated EB without bowel dilation and the 15 fetuses with EB and bowel dilation, 93% to 94% had no additional major pathology identified after birth. The group at greatest risk of demise was composed of fetuses whose EB was accompanied by fetal growth restriction. At intermediate risk of fetal mortality were those with EB accompanied by evidence of a major congenital anomaly or more than 2 less-severe abnormalities, and these infants were at greatest risk of major postnatal morbidity. The relatively reassuring data concerning fetuses with isolated EB, with or without bowel dilation, will prove highly valuable to those engaged in antenatal counseling and fetal and neonatal management and, hopefully, will lead to lower rates of iatrogenic preterm birth among this population of infants.

L. J. Van Marter, MD, MPH

2 Epidemiology and Pregnancy Complications

Pregnancy complications among women born preterm
Boivin A, Luo Z-C, Audibert F, et al (Univ of Montréal, Québec, Canada; et al)
CMAJ 184:1777-1784, 2012

Background.—Adults who were born with low birth weights are at increased risk of cardiovascular and metabolic conditions, including pregnancy complications. Low birth weight can result from intrauterine growth restriction, preterm birth or both. We examined the relation between preterm birth and pregnancy complications later in life.

Methods.—We conducted a population-based cohort study in the province of Quebec involving 7405 women born preterm (554 <32 weeks, 6851 at 32–36 weeks) and a matched cohort of 16 714 born at term between 1976 and 1995 who had a live birth or stillbirth between 1987 and 2008. The primary outcome measures were pregnancy complications (gestational diabetes, gestational hypertension, and preeclampsia or eclampsia).

Results.—Overall, 19.9% of women born at less than 32 weeks, 13.2% born at 32–36 weeks and 11.7% born at term had at least 1 pregnancy complication at least once during the study period ($p < 0.001$). Women born small for gestational age (both term and preterm) had increased odds of having at least 1 pregnancy complication compared with women born at term and at appropriate weight for gestational age. After adjustment for various factors, including birth weight for gestational age, the odds of pregnancy complications associated with preterm birth was elevated by 1.95-fold (95% confidence interval [CI] 1.54–2.47) among women born before 32 weeks' gestation and 1.14-fold (95% CI 1.03–1.25) among those born at 32–36 weeks' gestation relative to women born at term.

Interpretation.—Being born preterm, in addition to, and independent of, being small for gestational age, was associated with a significantly increased risk of later having pregnancy complications.

▶ Women born with either low birth weight or who were preterm are at increased risk of pregnancy-induced hypertension, preeclampsia, and gestational diabetes.[1,2] In the above observational study, the investigators examined the effects of maternal preterm birth and intrauterine growth restriction separately on later pregnancy complications. In addition, they examined whether there is a dose-response relationship, with the more prematurely born women having the greatest risk of pregnancy complications (ie, gestational diabetes, pregnancy-induced hypertension, or preeclampsia/eclampsia).

The study was based on record linkage of administrative birth-related data files from 3 separate databases. Women born preterm were matched 1:2 with a cohort of women who were born at term according to year of birth and singleton vs twin status. Maternal gestational age at birth was collected from birth certificates and weight percentile for gestational age was calculated using Canadian reference charts. Women born preterm were stratified into 2 gestational age categories, less than 32 weeks and 32 to 36 weeks.

The percentage of women with at least one pregnancy complication increased significantly with decreasing gestational age at their own birth ($P < .001$ for trend). Restricting the analysis to singleton women with a singleton first live delivery yielded similar results. Chronic medical conditions, such as hypertension and type 2 diabetes, were significantly increased in the cohort of preterm women (adjusted odds ratio [OR], 1.70; 95% confidence interval [CI], 1.32–2.20 and adjusted OR 1.75, 95% CI, 1.12–2.73, respectively), and these conditions were, in turn, associated with a significantly increased risk of pregnancy complications. Among women born small for gestational age, the occurrence and OR of a least one pregnancy complication was increased but was essentially the same for the preterm and term cohorts. Although the study does not include data regarding the outcomes of the pregnancies, most likely there was an increased risk of neonatal complications among infants delivered to women born preterm. The results of the study suggest that a woman's gestational age at birth needs to be taken into account when planning her obstetric care.

L. A. Papile, MD

References

1. Zetterström K, Lindberg S, Haglund B, Magnuson A, Hanson U. Being born small for gestational age increases the risk of severe pre-eclampsia. *BJOG*. 2007;114:319-324.
2. Innes KE, Marshall JA, Byers TE, Calonge N. A woman's own birth weight and gestational age predict her later risk of developing preeclampsia, a precursor of chronic disease. *Epidemiology*. 1999;10:153-160.

Cerclage Pessary for Preventing Preterm Birth in Women with a Singleton Pregnancy and a Short Cervix at 20 to 24 Weeks: A Randomized Controlled Trial

Hui SA, Chor CM, Lau TK, et al (The Chinese Univ of Hong Kong, China; Paramount Clinic, Hong Kong SAR, China)
Am J Perinatol 30:283-288, 2013

Objective.—To determine the effectiveness of cerclage pessary in the prevention of preterm birth in asymptomatic Chinese women with a short cervix at 20 to 24 weeks.

Methods.—Low-risk women carrying singleton pregnancies were screened with transvaginal ultrasound, and those with a cervical length <25 mm at 20 to 24 weeks were recruited into a randomized controlled trial, comparing the prophylactic use of cerclage pessary with expectant management. The analysis was by intent-to-treat. The primary outcome measure was preterm delivery before 34 weeks.

Results.—Among 4438 screened women, 203 women (4.6%) met the inclusion criteria and 108 (58%) consented for the study. A total of 53 and 55 women were allocated to pessary and control groups, respectively. There was no difference in background demographics, including the mean cervical length (19.6 mm versus 20.5 mm) and the mean gestational age at randomization (both 21.9 weeks). Delivery before 34 weeks occurred in 9.4% and 5.5% ($p = 0.46$) in the pessary and the control groups, respectively. No differences in major side effects were noted between the groups.

Conclusion.—In our population, <5% had a cervical length of less than 25 mm at 20 to 24 weeks' gestation. The prophylactic use of cerclage pessary did not reduce the rate of preterm delivery before 34 weeks.

▶ Preterm birth (delivery at less than 37 weeks of gestation) is the leading cause of infant mortality worldwide. Despite our best efforts, the rates of prematurity have declined very slowly. Because many of the preterm births are late preterm (70 + %) there is hope that major progress will be made in the near future.

Preterm labor is a multifactorial problem. The current treatment options are symptomatic, rather than causally directed, and the primary objective is to delay delivery long enough for a full course of antenatal corticosteroids to be administered. This has been accomplished with several tocolytic drugs with different mechanisms of action (betamimetics, oxytocin antagonists, calcium-channel blockers). Preventive treatment with progesterone can lower the rate of preterm birth in selected high-risk groups by more than 30%. Premature rupture of the membranes is an indication for antibiotics.

The abstract from Hui et al is yet another failed trial for prevention of preterm labor in an identified high-risk population. It has become fashionable to treat a short cervix with rest and progesterone, but the results there too have been inconsistent. It is time to try new approaches, and the application of the human genome is the logical step.

Data are now accumulating on the important role for genetics in the timing of the onset of human labor. The use of modern genomic approaches, such as genomewide association studies, rare variant analyses using whole exome or genome sequencing, and family-based designs, holds enormous potential.[1] Some progress has been made in the search for causative genes and variants associated with preterm birth, but, and it is a big "but," the major genetic determinants remain to be identified. Further advances will depend on the identification of biomarkers for earlier detection of preterm labor as well as the development of effective therapeutic agents to inhibit labor when fetal compromise is not an issue.

A. A. Fanaroff, MBBCh, FRCPE

Reference

1. Bezold KY, Karjalainen MK, Hallman M, Teramo K, Muglia LJ. The genomics of preterm birth: from animal models to human studies. *Genome Med.* 2013;5:34.

Tocolytic therapy for preterm delivery: systematic review and network meta-analysis

Haas DM, Caldwell DM, Kirkpatrick P, et al (Indiana Univ School of Medicine, Indianapolis; Univ of Bristol, UK)
BMJ 345:e6226, 2012

Objective.—To determine the most effective tocolytic agent at delaying delivery.

Design.—Systematic review and network meta-analysis.

Data Sources.—Cochrane Central Register of Controlled Trials, Medline, Medline In-Process, Embase, and CINAHL up to 17 February 2012.

Study Selection.—Randomised controlled trials of tocolytic therapy in women at risk of preterm delivery.

Data Extraction.—At least two reviewers extracted data on study design, characteristics, number of participants, and outcomes reported (neonatal and maternal). A network meta-analysis was done using a random effects model with drug class effect. Two sensitivity analyses were carried out for the primary outcome; restricted to studies at low risk of bias and restricted to studies excluding women at high risk of preterm delivery (those with multiple gestation and ruptured membranes).

Results.—Of the 3263 titles initially identified, 95 randomized controlled trials of tocolytic therapy were reviewed. Compared with placebo, the probability of delivery being delayed by 48 hours was highest with prostaglandin inhibitors (odds ratio 5.39, 95% credible interval 2.14 to 12.34) followed by magnesium sulfate (2.76, 1.58 to 4.94), calcium channel blockers (2.71, 1.17 to 5.91), beta mimetics (2.41, 1.27 to 4.55), and the oxytocin receptor blocker atosiban (2.02, 1.10 to 3.80). No class of tocolytic was significantly superior to placebo in reducing neonatal respiratory distress syndrome. Compared with placebo, side effects requiring a change of medication were significantly higher for beta mimetics (22.68, 7.51 to 73.67), magnesium sulfate (8.15, 2.47 to 27.70), and calcium channel blockers (3.80, 1.02 to 16.92). Prostaglandin inhibitors and calcium channel blockers were the tocolytics with the best probability of being ranked in the top three medication classes for the outcomes of 48 hour delay in delivery, respiratory distress syndrome, neonatal mortality, and maternal side effects (all cause).

Conclusions.—Prostaglandin inhibitors and calcium channel blockers had the highest probability of delaying delivery and improving neonatal and maternal outcomes.

▶ Efforts to inhibit labor have been in progress for more than 40 years. Fortunately, we are long past the use of alcohol as an inhibitor of labor and no longer have to witness drunk, puking women delivering prematurely. The initial goals of tocolysis were to inhibit premature labor with the hope that the pregnancy would continue to term. Unfortunately, this has not been the case, and the current goals are more modest; namely, to delay preterm delivery so that antenatal corticosteroids can be administered to improve neonatal outcomes. The authors have done an excellent literature review and meta-analysis. In a prior publication[1] they reported that of the 3197 titles initially identified, 89 randomized, controlled trials of tocolytic therapy were reviewed. Of the 6 quality areas, 10 trials (11.2%) satisfied all areas. Overall, 52 of the 89 trials (58.4%) achieved high-quality categorization. They concluded that the "larger trials, more recent trials and placebo-controlled trials were associated with higher quality scores." Caritis had commented: "In the absence of a single high quality, randomized, controlled trial comparing all tocolytic therapies, uncertainty remains about which is the most effective at delaying preterm delivery."[2] In their network meta-analysis of tocolytic therapy, prostaglandin inhibitors and calcium channel blockers had the highest probability of delaying delivery and improving neonatal outcomes.

It is somewhat distressing that most of the trials reviewed did not have much information on neonatal morbidity or mortality, and issues still need to be resolved regarding maternal and fetal safety. Haas' comment, "Reporting of clinically relevant outcome comparisons should be improved and made more consistent," is the obvious conclusion and is being addressed by the Maternal Fetal Network.

A. A. Fanaroff, MBBCh, FRCPE

References

1. Haas DM, Kirkpatrick P, McIntosh JJ, Caldwell DM. Assessing the quality of evidence for preterm labor tocolytic trials. *J Matern Fetal Neonatal Med.* 2012; 25:1646-1652.
2. Caritis SN. Metaanalysis and labor inhibition therapy. *Am J Obstet Gynecol.* 2011;204:95-96.

"Early" versus "late" 23-week infant outcomes
Nguyen TP, Amon E, Al-Hosni M, et al (Saint Louis Univ School of Medicine, MO)
Am J Obstet Gynecol 207:226.e1-226.e6, 2012

Objective.—To determine whether survival is different in "early" ($23^{0/7}$-$23^{3/7}$ weeks) vs "late" ($23^{4/7}$-$23^{6/7}$ weeks) infants.

Study Design.—Records of 126 consecutive liveborn infants delivered at $23^{0/7}$ to $23^{6/7}$ weeks' gestation from 2001-2010 were examined using the Vermont Oxford Network database. Infants born at 23 0/7 to 23 3/7 weeks were grouped into "early" and those at 23 4/7 to 23 6/7 weeks were "late." Clinical characteristics were compared between groups and multivariate analyses were used to predict survival.

Results.—Seventy-two infants were early and 54 were late. Survival was 25% vs 56%, respectively ($P < .001$). The early group was less likely to receive steroids (43% vs 65%; $P = .016$) and had a lower mean birthweight (547 g vs 596 g; $P < .001$). No difference in other factors was seen between groups. No change in survival was observed during the study period in either group.

Conclusion.—Late 23-week infants have improved survival compared with early infants. Delaying delivery as little as 24-96 hours may improve survival for 23-week infants.

▶ As mortality rates among extremely low-birth-weight infants have declined over the last 3 or 4 decades, the perceived "threshold of viability" has slowly migrated to earlier and earlier gestational ages. Recent data have shown the potential for survival after only 22 completed weeks and significant benefit from antenatal steroid administration for neonates born as early as 23 weeks of gestation.[1] Survival rates increase steeply with gestational age at this new threshold of viability, increasing from less than 20% at 22 weeks to approximately 50% at 24 weeks. Infants born at 23 weeks fare only slightly better than those born at 22 weeks, with about 10% surviving without neurodevelopmental impairment. These authors address the important question of whether there is a gradient of outcomes within this transitional group. Examining data accrued at a single center during the last decade, they identify a substantially greater survival rate among infants born late (23-4/7—23-6/7 weeks; 56% survival rate) compared with those delivered early (23-0/7—23-3/7 weeks; 25% survival rate). Overall survival rate of 38% is similar to those of other reports from that period. Morbidity among survivors (particularly chronic lung disease; rates of neurosensory impairment were not reported) was essentially universal, however, and did not differ between the early and late groups. It is not clear whether prolongation of pregnancy with tocolytic therapy will similarly improve survival rates when preterm birth is threatened soon after completion of the 23rd week, as these authors suggest, or if the ultimate outcomes will fulfill the hopes of parents. It is clear, however, that accurate counseling of parents at this critical point in gestation now requires outcome statistics that are more granular than those provided using the traditional 1-week gestational age strata.

W. E. Benitz, MD

Reference

1. Carlo WA, McDonald SA, Fanaroff AA, et al. Association of antenatal corticosteroids with mortality and neurodevelopmental outcomes among infants born at 22 to 25 weeks' gestation. *JAMA*. 2011;306:2348-2358.

Very Low Birth Weight Hospital Volume and Mortality: An Instrumental Variables Approach

Wehby GL, Ullrich F, Xie Y (Univ of Iowa, Iowa City; Merck and Co. Inc, Whitehouse Station, NJ)
Med Care 50:714-721, 2012

Background.—Previous studies of very low birth weight (VLBW) hospital volume effects on in-hospital mortality have used standard risk-adjusted models that only account for observable confounders but not for self-selection bias due to unobservable confounders.

Objective.—To assess the effects of hospital volume of VLBW infants on in-hospital mortality while explicitly accounting for unobservable confounders and self-selection bias using an instrumental variables (IV) model.

Methods.—The sample includes 4553 VLBW infants born in 63 hospitals in 2000—2004 in New Jersey. We use IV analysis with the differences between the patient's distances to the nearest low (<50 VLBW infants annually), moderate (51—100 infants annually), and high (>100 VLBW infants annually)-volume hospitals as instruments. We evaluate several volume measures and adjusted for observable infant and hospital characteristics.

Results.—We find beneficial volume effects on survival that are significantly underestimated in classic risk-adjusted models, under which low and moderate volumes compared with high volumes increase mortality odds by 1.8 and 1.88 times, respectively (risk ratios of 1.4 and 1.5, respectively). However, using the IV approach, we find that low and moderate volumes increase mortality odds by 5.42 and 3.51 times, respectively (risk ratios of 2.76 and 2.21, respectively). These findings suggest unobservable confounders that increase the selection of infants at a greater mortality risk into higher-volume hospitals.

Conclusions.—Accounting for unobserved self-selection bias reveals large survival benefits from delivering and treating VLBW infants at high-volume hospitals. This supports policies regionalizing the delivery and care for pregnancies at risk for VLBW at high-volume hospitals.

▶ For nearly 2 decades, we have had data from California showing an increased risk of mortality among very-low-birth-weight (VLBW) infants born at facilities with low-volume neonatal intensive care units, as identified by either average daily census less than 15[1] or admission of fewer than 100 VLBW infants per year.[2] This new analysis of statewide data from New Jersey for infants born between 2000 and 2004 replicates those results and suggests that the magnitude of the risk has been underestimated. Like others before them, the authors conclude that the results support regionalizing delivery of VLBW infants at high-volume hospitals (> 100 VLBW infants annually), noting that 225 (58%) of the 386 observed deaths could have been avoided had all infants been delivered at high-volume hospitals. Because preterm delivery is much less predictable than surgical anomalies, which often can be identified by ultrasonography and referred for delivery at a specialty center, this likely would require consolidation of entire delivery services, not merely selection of high-risk pregnancies for delivery at high-volume prematurity facilities. Geography and access to the site of delivery within 20 minutes of the place of residence for all pregnant women may prevent simple consolidation of small delivery centers to create high-volume centers, but the data from California—a state with nonurban areas much larger than those in New Jersey—indicate that 92% of VLBW infants are born in urban areas, but only 25% are delivered at high-volume centers.[2] The barriers to consolidation, therefore, are not simply geographic but likely relate to factors such as competition between hospitals (each of which may feel the need to provide level III neonatal intensive care unit services), compartmentalization of the health care system (such that separate facilities serve patients who are indigent or publically insured, those who are enrolled in integrated health maintenance organizations, and those covered by more traditional third-party payors), or a need to meet requirements for accreditation of training programs (such as residency programs in pediatrics or obstetrics and gynecology). Overcoming such barriers will likely require comprehensive reform of the American health care system, which does not appear to be on the horizon. The immediate challenge, then, appears to be gaining an understanding of why low-volume units perform worse, so that their outcomes can be raised to the level of the higher-volume units.

W. E. Benitz, MD

References

1. Phibbs CS, Bronstein JM, Buxton E, Phibbs RH. The effects of patient volume and level of care at the hospital of birth on neonatal mortality. *JAMA*. 1996;276: 1054-1059.
2. Phibbs CS, Baker LC, Caughey AB, Danielsen B, Schmitt SK, Phibbs RH. Level and volume of neonatal intensive care and mortality in very-low-birth-weight infants. *N Engl J Med*. 2007;356:2165-2175.

Causes of death in infants admitted to Australian neonatal intensive care units between 1995 and 2006
Feng Y, On behalf of the Neonatal Intensive Care Units (NICUS) Group of New South Wales and the Australian Capital Territory, Australia (Univ of New South Wales, Kensington, Australia; et al)
Acta Paediatr 102:e17-e23, 2013

Aim.—To compare causes and rates of mortality among infants admitted to 10 Australian neonatal intensive care units (NICUs) between 1995 and 2006.

Methods.—De-identified perinatal data from the Neonatal Intensive Care Units' (NICUS) Data Collection for 24 131 infants were examined for causes and rates of death. The study period was divided into two epochs: I (1995–2000, n = 11 185 infants) and II (2001–2006, n = 12 946 infants).

Results.—A total of 2224 (9.2%) infants died in hospital. Mortality decreased from 10.3% (1152/11 185) in epoch I to 8.3% (1072/12 946) in epoch II ($p < 0.001$) due to improved survival in term infants. Extreme

TABLE 2.—Causes of Death Between Different Groups of Infants

Conditions	Epoch I (n = 1152)	Epoch II (n = 1072)	p-value	Preterm (n = 1592)	Term (n = 632)	p-value	Outborn (n = 552)	Inborn (n = 1672)	p-Value
Cardiovascular failure	56 (4.9)	36 (3.4)	0.087	62 (3.9)	30 (4.7)	0.408	25 (4.5)	67 (4.0)	0.453
Chronic lung disease	25 (2.2)	21 (2.0)	0.767	45 (2.8)	1 (0.2)	<0.001	4 (0.7)	42 (2.5)	0.013
Congenital problems	252 (21.9)	226 (21.1)	0.679	221 (13.9)	257 (40.7)	<0.001	134 (24.3)	344 (20.6)	0.015
Extreme prematurity	118 (10.2)	76 (7.1)	0.008	194 (12.2)	—	—	21 (3.8)	173 (10.3)	<0.001
Haematological disorders	8 (0.7)	4 (0.4)	0.390	9 (0.6)	3 (0.5)	1	3 (0.5)	9 (0.5)	1
HIE	128 (11.1)	129 (12.0)	0.507	78 (4.9)	179 (28.3)	<0.001	139 (25.2)	118 (7.1)	<0.001
Infection	136 (11.8)	116 (10.8)	0.503	216 (13.6)	36 (5.7)	<0.001	42 (7.6)	210 (12.6)	0.004
IVH	80 (6.9)	112 (10.4)	0.003	189 (11.9)	3 (5.7)	<0.001	29 (5.3)	163 (9.7)	0.002
Maternal	3 (0.3)	6 (0.6)	0.327	8 (0.5)	1 (0.2)	0.459	1 (0.2)	8 (0.5)	0.695
NEC	47 (4.1)	58 (5.4)	0.161	98 (6.2)	7 (1.1)	<0.001	16 (2.9)	89 (5.3)	0.034
Neoplasm	6 (0.5)	8 (0.7)	0.596	10 (0.6)	4 (0.6)	1	6 (1.1)	8 (0.5)	0.112
Renal failure	19 (1.6)	20 (1.9)	0.748	28 (1.8)	11 (1.7)	1	6 (1.1)	33 (2.0)	0.102
Respiratory failure	217 (18.8)	188 (17.5)	0.441	338 (21.2)	67 (10.6)	<0.001	80 (14.5)	325 (19.4)	0.038
SIDS	13 (1.1)	14 (1.3)	0.704	24 (1.5)	3 (0.3)	0.051	9 (14.5)	18 (1.1)	0.256
Trauma	4 (0.3)	5 (0.5)	0.745	4 (0.3)	6 (0.9)	0.036	5 (0.9)	35 (0.3)	0.064
Unspecified	14 (1.2)	11 (1.0)	0.693	20 (12.5)	5 (0.8)	0.503	7 (1.3)	18 (1.1)	0.637

Data are presented as n (%).
HIE denotes hypoxic ischaemic encephalopathy; IVH, intraventricular haemorrhage; NEC, necrotizing enterocolitis and SIDS, sudden infant death syndrome.

prematurity also decreased as a primary cause of death (118 (10.2%) vs 76 (7.1%), $p = 0.008$). No infant > 42-week gestation was admitted in epoch II. Congenital abnormalities were the most common cause of death (>20%) in both epochs, mostly in term rather than preterm infants (40.7% vs 13.9%, $p < 0.001$). Age of death was unchanged between the two epochs (median 4, 1st, 3rd quartiles: 1,16 days).

Conclusion.—Mortality rates have continued to decrease but improvement is predominantly due to improved survival of term infants and prevention of postdate deliveries. Congenital abnormalities continue to be the most common cause of death (Table 2).

▶ National data trump regional data, which in turn trump local data. This impressive data analysis from Australia covers 2 epochs in the postsurfactant era. It is revealing in that it reaffirms reports that survival in very immature infants has essentially reached a plateau.[1,2] The improved mortality rates can be attributed to the elimination of postdate deliveries (beyond 42 weeks) and better outcomes for term and late preterm deliveries. In the developed world, congenital malformations have become the leading cause of neonatal mortality, surpassing disorders of short gestation and respiratory distress. As reported by Heron,[3] in the United States in 2008, the leading causes of infant death were, in rank order, congenital malformations, deformations, and chromosomal abnormalities; disorders related to short gestation and low birth weight, not elsewhere classified; sudden infant death syndrome; newborns affected by maternal complications of pregnancy; accidents (unintentional injuries); newborns affected by complications of placenta, cord, and membranes; bacterial sepsis of newborns; respiratory distress of newborns; diseases of the circulatory system; and neonatal hemorrhage. These data are very similar to the Australian data (Table 2) and have changed little since 2007.[4]

The take-home message is that there is still much work to be done to reduce neonatal mortality. Every effort must be exerted to reduce those conditions that can be prevented, such as birth asphyxia, birth trauma, and early onset infections. Avoidance of the major morbidities in preterm infants remains a daunting task, but we must be up to that challenge.

A. A. Fanaroff, MBBCh, FRCPE

References

1. Stoll BJ, Hansen NI, Bell EF, et al; Eunice Kennedy Shriver National Institute of Child Health and Human Development Neonatal Research Network. Neonatal outcomes of extremely preterm infants from the NICHD Neonatal Research Network. *Pediatrics.* 2010;126:443-456.
2. Horbar JD, Carpenter JH, Badger GJ, et al. Mortality and neonatal morbidity among infants 501 to 1500 grams from 2000 to 2009. *Pediatrics.* 2012;129: 1019-1026.
3. Heron M. Deaths: leading causes for 2008. *Natl Vital Stat Rep.* 2012;60:1-94.
4. Heron M. Deaths: leading causes for 2007. *Natl Vital Stat Rep.* 2011;59:1-95.

3 Genetics and Teratology

Clinical Diagnosis by Whole-Genome Sequencing of a Prenatal Sample
Talkowski ME, Ordulu Z, Pillalamarri V, et al (Massachusetts General Hosp, Boston; Brigham and Women's Hosp and Harvard Med School, Boston, MA; et al)
N Engl J Med 367:2226-2232, 2012

Conventional cytogenetic testing offers low-resolution detection of balanced karyotypic abnormalities but cannot provide the precise, gene-level knowledge required to predict outcomes. The use of high-resolution whole-genome deep sequencing is currently impractical for the purpose of routine clinical care. We show here that whole-genome "jumping libraries" can offer an immediately applicable, nucleotide-level complement to conventional genetic diagnostics within a time frame that allows for clinical action. We performed large-insert sequencing of DNA extracted from amniotic-fluid cells with a balanced de novo translocation. The amniotic-fluid sample was from a patient in the third trimester of pregnancy who underwent amniocentesis because of severe polyhydramnios after multiple fetal anomalies had been detected on ultrasonography. Using a 13-day sequence and analysis pipeline, we discovered direct disruption of *CHD7*, a causal locus in the CHARGE syndrome (coloboma of the eye, heart anomaly, atresia of the choanae, retardation, and genital and ear anomalies). Clinical findings at birth were consistent with the CHARGE syndrome, a diagnosis that could not have been reliably inferred from the cytogenetic breakpoint. This case study illustrates the potential power of customized whole-genome jumping libraries when used to augment prenatal karyotyping.

▶ The future is here: genome sequencing in the neonatal intensive care unit (NICU)! Well, in truth, this report focuses more on the obstetric suite than the NICU, describing the application of a genomic evaluation using whole genome jumping libraries for timely prenatal diagnosis of a specific defective chromosomal locus, confirming CHARGE syndrome (coloboma of the eye, heart anomaly, atresia of the choanae, retardation, and genital and ear anomalies) in a fetus for whom the diagnosis was suspected based on prenatal ultrasonographic findings. Such powerful, high-resolution diagnostic techniques are sure to provoke discussion, not only of the extraordinary relevant science, but also of the more mundane clinical aspects: defining appropriate use, implications for health care costs, and the ethical considerations relevant to genomic testing and other advanced diagnostic technologies.

L. J. Van Marter, MD, MPH

Chromosomal Microarray versus Karyotyping for Prenatal Diagnosis
Wapner RJ, Martin CL, Levy B, et al (Columbia Univ Med Ct, NY; Emory Univ School of Medicine, Atlanta, GA; et al)
N Engl J Med 367:2175-2184, 2012

Background.—Chromosomal microarray analysis has emerged as a primary diagnostic tool for the evaluation of developmental delay and structural malformations in children. We aimed to evaluate the accuracy, efficacy, and incremental yield of chromosomal microarray analysis as compared with karyotyping for routine prenatal diagnosis.

Methods.—Samples from women undergoing prenatal diagnosis at 29 centers were sent to a central karyotyping laboratory. Each sample was split in two; standard karyotyping was performed on one portion and the other was sent to one of four laboratories for chromosomal microarray.

Results.—We enrolled a total of 4406 women. Indications for prenatal diagnosis were advanced maternal age (46.6%), abnormal result on Down's syndrome screening (18.8%), structural anomalies on ultrasonography (25.2%), and other indications (9.4%). In 4340 (98.8%) of the fetal samples, microarray analysis was successful; 87.9% of samples could be used without tissue culture. Microarray analysis of the 4282 nonmosaic samples identified all the aneuploidies and unbalanced rearrangements identified on karyotyping but did not identify balanced translocations and fetal triploidy. In samples with a normal karyotype, microarray analysis revealed clinically relevant deletions or duplications in 6.0% with a structural anomaly and in 1.7% of those whose indications were advanced maternal age or positive screening results.

Conclusions.—In the context of prenatal diagnostic testing, chromosomal microarray analysis identified additional, clinically significant cytogenetic information as compared with karyotyping and was equally efficacious in identifying aneuploidies and unbalanced rearrangements but did not identify balanced translocations and triploidies. (Funded by the Eunice Kennedy Shriver National Institute of Child Health and Human Development and others; ClinicalTrials.gov number, NCT01279733.)

▶ This data set represents a significant contribution to the ever-expanding field of fetal diagnosis. Before this report, microarray analysis for prenatal studies had been confined to small studies of selected pregnancies at high risk for chromosomal anomalies. This large, masked trial tested the ability of microarray to detect the common abnormal karyotypes but also to see whether additional information would emerge. Microarray analysis was performed in a manner equivalent to standard karyotype analysis for the prenatal diagnosis of common aneuploidies and unbalanced rearrangements. In some regard, chromosome microarray analysis was superior and provided additional, clinically significant cytogenetic information compared with the standard karyotype but did not identify balanced translocations and triploidies. No doubt the chromosomal microarray will soon be a standard part of prenatal testing; however, we anticipate that the noninvasive approach, using maternal plasma, will gain traction and ultimately become the standard of care.[1-3] The authors were careful to point out that many variants now being recognized with these advanced technologies are of uncertain clinical significance and represent "a challenge for counseling and cause anxiety."

The ultimate goal is to discover genetic information about the fetus without incurring a health risk, that is, noninvasively. Kitzman et al[2] and Fan et al[3] showed that molecular counting of parental haplotypes in maternal plasma by shotgun sequencing of maternal plasma DNA allows the inherited fetal genome to be deciphered noninvasively. They also applied the counting principle directly to each allele in the fetal exome by performing exome capture on maternal plasma DNA before shotgun sequencing. They speculate that noninvasive determination of the fetal genome may ultimately facilitate the diagnosis of all inherited and de novo genetic disease. We eagerly anticipate that time.

A. A. Fanaroff, MBBCh, FRCPE

References

1. Bodurtha J, Strauss JF III. Genomics and perinatal care. *N Engl J Med*. 2012;366: 64-73.
2. Kitzman JO, Snyder MW, Ventura M, et al. Noninvasive whole-genome sequencing of a human fetus. *Sci Transl Med*. 2012;4:137ra76.
3. Fan HC, Gu W, Wang J, Blumenfeld YJ, El-Sayed YY, Quake SR. Non-invasive prenatal measurement of the fetal genome. *Nature*. 2012;487:320-324.

Reproductive Technologies and the Risk of Birth Defects
Davies MJ, Moore VM, Willson KJ, et al (Univ of Adelaide, South Australia, Australia)
N Engl J Med 366:1803-1813, 2012

Background.—The extent to which birth defects after infertility treatment may be explained by underlying parental factors is uncertain.

Methods.—We linked a census of treatment with assisted reproductive technology in South Australia to a registry of births and terminations with a gestation period of at least 20 weeks or a birth weight of at least 400 g and registries of birth defects (including cerebral palsy and terminations for defects at any gestational period). We compared risks of birth defects (diagnosed before a child's fifth birthday) among pregnancies in women who received treatment with assisted reproductive technology, spontaneous pregnancies (i.e., without assisted conception) in women who had a previous birth with assisted conception, pregnancies in women with a record of infertility but no treatment with assisted reproductive technology, and pregnancies in women with no record of infertility.

Results.—Of the 308,974 births, 6163 resulted from assisted conception. The unadjusted odds ratio for any birth defect in pregnancies involving assisted conception (513 defects, 8.3%) as compared with pregnancies not involving assisted conception (17,546 defects, 5.8%) was 1.47 (95% confidence interval [CI], 1.33 to 1.62); the multivariate-adjusted odds ratio was 1.28 (95% CI, 1.16 to 1.41). The corresponding odds ratios with in vitro fertilization (IVF) (165 birth defects, 7.2%) were 1.26 (95% CI, 1.07 to 1.48) and 1.07 (95% CI, 0.90 to 1.26), and the odds ratios with intracytoplasmic sperm injection (ICSI) (139 defects, 9.9%) were 1.77 (95% CI, 1.47 to 2.12) and 1.57 (95% CI, 1.30 to 1.90). A history of infertility, either with or without assisted conception, was also significantly associated with birth defects.

Conclusions.—The increased risk of birth defects associated with IVF was no longer significant after adjustment for parental factors. The risk of birth defects associated with ICSI remained increased after multivariate adjustment, although the possibility of residual confounding cannot be excluded. (Funded by the National Health and Medical Research Council and the Australian Research Council.)

▶ I had the pleasure of attending the birth of the first test tube baby born in Boston—a lovely, healthy, full-term girl, and that exciting and heartwarming experience consolidated my fascination with the science and potential of assisted reproductive technologies (ART). One of the questions often posed is whether, multiple gestations notwithstanding, babies born after ART are as healthy as their peers born after natural conception. Miraculously, most infants born after assisted conception are healthy. In a study of a South Australian population, Davies et al linked census data on treatment with ART and a registry of births and terminations at or beyond 20 weeks of gestation, finding increased risk of birth defects associated with assisted conception. Specific subcategories of birth defects were associated with ART in analyses adjusted for parental risk, including cerebral palsy and anomalies of the cardiovascular, musculoskeletal, urogenital, and gastrointestinal systems. In analyses adjusted for parental risk factors, the association between birth defects and intracytoplasmic sperm injection (ICSI) persisted but was no longer evident for in vitro fertilization (IVF). A somewhat counterintuitive finding is that both for IVF and ICSI, the risk of birth defects also was found to be reduced with frozen, compared with fresh, embryo cycles. This study might be criticized for grouping cerebral palsy (CP) together with congenital anomalies as birth defects and for omitting from multivariable models of CP some important potential confounding variables (eg, gestational age, condition at birth, neonatal comorbidities), yet this is a powerful, single-registry study that offers a thorough and detailed analysis of the relationship of ART to birth defects.

L. J. Van Marter, MD, MPH

Chromosomal Microarray versus Karyotyping for Prenatal Diagnosis

Wapner RJ, Martin CL, Levy B, et al (Columbia Univ Med Ctr, NY; Emory Univ School of Medicine, Atlanta, GA; et al)
N Engl J Med 367:2175-2184, 2012

Background.—Chromosomal microarray analysis has emerged as a primary diagnostic tool for the evaluation of developmental delay and structural malformations in children. We aimed to evaluate the accuracy, efficacy, and incremental yield of chromosomal microarray analysis as compared with karyotyping for routine prenatal diagnosis.

Methods.—Samples from women undergoing prenatal diagnosis at 29 centers were sent to a central karyotyping laboratory. Each sample was split in two; standard karyotyping was performed on one portion and the other was sent to one of four laboratories for chromosomal microarray.

Results.—We enrolled a total of 4406 women. Indications for prenatal diagnosis were advanced maternal age (46.6%), abnormal result on Down's syndrome screening (18.8%), structural anomalies on ultrasonography (25.2%), and other indications (9.4%). In 4340 (98.8%) of the fetal samples, microarray analysis was successful; 87.9% of samples could be used without tissue culture. Microarray analysis of the 4282 nonmosaic samples identified all the aneuploidies and unbalanced rearrangements identified on karyotyping but did not identify balanced translocations and fetal triploidy. In samples with a normal karyotype, microarray analysis revealed clinically relevant deletions or duplications in 6.0% with a structural anomaly and in 1.7% of those whose indications were advanced maternal age or positive screening results.

Conclusions.—In the context of prenatal diagnostic testing, chromosomal microarray analysis identified additional, clinically significant cytogenetic information as compared with karyotyping and was equally efficacious in identifying aneuploidies and unbalanced rearrangements but did not identify balanced translocations and triploidies. (Funded by the Eunice Kennedy Shriver National Institute of Child Health and Human Development and others; ClinicalTrials.gov number, NCT01279733.)

▶ The development of array-based molecular cytogenetic techniques has introduced a powerful new diagnostic tool into perinatal and neonatal medicine. In this benchmark report, Wapner et al compare chromosomal microarray analysis, sometimes referred to as *comparative genomic hybridization,* with conventional karyotyping for prenatal diagnosis of chromosomal anomalies using samples collected by amniocentesis or chorionic villus sampling. In a series of 4340 pregnancies in which both karyotype and microarray results were obtained, microarray analysis identified all 374 fetuses that had autosomal or sex-chromosome aneuploidy, showing a sensitivity of 100% (lower 95% confidence limit, 99%). Unbalanced translocations were also reliably detected (sensitivity, 100%; lower 95% confidence limit, 87%), but neither balanced translocations nor triploidies were identified (sensitivity 0%). Samples exhibiting mosaicism on karyotype were excluded, so information on microarray detection of such anomalies is not provided. As a bonus, however, microarray analysis also detected segmental copy number variants (CNV, consisting of microdeletions or duplications) in more than one-third of the samples (1399 of 3822). Most (1234) of these findings were deemed clinically inconsequential; of the remainder, 69 (4.9% of positive results) were likely to be benign, 61 (4.3% of positive results) potentially clinically significant, and only 35 (2.5% of positive results) definitely pathogenic. The failure rate for microarray analysis was less than 2%, which is comparable to that for karyotyping.

The potential for this testing to enhance quality of life is counterbalanced by new challenges, as this information is incorporated into clinical practice. The implications of trisomies, monosomies, and many translocations and deletions are already known, with well-defined phenotypic characteristics, penetrance, and expressivity. For some CNV, such as the diGeorge deletion, there is also ample experience to guide counseling. That is not true of many copy number variants, however, so the diagnostic and prognostic implications of these findings may remain uncertain. The significance of novel or rarely observed CNV will be unknown until similar experience accrues, so capture of genotype-phenotype correlations into a database—even (perhaps especially) if the phenotype is normal—will be essential, yet this may raise concerns about privacy. CNV discovered by screening may not have the same prognostic meaning as similar or identical findings drawn from patients with known disease, which likely reflect the more severe portion of the phenotypic range (availability of Fluorescence in situ hybridization for detection of the diGeorge deletion has illuminated the broad range of phenotypes in individuals with that CNV, for example), so the significance of CNV with known disease associations may be ambiguous. Documentation of the identical CNV in an apparently healthy parent cannot guarantee similar good health for the fetus or newborn, as the potential for phenotypic variation or for adult-onset disease remains. Parental confirmatory testing after discovery of a fetal CNV associated with adult-onset disease may lead to a diagnosis of a latent condition in a parent that he or she does not wish to know about. Uncertainty about CNV findings may lead to substantial anxiety, warranted or not, with unpredictable effects on parent-child interactions. Results of these tests, whether obtained for prenatal testing or after babies arrive in our nurseries, will increasingly be coming our way. We must approach discussions of these findings with parents with great circumspection, basing prognostic estimates on current access to the rapidly developing reservoir of phenotype-genotype correlations. These challenges will only be amplified by availability of whole genome sequencing as that technology moves into clinical application. Optimal care for these patients will require collaboration with our colleagues in genetics and genetic counseling, who will be very busy.

W. E. Benitz, MD

Clinical Genomic Database

Solomon BD, Nguyen A-D, Bear KA, et al (Natl Insts of Health, Bethesda, MD)
Proc Natl Acad Sci U S A 110:9851-9855, 2013

Technological advances have greatly increased the availability of human genomic sequencing. However, the capacity to analyze genomic data in a clinically meaningful way lags behind the ability to generate such data. To help address this obstacle, we reviewed all conditions with genetic causes and constructed the Clinical Genomic Database (CGD) (http:// research.nhgri.nih.gov/CGD/), a searchable, freely Web-accessible database of conditions based on the clinical utility of genetic diagnosis and the availability of specific medical interventions. The CGD currently includes a total of 2,616 genes organized clinically by affected organ systems and interventions (including preventive measures, disease surveillance, and medical or surgical interventions) that could be reasonably warranted by the identification of pathogenic mutations. To aid independent analysis and optimize new data incorporation, the CGD also includes all genetic conditions for which genetic knowledge may affect the selection of supportive care, informed medical decision-making, prognostic considerations, reproductive decisions, and allow avoidance of unnecessary testing, but for which specific interventions are not otherwise currently available. For each entry, the CGD includes the gene symbol, conditions, allelic conditions, clinical categorization (for both manifestations and interventions), mode of inheritance, affected age group, description of interventions/ rationale, links to other complementary databases, including databases of variants and presumed pathogenic mutations, and links to PubMed references (>20,000). The CGD will be regularly maintained and updated to keep pace with scientific discovery. Further content-based expert opinions are actively solicited. Eventually, the CGD may assist the rapid curation of individual genomes as part of active medical care (Table 1).

▶ The finished sequence of the Human Genome Project, published 50 years after Watson and Crick's seminal report on the structure of DNA, has made human genetics visible to the public eye and ushered in the genomic era. DNA sequencing technologies have grown at an astonishing rate and have become more standardized, automated, and capable of higher throughput. The costs continue to decline. Next-generation sequencing (NGS) approaches, such as whole-exome sequencing[1] and whole-genome sequencing, are rapidly becoming affordable genetic testing strategies for the clinical laboratory.

This article is not confined to neonatal perinatal medicine but was included because it can serve as a useful reference and resource. Remarkably, more than 2500 single gene disorders have been identified, and half of these are amenable to therapy (Table 1). One could be depressed by this statistic; however, I am encouraged, as I am of the opinion that more therapies will evolve as these disorders are better understood. Indeed, the new genetics not only leads to the identification of new causes of disease but is changing the way disease is classified and subsequently treated. "A single test can now provide vast amounts of health

TABLE 1.—Organization of the 2,616 Genes Included in the by Manifestation Categories and Intervention Categories

Category	Number of Genes in Manifestation Categories*	Number of Genes in Intervention Categories[†]
Allergy/Immunology/Infectious	272	251
Audiologic/Otolaryngologic	273	150
Biochemical	452	175
Cardiovascular	486	267
Craniofacial	384	0
Dental	95	0
Dermatologic	391	33
Endocrine	300	153
Gastrointestinal	393	106
General	45	1,291
Genitourinary	183	27
Hematologic	326	247
Musculoskeletal	801	43
Neurologic	1183	46
Obstetric	38	35
Oncologic	230	229
Ophthalmologic	566	51
Pharmacogenomic	0[‡]	186
Pulmonary	96	60
Renal	355	133

Values shown may differ from updated versions available on the CGD website. To reflect the multisystemic nature of many genetic disorders and to allow comprehensive browsing, each entry may be listed under multiple categories.

*Manifestation categories include organ systems that are primarily affected by mutations in the corresponding gene. Recognition of these affected systems may aid in condition recognition, as well as supportive care. Genes not categorized by organ systems within the Manifestation categories are included in the General category here.

[†]Intervention categories include organ systems for which specific medical interventions are available. Genes not meeting the described criteria for these specific interventions (see *Materials and Methods*) are included in the General category here.

[‡]Pharmacogenomic-related genes are all categorized under the Intervention categories rather than Manifestation categories.

information pertaining not only to the disease of interest, but information that may also predict adult-onset disease, reveal carrier status for a rare disease and predict drug responsiveness. The issue of what to do with these incidental findings, along with questions pertaining to NGS testing strategies, data interpretation and storage, and applying genetic testing results into patient care, remains without a clear answer."[2]

The clinical genomic database (CGD) will serve to disseminate information but is meant to be a live document with continual input from experts studying relevant genes and conditions.

"The first long-term objective is the establishment of a user friendly resource relevant to a wide group of clinicians that can be used as a reference resource in a variety of situations. Eventually, in addition to serving as a reference tool, the CGD may be used as a filter superimposed on automated binning algorithms to help allow efficient, clinically relevant annotation of human genomes." This is an important and relevant new database.

A. A. Fanaroff, MBBCh, FRCPE

References

1. Bamshad MJ, Ng SB, Bigham AW, et al. Exome sequencing as a tool for Mendelian disease gene discovery. *Nat Rev Genet.* 2011;12:745-755.
2. Williams ES, Hegde M. Implementing genomic medicine in pathology. *Adv Anat Pathol.* 2013;20:238-244.

Single *ABCA3* Mutations Increase Risk for Neonatal Respiratory Distress Syndrome

Wambach JA, Wegner DJ, DePass K, et al (Washington Univ School of Medicine, St Louis, MO; et al)
Pediatrics 130:e1575-e1582, 2012

Background and Objective.—Neonatal respiratory distress syndrome (RDS) due to pulmonary surfactant deficiency is heritable, but common variants do not fully explain disease heritability.

Methods.—Using next-generation, pooled sequencing of race-stratified DNA samples from infants ≥34 weeks' gestation with and without RDS ($n = 513$) and from a Missouri population-based cohort ($n = 1066$), we scanned all exons of 5 surfactant-associated genes and used in silico algorithms to identify functional mutations. We validated each mutation with an independent genotyping platform and compared race-stratified, collapsed frequencies of rare mutations by gene to investigate disease associations and estimate attributable risk.

Results.—Single *ABCA3* mutations were overrepresented among European-descent RDS infants (14.3% of RDS vs 3.7% of non-RDS; $P = .002$) but were not statistically overrepresented among African-descent RDS infants (4.5% of RDS vs 1.5% of non-RDS; $P = .23$). In the Missouri population-based cohort, 3.6% of European-descent and 1.5% of African-descent infants carried a single *ABCA3* mutation. We found no mutations among the RDS infants and no evidence of contribution to population-based disease burden for *SFTPC, CHPT1, LPCAT1,* or *PCYT1B.*

Conclusions.—In contrast to lethal neonatal RDS resulting from homozygous or compound heterozygous *ABCA3* mutations, single *ABCA3* mutations are overrepresented among European-descent infants ≥34 weeks' gestation with RDS and account for ~10.9% of the attributable risk among term and late preterm infants. Although *ABCA3* mutations are individually rare, they are collectively common among European-and African-descent individuals in the general population.

▶ Complex genetic traits, such as an individual's risk for neonatal respiratory distress syndrome (RDS), are determined by multiple gene variants, environmental effects (ie, gestational age), and interactions between genes and the environment. Recently, improvements in genotyping technology have allowed for the investigation of the role of millions of common genetic variants in human disease. Although many new variants have been discovered in these studies, most have failed to identify mutations that determine a significant portion of an individual's genetic risk for a disease.[1] Currently, studies are focusing on the role of uncommon or rare variants that can be identified through DNA sequencing or specialized genotyping but are usually not detected in common variant-based genomewide association studies. These mutations are present in the population at frequencies less than 1% to 5%.

Wambach et al collected data from a cohort of late preterm infants with and without RDS and focused their analysis on rare variants in 5 candidate genes that have been previously linked to lethal neonatal RDS. The authors used an innovative approach to next-generation DNA sequencing, in which target DNAs were sequenced in pooled cohorts (cases vs controls). The frequency of damaging mutations was compared in aggregate tests to see if they were more likely to be present in cases vs controls. The authors also examined data in the National Heart, Lung, and Blood Institute's Exome Sequencing Project to determine allele frequencies in an unselected population.[2] Using this approach, the authors identified an overabundance of heterozygous deleterious mutations in *ABCA3* in the European RDS case cohort. Thus, haploinsufficiency of *ABCA3* (loss of one functional copy of a gene) seems to be a significant risk factor for RDS.

Although the findings in this study are statistically significant, this study should be considered as preliminary evidence that will require replication in independent cohorts. The primary limitations of the study are its small sample size and candidate gene approach. The overall size of this study is small (N = 112 cases), and the results need replication in a larger cohort for validation. Additionally, the authors recruited only late preterm infants with gestational ages greater than 34 weeks to limit the environmental effect of gestational age. Therefore, it is unclear what role these *ABCA3* mutations play in most infants (< 34 weeks) who have RDS.

Finally, promising results of many candidate gene studies have been subsequently invalidated by adequately powered genomewide studies. False-positive results in candidate gene studies may occur from the presence of cryptic population substructure. This may be particularly important in rare variants studies.[3] As the authors suggest, genomewide investigation, in a well-powered cohort, may provide a more accurate estimation of the role of *ABCA3* in neonatal RDS.

K. Desch, MD

References

1. Goldstein DB. Common genetic variation and human traits. *N Engl J Med.* 2009; 360:1696-1698.
2. Exome Variant Server NHLBI GO Exome Sequencing Project (ESP) Seattle, WA (URL: http://evs.gs.washington.edu/EVS/)
3. Liu Q, Nicolae DL, Chen LS. Marbled inflation from population structure in gene-based association studies with rare variants. *Genet Epidemiol.* 2013;37:286-292.

Evidence From Human and Zebrafish That *GPC1* Is a Biliary Atresia Susceptibility Gene

Cui S, Leyva-Vega M, Tsai EA, et al (Univ of Pennsylvania, Philadelphia; et al)
Gastroenterology 144:1107-1115.e3, 2013

Background & Aims.—Biliary atresia (BA) is a progressive fibroinflammatory disorder of infants involving the extrahepatic and intrahepatic biliary tree. Its etiology is unclear but is believed to involve exposure of a genetically susceptible individual to certain environmental factors. BA occurs exclusively in the neonatal liver, so variants of genes expressed during hepatobiliary development could affect susceptibility. Genome-wide association studies previously identified a potential region of interest at 2q37. We continued these studies to narrow the region and identify BA susceptibility genes.

Methods.—We searched for copy number variants that were increased among patients with BA (n = 61) compared with healthy individuals (controls; n = 5088). After identifying a candidate gene, we investigated expression patterns of orthologues in zebrafish liver and the effects of reducing expression, with morpholino antisense oligonucleotides, on biliary development, gene expression, and signal transduction.

Results.—We observed a statistically significant increase in deletions at 2q37.3 in patients with BA that resulted in deletion of one copy of *GPC1*, which encodes glypican 1, a heparan sulfate proteoglycan that regulates Hedgehog signaling and inflammation. Knockdown of *gpc1* in zebrafish led to developmental biliary defects. Exposure of the *gpc1* morphants to cyclopamine, a Hedgehog antagonist, partially rescued the *gpc1*-knockdown phenotype. Injection of zebrafish with recombinant Sonic Hedgehog led to biliary defects similar to those of the *gpc1* morphants. Liver samples from patients with BA had reduced levels of apical *GPC1* in cholangiocytes compared with samples from controls.

Conclusions.—Based on genetic analysis of patients with BA and zebrafish, *GPC1* appears to be a BA susceptibility gene. These findings also support a role for Hedgehog signaling in the pathogenesis of BA.

▶ This study is a nice example of how genomic studies in humans that identify candidate genes for a disease can be meshed with genetic knockout and restoration studies in an animal model to support that the candidate gene is, in fact, mechanistically related to development of the disease. In congenital biliary atresia, the common bile duct between the liver and the small intestine is blocked or absent. In this study, genewide association analysis was done on 61 patients with biliary atresia compared with 5088 controls. An association with the gene *GPC1*, which encodes a glypican-1a heparan sulfate proteoglycan, was found. This gene is located on the long arm of chromosome 2 (2q37). This gene is involved in the regulation of the gene Hedgehog and also of inflammation. To support the concept that this gene is involved in the pathogenesis of biliary atresia, morpholino knockdown experiments were performed. Morpholino oligomers are antisense molecules that block access of other molecules to specific sequences within nucleic acid. Morpholinos block small (approximately 25 base) regions of the base-pairing surfaces of ribonucleic acid. Most morpholinos are used as research tools for reverse genetics by knocking down gene function. In this case, morpholinos to *GPC1* were used in zebrafish and were shown to develop lesions similar to biliary atresia in the liver. The *GPC1* gene deficiency has been found to affect an important signaling pathway called *Hedgehog*. Inhibitors of this pathway were used in the zebrafish morpholino knockdowns and were shown to ameliorate the features in the mutated fish and the addition of Hedgehog to normal fish-produced lesions.

This is an important study in that it shows feasibility of testing results of human genomic studies in a readily available animal platform (zebrafish) that can provide mechanistic support that a genetic variant may, in fact, be causally related to a disease by recapitulating the disease in the animal model.

J. Neu, MD

Trends in Survival Among Children With Down Syndrome in 10 Regions of the United States
Kucik JE, for the Congenital Anomaly Multistate Prevalence and Survival Collaborative (Ctrs for Disease Control and Prevention, Atlanta, GA; et al)
Pediatrics 131:e27-e36, 2013

Objective.—This study examined changes in survival among children with Down syndrome (DS) by race/ethnicity in 10 regions of the United States. A retrospective cohort study was conducted on 16 506 infants with DS delivered during 1983–2003 and identified by 10 US birth defects monitoring programs. Kaplan-Meier survival probabilities were estimated by select demographic and clinical characteristics. Adjusted hazard ratios (aHR) were estimated for maternal and infant characteristics by using Cox proportional hazard models.

Results.—The overall 1-month and 1-, 5-, and 20-year survival probabilities were 98%, 93%, 91%, and 88%, respectively. Over the study period, neonatal survival did not improve appreciably, but survival at all other ages improved modestly. Infants of very low birth weight had 24 times the risk of dying in the neonatal period compared with infants of normal birth weight (aHR 23.8; 95% confidence interval [CI] 18.4–30.7). Presence of a heart defect increased the risk of death in the postneonatal period nearly fivefold (aHR 4.6; 95% CI 3.9–5.4) and continued to be one of the most significant predictors of mortality through to age 20. The postneonatal aHR among non-Hispanic blacks was 1.4 (95% CI 1.2–1.8) compared with non-Hispanic whites and remained elevated by age 10 (2.0; 95% CI 1.0–4.0).

Conclusions.—The survival of children born with DS has improved and racial disparities in infant survival have narrowed. However, compared with non-Hispanic white children, non-Hispanic black children have lower survival beyond infancy. Congenital heart defects are a significant risk factor for mortality through age twenty.

▶ One of the most troubling aspects of health care in the United States is the persistence of disparities in health outcomes across socioeconomic and racial groups. Such data commonly show higher rates of adverse health outcomes among individuals who are of black race or economically disadvantaged. In this large, population-based study of birth defects, a retrospective assessment of survival probabilities showed overall survival among individuals with Down syndrome improved over the 20 years studied (1983—2003), currently averaging 94% among the regions studied. However, infants with Down syndrome were more often born with low birth weight, and, among low-birth-weight infants, the presence of Down syndrome held a 2.5 times greater risk of mortality compared with infants of normal chromosomal makeup. There was a stepwise decline in survival for children born with Down syndrome from age 1 month (98%) to 20 years (88%). Cox regression adjusted hazard ratios identified as most strongly associated with increased mortality, low birth weight, the presence of a heart defect, and non-Hispanic black race. Survival improved within every age range, except the neonatal period. Among neonates, low birth weight was the greatest factor attributable to mortality whereas among children of other age groups, congenital heart disease was the leading risk factor. This study adds to the growing body of evidence underscoring the importance of identifying and eradicating the underlying causes of disparities in health outcomes—be they biological, systems based, or socioeconomic—and ensuring optimal health outcomes among all racial groups.

L. J. Van Marter, MD, MPH

4 Labor and Delivery

Effect of umbilical cord milking in term and near term infants: randomized control trial

Upadhyay A, Gothwal S, Parihar R, et al (LLRM Med College, Meerut, India)
Am J Obstet Gynecol 208:120.e1-120.e6, 2013

Objective.—The objective of the study was to investigate the effect of umbilical cord milking as compared with early cord clamping on hematological parameters at 6 weeks of age among term and near term neonates.

Study Design.—This was a randomized control trial. Eligible neonates (>35 weeks' gestation) were randomized in intervention and control groups (100 each). Neonates of both groups got early cord clamping (within 30 seconds). The cord of the experimental group was milked after cutting and clamping at 25 cm from the umbilicus, whereas in control group cord was clamped near (2-3 cm) the umbilicus and not milked. Both groups got similar routine care. Unpaired Student t and Fisher exact tests were used for statistical analysis.

Results.—Baseline characteristics were comparable in the 2 groups. Mean hemoglobin (Hgb) (11.9 [1.5] g/dL and mean serum ferritin 355.9 [182.6] μg/L) were significantly higher in the intervention group as compared with the control group (10.8 [0.9] g/dL and 177.5 [135.8] μg/L), respectively, at 6 weeks of age. The mean Hgb and hematocrit at 12 hours and 48 hours was significantly higher in intervention group ($P = .0001$). The mean blood pressure at 30 minutes, 12 hours, and 48 hours after birth was significantly higher but within normal range. No significant difference was observed in the heart rate, respiratory rate, polycythemia, serum bilirubin, and need of phototherapy in the 2 groups.

Conclusion.—Umbilical cord milking is a safe procedure and it improved Hgb and iron status at 6 weeks of life among term and near term neonates.

▶ The optimal time to clamp the umbilical cord after birth has garnered much interest recently. In December 2012, the American Congress of Obstetricians and Gynecologists, with the American Academy of Pediatrics, recommended delayed cord clamping for preterm infants although not for term infants.[1] Systematic reviews of available data showed that although delayed cord clamping for preterm infants had numerous beneficial effects, including nearly a 40% reduction in intraventricular hemorrhage, the benefits for term infants in industrialized countries do not outweigh the possibility of more infants having jaundice and needing phototherapy, especially in settings in which early discharge is commonly practiced.[2,3]

In the above clinical trial, an alternative to delayed cord clamping was used to increase systemic blood volume, namely, milking the umbilical cord. Rather than the passive transfer of blood from the cord to the infant that occurs with delayed cord clamping, this technique uses the active movement of cord contents toward the infant. The technique involves cutting the cord about 25 cm from the umbilicus within 30 seconds of birth and then milking the cord toward the infant 3 times with speed at 10 cm/s (http://www.videos.med.usdy.edu.au/unitube/videos/file19). The technique is appealing because it does not interfere with the assessment of the newborn immediately after delivery. However, it should be noted that infants in this study were near term and at term. Currently, there are insufficient data regarding the potential benefits and risks of umbilical cord milking in preterm infants.[4]

L. A. Papile, MD

References

1. Committee on Obstetric Practice, American College of Obstetricians and Gynecologists. Committee Opinion No.543: timing of umbilical cord clamping after birth. *Obstet Gynecol.* 2012;120:1522-1526.
2. Rabe H, Diaz-Rossello JL, Duley L, Dowswell T. Effect of timing of umbilical cord clamping and other strategies to influence placental transfusion at preterm birth on maternal and infant outcomes. *Cochrane Data Base Syst Rev.* 2012;(8):CD003248.
3. McDonald SJ, Middleton P. Effect of timing of umbilical cord clamping of term infants on maternal and neonatal outcomes. *Cochrane Database Syst Rev.* 2008;(2):CD004074.
4. Takami T, Suganami Y, Sunohara D, et al. Umbilical cord milking stabilizes cerebral oxygenation and perfusion in infants born before 29 weeks of gestation. *J Pediatr.* 2012;161:742-747.

Obstetric outcome after intervention for severe fear of childbirth in nulliparous women — randomised trial
Rouhe H, Salmela-Aro K, Toivanen R, et al (Helsinki Univ Central Hosp, Finland; Univ of Helsinki, Finland)
BJOG 120:75-84, 2013

Objective.—To compare the numbers of vaginal deliveries and delivery satisfaction among women with fear of childbirth randomised to either psychoeducation or conventional surveillance during pregnancy.

Design.—Randomised controlled trial.

Setting.—Maternity unit of Helsinki University Central Hospital.

Population.—Fear of childbirth was screened during early pregnancy by the Wijma Delivery Expectancy Questionnaire (W-DEQ-A). Of 4575 screened nulliparous women, 371 (8.1%) scored ≥100, showing severe fear of childbirth.

Methods.—Women with W-DEQ-A ≥100 were randomised to intervention (*n* = 131) (psychoeducative group therapy, six sessions during pregnancy and one after childbirth) or control (*n* = 240) (care by community nurses and referral if necessary) groups. Obstetric data were collected from patient records and delivery satisfaction was examined by questionnaire.

Main Outcome Measures.—Delivery mode and satisfaction.

Results.—Women randomised to the intervention group more often had spontaneous vaginal delivery (SVD) than did controls (63.4% versus 47.5%, $P = 0.005$) and fewer caesarean sections (CSs) (22.9% versus 32.5%, $P = 0.05$). SVD was more frequent and CSs were less frequent among those who actually participated in intervention ($n = 90$) compared with controls who had been referred to consultation ($n = 106$) (SVD: 65.6% versus 47.2%, $P = 0.014$; CS: 23.3% versus 38.7%, $P = 0.031$). Women in intervention more often had a very positive delivery experience (36.1% versus 22.8%, $P = 0.04$, $n = 219$).

Conclusions.—To decrease the number of CSs, appropriate treatment for fear of childbirth is important. This study shows positive effects of psychoeducative group therapy in nulliparous women with severe fear of childbirth in terms of fewer CSs and more satisfactory delivery experiences relative to control women with a similar severe fear of childbirth.

▶ It is estimated that 6% to 10% of all pregnant women manifest a severe fear of childbirth, which has been associated with a high rate of operative delivery.[1,2] The goal of the above Finnish study was to examine the effect of psychoeducative group therapy for primary fear of childbirth on pregnancy outcomes, primarily the rate of vaginal deliveries. Eligible pregnant women were those who scored greater than the 95th percentile on a validated screening tool for fear of childbirth. The control group received a letter encouraging them to discuss their fears with the primary health care provider whereas the intervention group was offered a series of 6 group psychotherapeutic intervention sessions during pregnancy and one session 6 to 8 weeks after delivery. Although the rate of spontaneous vaginal delivery was significantly greater and the rate of operative delivery significantly lower in the intervention group, the operative delivery rate in the intervention group was approximately 1.5 times higher than that for Finland as a whole (22.9% vs 16.3%). Of note, more than 40% of women in either group who underwent an operative delivery did so by maternal request, accounting for approximately 10% of all deliveries. Elective operative delivery is essentially disallowed in the United States at this time. Thus, it is essential to identify early and support pregnant women who fear childbirth to provide counseling and therapy before the onset of labor.

L. A. Papile, MD

References

1. Rouhe H, Salmela-Aro K, Halmesmaki E, Saisto T. Fear of childbirth according to parity, gestational age, and obstetric history. *BJOG.* 2009;116:67-73.
2. Nieminen K, Stephansson O, Ryding EL. Women's fear of childbirth and preference for cesarean section—a cross-sectional study at various stages in pregnancy. *Acta Obstet Gynecol Scand.* 2009;88:807-813.

Outcome of extremely low gestational age newborns after introduction of a revised protocol to assist preterm infants in their transition to extrauterine life

Mehler K, Grimme J, Abele J, et al (Univ of Cologne, Germany)
Acta Paediatr 101:1232-1239, 2012

Aim.—To evaluate the outcome of a cohort of extremely low gestational age newborn infants (ELGAN) below 26-week gestation who were treated following a revised, gentle delivery room protocol to assist them in the transition and adaptation to extrauterine life.

Methods.—A cohort of infants with a gestational age (GA) below 26 weeks (study group; n = 164) was treated according to a revised delivery room protocol. The protocol included an optimized prenatal management, strict use of continuous positive airway pressure (CPAP), avoiding mechanical ventilation and early administration of surfactant without intubation. The parameters management of respiratory distress syndrome, survival, neonatal morbidity and neurodevelopmental outcome were compared with a historical control group (n = 44).

Results.—Seventy-four per cent of the study group infants were initially treated with CPAP and surfactant administration without intubation. In comparison with the control group, significantly less children were intubated in the delivery room (24% vs. 41%) and needed mechanical ventilation (51% vs. 72%; both $p < 0.05$). Furthermore, compared with the historical control overall mortality (20% vs. 39%), rate of bronchopulmonary dysplasia (18% vs. 37%) and IVH > II° (10% vs. 33%) in survivors were significantly lower during the observational period (all $p < 0.05$). Neurodevelopmental outcome was normal in 70% of examined study group infants.

Conclusions.—A revised delivery room management protocol was applied safely to infants with a GA below 26 completed weeks with improved rates of survival and morbidity.

▶ Over the last several years there has been a plethora of single-center retrospective observational studies describing what has been termed "less aggressive" approaches to the delivery room management of extremely preterm infants than those that were customary in the early 2000s. The intent of this gentle approach is to assist very immature preterm infants in their adaptation from intrauterine to extrauterine existence rather than resuscitate them.

In the above study from Germany, this less-aggressive approach included operative delivery under regional anesthesia, extracting the infant en caul, when possible, initiating continuous positive airway pressure (CPAP) via a face mask at 8 cm H_2O and incrementally increasing CPAP to 14 cm H_2O before considering intubation. In addition, all spontaneously breathing infants who were not intubated at 10 minutes of age, but who were considered to have respiratory distress, received surfactant through a catheter placed in the trachea. The authors noted significant improvement in survival without an increase in neonatal morbidity using this approach. However, the wide gap between the birth date of the control infants and most of the study infants, as well as the inherent bias in a single-center study, makes it difficult to draw any conclusions regarding the usefulness of this approach. Additionally, the authors do not report data on the rate of pneumothorax, a potential complication of the high CPAP pressure that was used.

L. A. Papile, MD

Outcome of extremely low gestational age newborns after introduction of a revised protocol to assist preterm infants in their transition to extrauterine life

Mehler K, Grimme J, Abele J, et al (Univ of Cologne, Germany)
Acta Paediatr 101:1232-1239, 2012

Aim.—To evaluate the outcome of a cohort of extremely low gestational age newborn infants (ELGAN) below 26-week gestation who were treated following a revised, gentle delivery room protocol to assist them in the transition and adaptation to extrauterine life.

Methods.—A cohort of infants with a gestational age (GA) below 26 weeks (study group; n = 164) was treated according to a revised delivery room protocol. The protocol included an optimized prenatal management, strict use of continuous positive airway pressure (CPAP), avoiding mechanical ventilation and early administration of surfactant without intubation. The parameters management of respiratory distress syndrome, survival, neonatal morbidity and neurodevelopmental outcome were compared with a historical control group (n = 44).

Results.—Seventy-four per cent of the study group infants were initially treated with CPAP and surfactant administration without intubation. In comparison with the control group, significantly less children were intubated in the delivery room (24% vs. 41%) and needed mechanical ventilation (51% vs. 72%; both p < 0.05). Furthermore, compared with the historical control overall mortality (20% vs. 39%), rate of bronchopulmonary dysplasia (18% vs. 37%) and IVH > II° (10% vs. 33%) in survivors were significantly lower during the observational period (all *p* < 0.05). Neurodevelopmental outcome was normal in 70% of examined study group infants.

Conclusions.—A revised delivery room management protocol was applied safely to infants with a GA below 26 completed weeks with improved rates of survival and morbidity (Fig 1).

▶ This is how quality improvement gets done: identify a process characterized by practice heterogeneity and potentially suboptimal results, standardize the practice, get all providers to commit to participate in implementation, track the outcomes of interest, make adjustments as guided by new information, and then build on that foundation to continue improvements. This report exemplifies each of those steps. Standardization is absolutely critical even though there may be little or no evidence to guide some of the choices that must be made. These

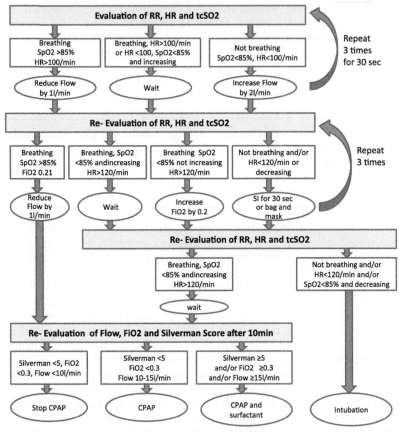

FIGURE 1.—Flow chart of delivery room management. FiO₂, inspired fraction of oxygen; SpO₂, oxygen saturation measured by pulse oximetry; HR, heart rate; RR, respiratory rate; CPAP, continuous positive airway pressure. (Reprinted from Mehler K, Grimme J, Abele J, et al. Outcome of extremely low gestational age newborns after introduction of a revised protocol to assist preterm infants in their transition to extrauterine life. *Acta Paediatr.* 2012;101:1232-1239, with permission from Acta Paediatrica and John Wiley and sons, www.interscience.wiley.com.)

authors compare outcomes of infants cared for before (44 infants) and after (176 infants) implementation of a new protocol for delivery room management of extremely-low-gestational-age (< 26 weeks) newborn infants. In the preintervention period, resuscitation followed Neonatal Resuscitation Program guidelines, including positive predictive value and chest compressions as indicated; if the infant was breathing, continuous positive airway pressure (CPAP) was the primary mode of support. Infants who required surfactant were intubated and supported with mechanical ventilation. Although the description of the new regimen in the abstract is terse ("strict use of continuous positive airway pressure, avoiding mechanical ventilation, and early administration of surfactant without intubation"), the text provides specific details regarding application of those measures in the delivery room as well as approaches to prenatal and postdelivery care. The authors provide an elegant flow diagram to guide decision making throughout the course of delivery room care (Fig 1). A critical component of this paradigm is early application of CPAP via a face mask using a Benveniste valve (a simple mechanical device with no moving parts, which utilizes gas flow to generate the applied distending pressure; it is not equivalent to high-flow nasal cannula). Management was initiated with a flow of 15 L/min, which generates a distending pressure of approximately 8 cm H_2O; as shown in Fig 1, flow (ie, pressure) was adjusted up or down according to the infant's response. If indicated, surfactant was given via a thin endotracheal catheter during spontaneous breathing while on CPAP, typically at about 30 min of age. Despite lower rates of intubation and mechanical ventilation, rates of mortality, bronchopulmonary dysplasia, and intraventricular hemorrhage were all lower after the practice change. In their discussion, the authors are very circumspect about generalizing these results to other centers, noting the retrospective study design, relatively small sample size, potential for confounding by other practice changes, and implementation of this regimen within the context of a broader "delivery room milieu." Accordingly, they stop short of advocating wholesale adoption of their regimen by other units. For those of us who practice in the United States, that would, in fact, be impossible, as the Benveniste valve is not available here. Nonetheless, these results support the concept of a more gentle approach to delivery room management of these most vulnerable infants. Even if we cannot all emulate these care practices exactly, we can look to this as an exemplar of effective quality improvement in delivery room care.

W. E. Benitz, MD

Evaluation of the Clinical Use of Magnesium Sulfate for Cerebral Palsy Prevention

Gibbins KJ, Browning KR, Lopes VV, et al (Brown Univ Alpert School of Medicine, Providence, RI)
Obstet Gynecol 121:235-240, 2013

Objective.—Clinical trials support the efficacy and safety of magnesium sulfate for cerebral palsy prevention. We evaluated the implementation of a clinical protocol for the use of magnesium for cerebral palsy prevention in our large women's hospital, focusing on uptake, indications, and safety.

Methods.—We performed a review of selected gravidas with threatened or planned delivery before 32 weeks of gestation from October 2007 to February 2011. The primary study outcome was the change in the rate of predelivery administration of magnesium sulfate over this time period.

Results.—Three hundred seventy-three patients were included. In 2007, before guideline implementation, 20% of eligible gravidas (95% confidence interval [CI] 9.1-35.6%) received magnesium before delivery compared with 93.9% (95% CI 79.8–99.3%) in the final 2 months of the study period ($P < .001$). Dosing did not vary significantly over the 4 study years: the median number of treatments was one, the total predelivery median dose ranged from 15 to 48 g, and the median duration of therapy ranged from 3 to 12 hours. After 3 years, magnesium administration was almost universal among patients diagnosed with preeclampsia, preterm labor, or preterm premature rupture of membranes (95.4%), whereas patients delivered preterm for fetal growth restriction were significantly less likely to receive predelivery magnesium (44%, $P < .001$). No maternal or perinatal magnesium-attributable morbidity was noted. Among patients eligible for the protocol who received magnesium, 84.2% delivered before 32 weeks of gestation.

Conclusion.—It is feasible to implement a magnesium sulfate cerebral palsy prevention protocol into clinical practice.

Level of Evidence.—III.

▶ In August 2008, the National Institute of Child Health and Human Development (NICHD) Maternal Fetal Research Network published the results of a large, randomized, clinical trial (RCT) indicating that magnesium sulfate before anticipated preterm birth was associated with an overall reduction in cerebral palsy.[1] Before the publication of the report, but after the results were known, Women and Children's Hospital of Rhode Island, a center that participated in the RCT, implemented an obstetric departmental guideline for the use of magnesium sulfate for the prevention of cerebral palsy modeled on the NICHD trial. The guideline was announced at a faculty meeting, but there was no formal implementation plan. The above study examines compliance with the guideline before and after the publication of the RCT and American College of Obstetricians and Gynecologists (ACOG) subsequent Practice Bulletin addressing the use of magnesium sulfate.

Before the guideline (2007), 40% of eligible women on the maternal-fetal medicine service received magnesium sulfate compared with 10% of eligible women on either the resident or private practice service. In the year after the publication of the RCT (2009), compliance with the guideline was 80% on both the maternal-fetal and resident service, whereas it was 55% on the private practice service. In March 2010, ACOG recommended that magnesium sulfate be used before anticipated early preterm birth for fetal neuroprotection.[2] Shortly thereafter, the compliance rate for the private practice service was identical to that of the other 2 services (80%). After 3 years, magnesium sulfate administration was universal among patients on the maternal-fetal and resident services but was only 88% on the private practice service with most of the noncompliance occurring in the group of women who were delivered for fetal growth restriction.

It is interesting to speculate that the publication of the RCT was a sufficient impetus to change practice on the university services, whereas ACOG endorsement was needed to improve compliance by private practitioners. If only American Academy of Pediatrics statements regarding neonatal care were as influential.

L. A. Papile, MD

References

1. Rouse DJ, Hirtz DG, Thom E, et al; Eunice Kennedy Shriver NICHD Maternal-Fetal Medicine Units Network. A randomized, controlled trial of magnesium sulfate for the prevention of cerebral palsy. *N Engl J Med.* 2008;359:895-905.
2. American College of Obstetricians and Gynecologists Committee on Obstetric Practice, Society for Maternal-Fetal Medicine. Committee Opinion No. 455: Magnesium sulfate before anticipated preterm birth for neuroprotection. *Obstet Gynecol.* 2010;115:669-671.

Why the term neonatal encephalopathy should be preferred over neonatal hypoxic-ischemic encephalopathy

Leviton A (Boston Children's Hosp and Harvard Med School, MA)
Am J Obstet Gynecol 208:176-180, 2013

The unresponsiveness of the full-term newborn is sometimes attributed to asphyxia, even when no severe physiologic disturbance occurred during labor and delivery. The controversy about whether to use the name "hypoxic-ischemic encephalopathy" or "newborn encephalopathy" has recently flared in publications directed toward pediatricians and neurologists. In this clinic opinion piece, I discuss the importance to obstetricians of this decision and explain why "newborn encephalopathy" should be the default term.

▶ This opinion article, which appeared in the obstetric literature, should also be directed to neonatologists and pediatricians. As the author correctly indicates, the depressed and unresponsive newborn is often described as suffering from hypoxic-ischemic encephalopathy (HIE), although the cause of the encephalopathy may be unknown or cannot be established.

This article focuses on five key points: what constitutes cause, multihit models of brain injury, etiologies of unresponsiveness at birth, evidence that intrapartum hypoxic-ischemic exposures result in encephalopathy, attribution of whether HIE is the best diagnosis, and the consequences of using the general term neonatal encephalopathy (NE) rather than HIE. The author makes valid points for all of these, but perhaps the most far-reaching is the medicolegal consequences when a newborn is labeled as having HIE, greatly increasing the risk of an allegation of medical malpractice. In addition, the diagnosis of HIE often results in truncating the search for other diagnostic entities capable of producing NE, which may not be avoidable or result in allegation of medical negligence. I concur that the default diagnosis should be neonatal encephalopathy until hypoxia ischemia can be reasonably established as the etiologic cause.

S. M. Donn, MD

Antecedents of Neonatal Encephalopathy in the Vermont Oxford Network Encephalopathy Registry

Nelson KB, Bingham P, Edwards EM, et al (Children's Hosp Natl Med Ctr, Washington, DC; Univ of Vermont, Burlington; et al)
Pediatrics 130:878-886, 2012

Background.—Neonatal encephalopathy (NE) is a major predictor of death and long-term neurologic disability, but there are few studies of antecedents of NE.

Objectives.—To identify antecedents in a large registry of infants who had NE.

Methods.—This was a maternal and infant record review of 4165 singleton neonates, gestational age of ≥36 weeks, meeting criteria for inclusion in the Vermont Oxford Network Neonatal Encephalopathy Registry.

Results.—Clinically recognized seizures were the most prevalent condition (60%); 49% had a 5-minute Apgar score of ≤3 and 18% had a reduced level of consciousness. An abnormal maternal or fetal condition predated labor in 46%; maternal hypertension (16%) or small for gestational age (16%) were the most frequent risk factors. In 8%, birth defects were identified. The most prevalent birth complication was elevated maternal temperature in labor of ≥37.5°C in 27% of mothers with documented temperatures compared with 2% to 3.2% in controls in population-based studies. Clinical chorioamnionitis, prolonged membrane rupture, and maternal hypothyroidism exceeded rates in published controls. Acute asphyxial indicators were reported in 15% (in 35% if fetal bradycardia included) and inflammatory indicators in 24%. Almost one-half had neither asphyxial nor inflammatory indicators. Although most infants with NE were observably ill since the first minutes of life, only 54% of placentas were submitted for examination.

Conclusions.—Clinically recognized asphyxial birth events, indicators of intrauterine exposure to inflammation, fetal growth restriction, and birth defects were each observed in term infants with NE, but much of NE in this large registry remained unexplained.

▶ The timing of an insult that leads to neonatal encephalopathy is a key feature of obstetrical and neonatal litigation. It is perhaps an unfortunate circumstance that our tort system is outcomes-based, and when an infant develops long-term neurologic sequelae, the first thought always seems to be "blame the obstetrician, the neo, or the hospital."

More than 100 years ago, Sigmund Freud suggested that depression at birth might actually be a reflection of an abnormal brain rather than the cause of it. We are, of course, in a difficult scientific situation, where the definitive trial can never be done, and thus we rely heavily on animal experimentation and human epidemiological evidence to try to answer this critical question.

Dr Nelson has been a prolific investigator in this area, beginning with the National Collaborative Perinatal Project a number of years ago, and she continues to shed light on this area. This article reviewed a large database compiled from the Vermont-Oxford Neonatal Encephalopathy Registry to examine possible antecedents of neonatal encephalopathy. Although we might quibble about the criteria chosen for selection—a notable absence was a disturbance in muscle tone—the results continue to demonstrate that in the large majority of cases, the encephalopathy is the aftermath of a prior event or events. An acute intrapartum sentinel event was recognized in only 15% of the cases. Maternal fever and inflammation, congenital anomalies, and maternal hypothyroidism are significant antecedents of neonatal encephalopathy. As the authors conclude, these are underresearched components of neonatal encephalopathy and need a lot more investigation. In the meantime, we should recognize that Freud was correct and should not jump to the conclusion that the encephalopathic newborn sustained an acute intrapartum asphyxial insult.

S. M. Donn, MD

Brachial Plexus Palsy and Shoulder Dystocia: Obstetric Risk Factors Remain Elusive
Ouzounian JG, Korst LM, Miller DA, et al (Univ of Southern California, Los Angeles)
Am J Perinatol 30:303-308, 2013

Objective.—Shoulder dystocia (SD) and brachial plexus palsy (BPP) are complications of childbirth that can result in significant long-term sequelae. The purpose of the present study was to analyze risk factors in cases of SD and BPP.

Methods.—We performed a retrospective study of laboring women who delivered a singleton, term, live-born infant at the Los Angeles County + University of Southern California Medical Center from 1995 to 2004. Multivariable logistic regression models were used to analyze risk factors among SD cases with and without BPP.

Results.—Of the 13,998 deliveries that met inclusion criteria, 221 (1.6%) had SD. Of these, 42 (19.0%) had BPP. After testing for association with multiple potential risk factors, including maternal demographic variables, diabetes, hypertension, prior cesarean delivery, uterine abnormalities, induction of labor, prolonged second stage (adjusted by parity and epidural use), assisted vaginal delivery, and neonatal birth weight, no statistical association of BPP with any specific risk factor was identified.

Conclusion.—In the present study, we were unable to identify any reliable risk factors for BPP among deliveries with or without SD. SD and BPP remain unpredictable complications of childbirth.

▶ The words shoulder dystocia (SD) and brachial plexus palsy (BPP) strike fear into the hearts of every obstetrician. They are a malpractice lawsuit waiting to happen. However, the findings of this retrospective study should partially allay some of the fear. Despite the limitations of a retrospective study, the large cohort reviewed lends credence to the findings that essentially reveal that the factors resulting in BPP are largely unknown. Risk factors for SD emerged (macrosomia, maternal diabetes and prolonged second stage), however, multivariate analysis failed to identify the factors responsible for BPP. Macrosomia is identified as a risk factor for SD and BPP, but in this series, almost half of the cases of SD and half of the cases of BPP occurred when birth weight was less than 4000 g. Among patients with SD, macrosomia (defined at 4000-g or 4500-g levels) was not associated with BPP.

The authors speculate that "it is possible that unmeasured factors (e.g., the propulsive forces of labor, intrauterine maladaptation, uterine abnormalities, and/or compression of the posterior shoulder against the sacral promontory), rather than the documented clinical characteristics of the patients and their labor and delivery, were responsible for the BPP."

These findings are in accord with the mega series of Foad et al[1] of 17 334 cases of neonatal BPP from 11 million births over a 3-year period in the United States where most had no identifiable risk factors. Unfortunately, information regarding important maternal characteristics (eg, duration of labor, epidural use) was not available in that series. Although SD is a rare event, the obstetric teams need to train and simulate such deliveries so they are ready when it presents itself. Indeed both Buerkle et al[2] and Inglis et al[3] reported that shoulder dystocia training was associated with a lower incidence of obstetrical brachial plexus injury.

A. A. Fanaroff, MBBCh, FRCPE

References

1. Foad SL, Mehlman CT, Ying J. The epidemiology of neonatal brachial plexus palsy in the United States. *J Bone Joint Surg Am.* 2008;90:1258-1264.
2. Buerkle B, Pueth J, Hefler LA, Tempfer-Bentz EK, Tempfer CB. Objective structured assessment of technical skills evaluation of theoretical compared with hands-on training of shoulder dystocia management: a randomized controlled trial. *Obstet Gynecol.* 2012;120:809-814.
3. Inglis SR, Feier N, Chetiyaar JB, et al. Effects of shoulder dystocia training on the incidence of brachial plexus injury. *Am J Obstet Gynecol.* 2011;204:322.e1-322.e6.

Effect of delivery room temperature on the admission temperature of premature infants: A randomized controlled trial
Jia Y-S, Lin Z-L, Lv H, et al (Yuying Children's Hosp of Wenzhou Med College, China; The Second Affiliated Hosp of Wenzhou Med College, China; et al)
J Perinatol 33:264-267, 2013

Objective.—To determine if increasing delivery room temperature to that recommended by the World Health Organization results in increased admission temperatures of preterm infants.

Study Design.—Admission rectal temperatures of newborns ≤32 weeks gestation delivered in rooms with temperature set at 24 to 26 °C were compared with those of similar newborns delivered in rooms with temperature set at 20 to 23 °C.

Result.—Premature newborns delivered in rooms with mean temperature 25.1 ± 0.6 °C ($n = 43$), compared with those delivered in rooms with mean temperature 22.5 ± 0.6 °C ($n = 48$), had a lower incidence (34.9% vs 68.8%, $P < 0.01$) of admission rectal temperature <36 °C and higher admission rectal temperatures (36.0 $\pm$ 0.9 °C vs 35.5 $\pm$ 0.8 °C, $P < 0.01$). This difference persisted after adjustment for birth weight and 5 min Apgar score.

Conclusion.—Increasing delivery room temperatures to that recommended by the World Health Organization decreases cold stress in premature newborns.

▶ Hypothermia on admission to neonatal units is a worldwide problem across all climates, particularly for small infants and those born prematurely. Immediate postnatal hypothermia is an independent risk factor for death in premature newborns, and every effort must be expended to prevent it. Even in highly sophisticated academic medical centers, fully aware of the consequences of hypothermia, admission temperatures below 36°C are recorded in almost half the babies.[1] Minimizing the heat loss in preterm infants during the initial stabilization and resuscitation in the delivery room is critical for improved outcome in those babies.

Despite recommendations from the Neonatal Resuscitation program and the World Health Organization to maintain the temperature in the delivery room at 25°C, this recommendation is largely ignored. In developed countries, the priority has been the comfort of the mother and medical staff rather than the critically important thermal environment of the preterm infant. This practice is intellectually justified by the assumption that the newborn's thermal needs will be met by a radiant warmer or incubator together with the immediate use of warmer pads or plastic bags. Indeed, the conclusion from a randomized trial that compared the efficacy of vinyl bags and thermal warming mattresses in preventing hypothermia during delivery room resuscitation and stabilization of extremely low-gestational-age neonates (ELGANs) was that they were equally effective in improving admission temperatures.[2] There are still many ELGANs admitted with low and high temperatures, and the authors speculated that the "improvements in other areas such as delivery room temperature may be needed to achieve the goal of preventing hypothermia in this vulnerable population." The absence of direct evidence from a large, randomized trial served as the impetus for Jia et al to undertake the trial evaluating the impact of delivery room temperature on the incidence of hypothermia in premature infants upon admission to the neonatal intensive care unit. They found a substantial benefit for the premature babies by warming the delivery room to 25.1 ± 0.6°C (approximately 77°F), with only 35% of admissions having temperatures less than 36°C, compared with 69% with admission temperatures less than 36°C when the delivery room temperature was 22.5 ± 0.6°C (approximately 73°F). These are unacceptably high rates of hypothermia, even in the warmer delivery room (DR) environment.

Preterm newborns transition from a warm intrauterine environment to the air-conditioned DR. They are ill equipped to deal with the thermal stress, devoid of metabolic reserves with minimal insulation, limited muscle mass, and inability to shiver. It comes as no surprise that so many of them become hypothermic. It is time to take the necessary steps to limit hypothermia and to set the temperature in the delivery room to benefit the babies. The temperature must not be set to satisfy the thermal needs of the medical staff. An increase in the DR temperature will greatly facilitate the maintenance of adequate core temperatures in the extremely low-birth-weight infant. This is in addition to the use of warming mattresses or vinyl bags.[2]

A. A. Fanaroff, MBBCh, FRCPE

References

1. Laptook AR, Salhab W, Bhaskar B; The Neonatal Research Network. Admission temperature of low birth weight infants: predictors and associated morbidities. *Pediatrics*. 2007;119:e643-e649.
2. Mathew B, Lakshminrusimha S, Sengupta S, Carrion V. Randomized controlled trial of vinyl bags versus thermal mattress to prevent hypothermia in extremely low-gestational-age infants. *Am J Perinatol*. 2013;30:317-322.

Meconium-stained amniotic fluid and the need for paediatrician attendance
Maayan-Metzger A, Leibovitch L, Schushan-Eisen I, et al (The Edmond and Lili Safra Children's Hosp, Ramat-Gan, Israel)
Acta Paediatr 102:e8-e12, 2013

Aim.—To determine perinatal parameters among term newborn infants born by vaginal delivery with meconium-stained amniotic fluid (MSAF) that needed paediatrician assistance.

Methods.—Paediatricians who were in attendance in the delivery room due to MSAF among term infants completed 775 reports regarding the infants' delivery conditions, and the assistance provided. We defined 'paediatrician attendance needed' for a subgroup of infants for whom we retrospectively determined that paediatrician attendance in the delivery room was required.

Results.—'Paediatrician attendance needed' was determined in 31 (4%) cases. Among cases with documented normal foetal monitor, only 10 (1.8%) were defined as 'paediatrician attendance needed', a percentage significantly lower than among infants born following non-reassuring foetal monitor: 21 (9.7%) ($p < 0.001$). 'Paediatrician attendance needed' was predicted by non-reassuring foetal monitor [OR 6.02 (CI 2.72–13.31), $p < 0.001$], maternal fever [OR 6.34 (1.92–20.92), $p = 0.002$] and younger maternal age (for every year) [OR 0.889 (CI 0.82–0.96), $p = 0.003$].

Conclusions.—Term newborn infants born by vaginal delivery with MSAF with documented normal tracing foetal monitor are at low risk of the need for paediatrician assistance. Paediatrician attendance in the delivery room in labour involving MSAF should be recommended when non-reassuring foetal monitor tracing is observed and should also be considered when maternal fever is recorded, and/or thick meconium is observed.

▶ The delivery room management of the meconium-stained infant has evolved dramatically since the publications of the mid-1970s, which urged us to suction every last vestige of mucus from the airway of affected newborns. This study takes the process a step further by attempting to use retrospectively collected data to create an a priori determination for the need for pediatrician attendance at delivery when meconium-stained amniotic fluid (MSAF) is found.

These authors had pediatricians attending deliveries complicated by MSAF complete a report to document the baby's condition at birth and the need for intervention. A review of the 775 cases found that pediatrician attendance was needed in only 4% of cases, and these were accompanied by a nonreassuring fetal heart rate on electronic monitoring, maternal fever, or younger maternal age.

The results of this study further help to refine the approach to the MSAF infant. In the age of cost containment and lean projects, it appears that routine attendance by physicians at deliveries complicated by MSAF is superfluous in 96% of cases. This has significant implications for deliveries performed in hospitals where pediatricians or family physicians have to be called in, either disrupting their office practice or a night's sleep, and adding unnecessary costs to health care. These data will be useful in establishing algorithms to define specific situations in which a physician should be requested to attend a delivery when MSAF is present.

S. M. Donn, MD

Proficiency and Retention of Neonatal Resuscitation Skills by Pediatric Residents
Patel J, Posencheg M, Ades A (Children's Hosp of Philadelphia, PA)
Pediatrics 130:515-521, 2012

Background.—The basic knowledge and skill base to resuscitate a newborn infant is taught in the Neonatal Resuscitation Program (NRP). We hypothesize that caregivers will perform below current acceptable standards before the recertification period of two years.

Methods.—This is a prospective descriptive study evaluating performance of pediatric residents' NRP knowledge and skills over time. NRP scores are used as baseline data. Follow-up is performed before the resident 's first NICU rotation. Differences in the mean scores are analyzed for degree of retention. Subset score analysis is also performed.

Results.—Eighty-eight subjects completed both evaluations. Knowledge scores maintained close to passing throughout the academic year. Subset evaluation revealed significant deficits within the intubation lesson. Alarming deficits were seen in skills evaluation starting at initial NRP certification with 39.1% residents having failing scores. Mean scores were below passing for every group on follow-up testing. Subgroup analysis of skills revealed deficits in the initial phases of resuscitation (lessons 1–3).

Conclusions.—Deterioration of skills is seen shortly after training. It appears that knowledge is generally better retained. Discrepancies between areas of knowledge and skill deterioration indicate that proficiency in one does not necessarily indicate proficiency of the other.

▶ This article re-demonstrates the previously described experience of learner decay in knowledge and skills taught in standardized courses such as the Neonatal Resuscitation Program (NRP). It documents the lack of competency of pediatric house officers (HO) in neonatal resuscitation. This problem has assumed special importance these days as HOs rotate less frequently in the neonatal intensive care unit (NICU). The findings of this article can be helpful to caregivers designing models of delivering safe and effective medical care in NICUs, including neonatal resuscitation. Although the study examined HOs, the described decay in skills and the concerns for incompetency also apply to practitioners who infrequently attend deliveries or use their NRP skills as part of their practice. The article achieved its objectives in describing variation in the timeline and the degree of deterioration in different components of NRP knowledge and skills.

The teaching methods for NRP certification courses have changed since this study was conducted. HOs now complete the knowledge portion using web-based modules prior to their hands-on skills sessions. In addition, more emphases are currently placed on teamwork during the debriefing part of the NRP simulation exercises. These changes might improve retention of NRP skills, but it is doubtful that these changes alone will prevent the serious and rapid deterioration in these skills that the HOs experience by the time that they need to use them.

Refresher sessions to review NRP skills and knowledge sound like what is needed during the rotations when HOs use NRP skills. However, as the authors correctly indicate, the optimal content and method of delivering these refresher sessions are yet to be determined.

M. A. Attar, MD

Influence of location of delivery on outcome in neonates with gastroschisis
Nasr A, Canadian Paediatric Surgery Network (Univ of Ottawa, Ontario, Canada; et al)
J Pediatr Surg 47:2022-2025, 2012

Background.—It is not clear in the literature whether infants with a prenatal diagnosis of gastroschisis should be delivered in a perinatal center with level 3 neonatal intensive care unit (NICU) and surgical facilities ("inborn") or if they could be safely delivered in a more local hospital and then transferred to a perinatal center ("outborn"). Our goal was to determine the impact of delivery site on outcomes for neonates diagnosed as having gastroschisis.

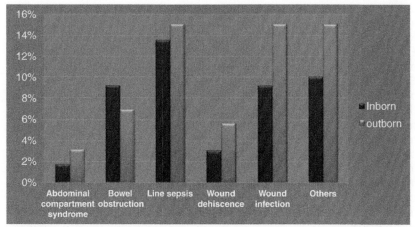

Others: include chylothorax, cholestasis, Necrotizing enterocolitis, bowel perforation, short bowel, renal insufficiency

FIGURE.—Complications. (Reprinted from Journal of Pediatric Surgery. Nasr A, Canadian Paediatric Surgery Network. Influence of location of delivery on outcome in neonates with gastroschisis. *J Pediatr Surg.* 2012;47:2022-2025, Copyright 2012, with permission from Elsevier.)

Methods.—Data were obtained from the Canadian Pediatric Surgery Network, covering the years 2005 to 2008 for 18 pediatric surgical centers. *Inborn* was defined as birth in a hospital with a NICU or connected to a NICU by a bridge or tunnel. *Outborn* was defined as requiring transfer by ambulance or flight. A P value less than .05 was considered significant.

Results.—Of 395 infants with prenatally diagnosed gastroschisis, 237 were inborn and 158 were outborn. Univariate analysis demonstrated no significant difference between groups with respect to gestational age, birth weight, days on total parenteral nutrition, or length of hospital stay. There was a significant difference with regard to Score for Neonatal Acute Physiology—Version II, complication rates, comorbidities, and age at final closure. Logistic regression showed that location of delivery was a significant independent predictor for incidence of complications, as were Score for Neonatal Acute Physiology—Version II, comorbidities, and presence of bowel atresia or necrosis. The odds ratio of developing a complication when outborn was 1.6 ($P = .05$).

Conclusions.—Delivery outside a perinatal center is a significant predictor of complications for infants born with gastroschisis (Fig).

▶ Among neonatologists, the advantage of birth at centers with high levels of neonatal care is an article of faith: a widely and deeply held belief developed many years ago in the absence of substantial empirical supporting evidence.[1] Although evidence of substantial survival advantages for low-birth-weight infants has steadily accrued, evidence of benefits for term infants and those with prenatally diagnosed congenital anomalies (who have been excluded from most such analyses) has been slower to develop. This article is the second from the Canadian Pediatric Surgery Network to examine the effects of location of birth on outcomes of neonates with surgical conditions. In the first of these,[2] authors representing the Network described higher risk-adjusted mortality rates for outborn infants with congenital diaphragmatic hernia (odds ratio 2.8, $P = .04$), although unadjusted mortality rates were similar. In the present report, outborn infants with gastroschisis had more complications (60% vs 48%, $P = .02$) and later achievement of final closure (4.2 vs 2.4 days, $P = .001$), despite having lower Score for Neonatal Acute Physiology version II (SNAP II) scores (6.8 vs 11.1, $P = .001$). Unadjusted mortality rates were low and did not differ between inborn and outborn cases (4.6 vs 2.5%, $P = .1$). After logistic regression adjustment for SNAP II, comorbidities, and presence of bowel atresia or necrosis, the odds ratio for complications (as described in the Fig) in outborn infants was 1.6 ($P = .05$). Adjusted odds ratios for other outcomes, including mortality rates, were not reported. These results are an important contribution to the empirical basis for recommendation that infants with congenital anomalies requiring early postnatal surgery should be delivered at a perinatal center whenever possible.

W. E. Benitz, MD

References

1. Sinclair JC, Torrance GW, Boyle MH, Horwood SP, Saigal S, Sackett DL. Evaluation of neonatal-intensive-care program. *N Engl J Med.* 1981;305:489-494.
2. Nasr A, Langer JC; Canadian Pediatric Surgery Network. Influence of location of delivery on outcome in neonates with congenital diaphragmatic hernia. *J Pediatr Surg.* 2011;46:814-816.

DNA methylation at imprint regulatory regions in preterm birth and infection

Liu Y, Hoyo C, Murphy S, et al (Duke Univ School of Medicine, Durham, NC)
Am J Obstet Gynecol 208:395.e1-395.e7, 2013

Objective.—To aid in understanding long-term health consequences of intrauterine infections in preterm birth, we evaluated DNA methylation at 9 differentially methylated regions that regulate imprinted genes by type of preterm birth (spontaneous preterm labor, preterm premature rupture of membranes, or medically indicated [fetal growth restriction and preeclampsia]) and infection status (chorioamnionitis or funisitis).

Study Design.—Data on type of preterm birth and infection status were abstracted from medical records and standardized pathology reports in 73 preterm infants enrolled in the Newborn Epigenetics Study, a prospective cohort study of mother-infant dyads in Durham, NC. Cord blood was collected at birth, and infant DNA methylation levels at the *H19, IGF2, MEG3, MEST, SGCE/PEG10, PEG3, NNAT,* and *PLAGL1* differentially methylated regions were measured using bisulfite pyrosequencing. One-way analyses of variance and logistic regression models were used to compare DNA methylation levels by type of preterm birth and infection status.

Results.—DNA methylation levels did not differ at any of the regions ($P > .20$) between infants born via spontaneous preterm labor (average n = 29), preterm premature rupture of membranes (average n = 17), or medically indicated preterm birth (average n = 40). Levels were significantly increased at *PLAGL1* in infants with chorioamnionitis (n = 10, 64.4%) compared with infants without chorioamnionitis (n = 63, 57.9%), $P < .01$. DNA methylation levels were also increased at *PLAGL1* for infants with funisitis (n = 7, 63.3%) compared with infants without funisitis (n = 66, 58.3%), $P < .05$.

Conclusion.—Dysregulation of *PLAGL1* has been associated with abnormal development and cancer. Early-life exposures, including infection/inflammation, may affect epigenetic changes that increase susceptibility to later chronic disease.

▶ The role of epigenetics and preterm birth remains to be established. Liu et al studied preterm infants (< 37 weeks of gestation) enrolled in the Newborn Epigenetics Study in North Carolina. They analyzed DNA methylation of CpG sites within 9 imprinted differentially methylated regions (DMRs) in cord blood samples from 73 infants. DNA methylation analyses were conducted using pyrosequencing of IGF2, H19, MEG3-IG, MEG3, PEG3, MEST, SGCE/PEG10, NNAT, and PLAGL1. The investigators examined whether the type of preterm birth (medically indicated, preterm premature rupture of membranes, and spontaneous preterm labor) or infection status (chorioamnionitis and funisitis) was associated with DNA methylation of these DMRs. Infant DNA methylation levels did not differ by type of preterm birth. Infants with pathologic evidence of chorioamnionitis had higher methylation of PLAGL1 ($P < .05$). This DMR is located at chromosome 6p24.2 and encodes a zinc-finger transcription factor involved in tumor development and growth via IGF2 signaling. Blood DNA is obtained largely from leukocytes, and DNA methylation patterns differ by cell type. While intriguing, the authors did not address whether DNA methylation differences persisted after adjustment for leukocyte subtype. Such adjustment is crucial, especially given the association with infection, which could affect the white blood cell population distribution. The failure to adjust for cell type leaves unanswered the question of whether DNA methylation of PLAGL1 is associated with both infection and preterm birth.

H. Burris, MD

5 Infectious Disease and Immunology

Limitations of the risk factor based approach in early neonatal sepsis evaluations
Flidel-Rimon O, Galstyan S, Juster-Reicher A, et al (Affiliated to the Hebrew Univ, Jerusalem, Israel)
Acta Paediatr 101:e540-e544, 2012

Aim.—Guidelines for detection of early neonatal sepsis employ a risk factor approach combined with laboratory parameters. In an era of increasing intrapartum antibiotic prophylaxis (IAP), we re-assessed the approach as a whole and each of the risk factors individually.

Method.—This retrospective study included infants with risk factors for sepsis or those treated with antibiotics or who had documented early sepsis. Safety of the protocol was assessed by the number of cases of either missed or partially treated late sepsis or meningitis and the sepsis-related mortality rate. Predictive value of each clinical and laboratory factor was calculated.

Results.—Of the 22 215 neonates, 2096 were assessed. IAP among infants with risk factors rose from 68% in 2005 to 78% in 2008 ($p = 0.001$). A total of 1662 asymptomatic infants had risk factors, 635 received antibiotics and one (0.06%) had sepsis. A total of 434 symptomatic infants were treated with antibiotics and of these 234 had risk factors and 20 (4.6%) had sepsis. No cases of partially treated or missed sepsis were detected. Poor predictive value was found for all risk factors except prematurity and leukopenia.

Conclusion.—The risk factor based approach in asymptomatic infants cannot be justified. In-hospital observation of asymptomatic infants for 2–3 days with antibiotic treatment being reserved only for symptomatic infants may be a reasonable alternative.

▶ Achievement of nearly universal intrapartum antibiotic prophylaxis for parturients whose babies are at increased risk has changed the landscape of early-onset neonatal infections. It is becoming evident that experiences from a prior era may no longer be germane, prompting re-evaluation of long-established paradigms for postnatal treatment of these infants. This report provides evidence that current practices may entail inefficient use of laboratory evaluations in many low-risk infants. From a birth cohort of more than 22 000 babies, the authors identified 2096 as at risk for sepsis. The analysis in the report primarily addresses the utility of clinical findings and blood counts in that patient group, but the key observation comes from the subset of 1662 infants who had risk factors but no clinical signs of illness. Of these, only one—a preterm infant whose mother had chorioamnionitis—had a positive blood culture. This attack rate is not statistically different from the overall rate in this birth cohort (1 per 1000 births), with an upper 95% confidence of only 3.3 per 1000. Complete blood counts (which did not include manual differential counts or immature/mature or immature/total granulocyte ratios) added nothing to the evaluation of these infants. Given this very low attack rate in asymptomatic infants, it is unlikely that any test will accurately identify the rare case of sepsis in that group. The utility of complete blood counts, therefore, might lie in exclusion of sepsis in babies with clinical signs of disease, but prior experience has found poor sensitivity of blood counts for that purpose. In this cohort, infected babies made themselves known by developing tachypnea (19 cases) or fever (3 cases) within the first 40 hours after birth. Others who have similar experiences with interventional approaches should be encouraged to share their data, as these authors have done, because further experience will guide evolution of practice in this area. Optimal management of asymptomatic infants with antenatal or intrapartum risk factors for sepsis might consist of close monitoring for clinical signs of illness—respiratory distress, in particular—rather than dependence on unreliable laboratory tests. We might begin by abandoning the traditional sepsis screen in term infants who appear to be well and consider extending this practice to preterm infants as its safety is demonstrated. At the least, this approach merits systematic evaluation, as these authors have recommended.

W. E. Benitz, MD

Use of the Complete Blood Cell Count in Late-Onset Neonatal Sepsis

Hornik CP, Benjamin DK, Becker KC, et al (Duke Univ, Durham, NC; Clemson Univ, SC; Duke Clinical Res Inst, Durham, NC; et al)

Pediatr Infect Dis J 31:803-807, 2012

Background.—Late-onset sepsis is an important cause of morbidity and mortality in infants. Diagnosis of late-onset sepsis can be challenging. The complete blood cell count and differential have been previously evaluated as diagnostic tools for late-onset sepsis in small, single-center reports.

Objective.—We evaluated the diagnostic accuracy of the complete blood cell count and differential in late-onset sepsis in a large multicenter population.

Study Design.—Using a cohort of all infants with cultures and complete blood cell count data from a large administrative database, we calculated odds ratios for infection, as well as sensitivity, specificity, positive and negative predictive values and likelihood ratios for various commonly used cutoff values.

Results.—High and low white blood cell counts, high absolute neutrophil counts, high immature-to-total neutrophil ratios and low platelet counts were associated with late-onset sepsis. Associations were weaker

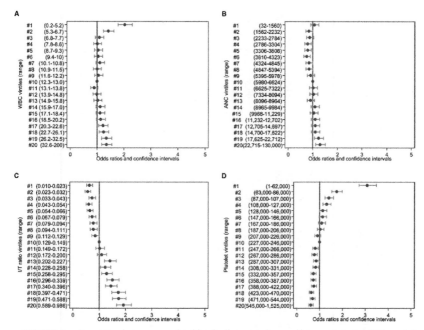

FIGURE 1.—Association between complete blood cell count indices and late-onset sepsis (>72 hours). A, WBC vintiles and ORs; B, ANC vintiles and ORs; C, I/T ratio vintiles and ORs; D, Platelet vintiles and ORs. (Reprinted from Hornik CP, Benjamin DK, Becker KC, et al. Use of the complete blood cell count in late-onset neonatal sepsis. *Pediatr Infect Dis J.* 2012;31:803-807, with permission from Lippincott Williams & Wilkins.)

with increasing postnatal age at the time of the culture. Specificity was highest for white blood cell counts < 1000/mm³ and >50,000/mm³ (>99%). Positive likelihood ratios were highest for white blood cell counts < 1000/mm³ (4.1) and platelet counts < 50,000/mm³ (3.5).

Conclusion.—No complete blood cell count index possessed adequate sensitivity to reliably rule out late-onset sepsis in this population (Fig 1, Table).

▶ Drawing on a truly enormous data set including more than 160 000 episodes of suspected sepsis, this report provides powerful confirmation of a well-established but insufficiently appreciated fact: blood counts are an unreliable diagnostic test for early-onset neonatal sepsis. The large size of this sample allows stratification of the data for each observation in vintiles (20 strata) while preserving narrow confidence intervals. Areas under receiver operating characteristic curves fell into a range (< 0.75) generally deemed to be not clinically useful: 0.668 for white blood cell (WBC) counts < 5000/mm³, 0.686 for I/T ratio, 0.586 for absolute neutrophil count (ANC), 0.554 for platelet counts, and 0.525 for WBC counts > 20 000/mm³; no confidence intervals are provided. Although the abstract describes negative predictive values (NPV) as > 99.8%, no further data are provided in the text or supplements to illuminate that observation. It is important to note that the prevalence of sepsis in this sample was

TABLE.—Supplemental Digital Content 3. Test Characteristics of Various WBC, ANC, I/T Ratio, and Platelet Count Values

	All				<34 weeks GA				34–36 weeks GA				>36 weeks GA			
	Sens (%)	Spec (%)	+LR	−LR	Sens (%)	Spec (%)	+LR	−LR	Sens (%)	Spec (%)	+LR	−LR	Sens (%)	Spec (%)	+LR	−LR
WBC, /mm³																
<1000	0.3	>99.9	19.4	1.0	0.3	>99.9	8.4	1.0	0.3	>99.9	19.4	1.0	0.4	>99.9	85.4	1.0
<5000	17.7	96.3	4.7	0.9	24.3	91.4	2.8	0.8	17.7	96.3	4.7	0.9	15.4	99.1	17.2	0.9
>20,000	18.4	79.3	0.9	1.0	12.6	91.0	1.4	1.0	18.4	79.3	0.9	1.0	23.7	61.9	0.6	1.2
>50,000	0.5	99.6	1.3	1.0	1.4	99.4	2.3	1.0	0.5	99.6	1.3	1.0	0.1	99.7	0.3	1.0
ANC, /mm³																
<100	0.8	>99.9	45.2	1.0	1.6	>99.9	34.2	1.0	0.8	>99.9	45.2	1.0	0.5	>99.9	229	1.0
<1000	11.7	97.8	5.4	0.9	20.4	94.5	3.7	0.8	11.7	97.8	5.4	0.9	7.6	99.6	19.2	0.9
<1500	18.8	95.2	3.9	0.9	30.0	88.1	2.5	0.8	18.8	95.2	3.9	0.9	13.8	99.2	16.4	0.9
I/T ratio																
>0.20	54.6	73.7	2.1	0.6	65.1	74.7	2.6	0.5	54.6	73.7	2.1	0.6	52.1	68.9	1.7	0.7
>0.25	47.9	81.7	2.6	0.6	56.2	82.3	3.2	0.5	47.9	81.7	2.6	0.6	46.8	77.6	2.1	0.7
>0.50	21.9	95.7	5.0	0.8	28.5	95.0	5.7	0.8	21.9	95.7	5.0	0.8	20.2	94.9	3.9	0.8
Platelet, /mm³																
<50,000	0.8	99.4	1.2	1.0	1.4	99.4	2.2	1.0	0.7	99.4	1.2	1.0	0.5	99.3	0.7	1.0
<70,000	1.7	98.7	1.3	1.0	3.4	98.7	2.6	1.0	1.7	98.7	1.3	1.0	0.9	98.5	0.6	1.0
<100,000	4.0	96.9	1.3	1.0	8.0	96.9	2.5	1.0	4.0	96.9	1.3	1.0	2.1	96.6	0.6	1.0
Other																
WBC <8000	34.0	84.4	2.2	0.8												
ANC <4134	41.5	74.3	1.6	0.8												
I/T ratio >0.24	49.2	80.6	2.5	0.6												
Platelet <147,000	14.6	90.1	1.5	1.0												

GA indicates gestational age; WBC, white blood cell; ANC, absolute neutrophil count; I/T, immature-to-total neutrophils; sens, sensitivity; spec, specificity; +LR, positive likelihood ratio; −LR, negative likelihood ratio.

only 1.3%, so even a useless test would have an NPV of 98.7%. Key test performance indicators are reported only in an online supplement, which does not include confidence intervals (Table). These shortcomings notwithstanding, the conclusions are compelling. Notably, only the most extreme values of WBC count, ANC, and I/T ratio were associated with odds ratios for early-onset sepsis that differed significantly from median result for each measurement (Fig 1). Those extreme values, consisting primarily of very low WBC and ANC and very high I/T ratios (Table), had high positive likelihood ratios and high specificities, but very poor sensitivities and inconsequential negative likelihood ratios. In brief, blood counts did not reliably predict either the presence or absence of sepsis. It is increasingly apparent that we continue to use blood counts only because of deeply ingrained habit rather than evidence of clinical utility.

W. E. Benitz, MD

Cerebrospinal Fluid Reference Ranges in Term and Preterm Infants in the Neonatal Intensive Care Unit
Srinivasan L, Shah SS, Padula MA, et al (The Children's Hosp of Philadelphia, PA; Cincinnati Children's Hosp Med Ctr, OH; et al)
J Pediatr 161:729-734, 2012

Objective.—To determine reference ranges of cerebrospinal fluid (CSF) laboratory findings in term and preterm infants in the neonatal intensive care unit.

Study Design.—Data were collected prospectively as part of a multisite study of infants aged < 6 months undergoing lumbar puncture for evaluation of suspected sepsis. Infants with a red blood cell count > 500 cells/μL or a known cause of CSF pleocytosis were excluded from the analysis.

Results.—A total of 318 infants met the inclusion criteria. Of these, 148 infants (47%) were preterm, and 229 (72%) received antibiotics before undergoing lumbar puncture. The upper reference limit of the CSF white blood cell (WBC) count was 12 cells/μL in preterm infants and 14 cells/μL in term infants. CSF protein levels were significantly higher in preterm infants (upper reference limit, 209 mg/dL vs 159 mg/dL in term infants; $P < .001$), and declined with advancing postnatal age in both groups (preterm, $P = .008$; term, $P < .001$). CSF glucose levels did not differ in term and preterm infants. Antibiotic exposure did not significantly affect CSF WBC, protein, or glucose values.

Conclusions.—CSF WBC counts are not significantly different in preterm and term infants. CSF protein levels are higher and decline more slowly with postnatal age in preterm infants compared with term infants. This study provides CSF reference ranges for hospitalized preterm and term infants, particularly in the first month of life (Fig).

▶ Bacterial meningitis is an infrequent but often devastating disease in the neonatal period, occurring in about 0.3 per 1000 live births or in 1% to 2% of infants evaluated for suspected neonatal sepsis.[1,2] Experience has shown that

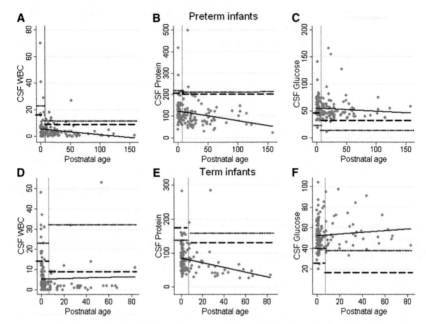

FIGURE.—Changes in **A** and **D**, CSF WBC count (**A** and **D**), CSF protein level **C** and **F**, and CSF glucose level with increasing postnatal age in preterm and term infants. The graphs exclude infants with unknown CSF WBC concentration (n = 1) or an extremely outlying value (n = 1; CSF WBC of 850), unknown CSF protein concentration (n = 4), and unknown CSF glucose concentration (n = 2). The *solid lines* represent the best linear fit for each laboratory test result; the *dashed lines* represent upper limits (for CSF WBC and protein) and lower limits (for CSF glucose) based on the addition or subtraction of 1.5 × IQR to the upper or lower limit of the IQR, respectively; and the *dotted lines* represent upper limits (for CSF WBC and protein) and lower limits (for CSF glucose) based on the 95th and 5th percentile values, respectively. The *vertical line* represents a postnatal age of 7 days. (Reprinted from Journal Pediatrics. Srinivasan L, Shah SS, Padula MA, et al. Cerebrospinal fluid reference ranges in term and preterm infants in the neonatal intensive care unit. *J Pediatr.* 2012;161:729-734, Copyright 2012, with permission from Elsevier.)

there is no substitute for analysis of cerebrospinal fluid (CSF) in diagnosis of this condition. In recent years, recognition that older studies of CSF analysis in neonates may not be representative of the populations now cared for in our nurseries, which include more very-low-birth-weight infants and much higher rates of prior antibiotic exposure, has renewed interest in characterization of normal CSF findings in neonates. This report addresses the question of normal values for CSF analytes in infants evaluated for and found not to have significant central nervous system pathology, including bacterial meningitis. Accordingly, infants with herpes simplex or enteroviral meningoencephalitis, ventriculoperitoneal shunts, seizures, bacteremia, or greater than 500 red blood cells per microliter of CSF were also excluded. Traditional boundaries for normal values may need some adjustment. However, inconsistencies in presentation of these data make it difficult to ascertain just what those adjustments should be. Inspection of the data (Fig) suggests a few reasonable conclusions. CSF white blood cell counts may be higher in the first postnatal week, but 95% appear to be less than 25 cells per microliter in both term and preterm (< 37 weeks of gestation) infants; after the first week, the 95th percentile is lower, at about 12 cells per microliter. CSF protein concentrations are higher in preterm than in term infants; in the first week, the 95th percentile appears to be about 210 mg/dL in preterm infants and 140 mg/dL in term infants. CSF protein concentrations decline with postnatal age in both groups, with the 95th percentile approximating 180 mg/dL in preterm and 150 mg/dL in term infants. A more detailed description of developmental evolution of CSF protein concentrations, both before and after term gestation, would be very useful. Normal concentrations of glucose in the CSF may be lower than suggested by established norms, which might be replaced by a fifth percentile of 33 mg/L for all preterms and for term infants for the first week; the widely used threshold of 40 mg/dL appears appropriate for term infants older than 7 days. (These visual estimates differ from those offered by the authors, and readers are urged to examine the data to reach their own conclusions.) CSF culture, which can confirm the diagnosis and provide critical guidance for selection and duration of antimicrobial therapy, remains the essential test for bacterial meningitis in neonates. Values that fall outside the boundaries suggested by these data may inform clinical judgments about management of infants with possible meningitis and negative cultures, but it must be remembered that these measurements are neither sensitive nor specific for diagnosis of bacterial meningitis.[1,2]

W. E. Benitz, MD

References

1. Garges HP, Moody MA, Cotten CM, et al. Neonatal meningitis: what is the correlation among cerebrospinal fluid cultures, blood cultures, and cerebrospinal fluid parameters? *Pediatrics.* 2006;117:1094-1100.
2. Smith PB, Garges HP, Cotton CM, Walsh TJ, Clark RH, Benjamin DK Jr. Meningitis in preterm neonates: importance of cerebrospinal fluid parameters. *Am J Perinatol.* 2008;25:421-426.

Group B *Streptococcus* and *Escherichia coli* Infections in the Intensive Care Nursery in the Era of Intrapartum Antibiotic Prophylaxis
Bauserman MS, Laughon MM, Hornik CP, et al (Univ of North Carolina, Chapel Hill; Duke Univ, Durham, NC; et al)
Pediatr Infect Dis J 32:208-212, 2013

Background.—Group B *Streptococcus* (GBS) and *Escherichia coli* cause serious bacterial infections (SBIs) and are associated with morbidity and mortality in newborn infants. Intrapartum antibiotic prophylaxis reduces early-onset SBIs caused by GBS. The effect of intrapartum antibiotic prophylaxis on late-onset SBIs caused by these organisms is unknown.

Methods.—We examined all blood, urine and cerebrospinal fluid culture results from infants admitted from 1997 to 2010 to 322 neonatal intensive care units managed by the Pediatrix Medical Group. We identified infants with positive cultures for GBS or *E. coli* and compared the incidence of early- and late-onset SBI for each organism in the time period before

(1997 to 2001) and after (2002 to 2010) universal intrapartum antibiotic prophylaxis recommendations.

Results.—We identified 716,407 infants with cultures, 2520 (0.4%) with cultures positive for GBS and 2476 (0.3%) with cultures positive for *E. coli.* The incidence of GBS early-onset SBI decreased between 1997 to 2001 and 2002 to 2010 from 3.5 to 2.6 per 1000 admissions, and the incidence for *E. coli* early-onset SBI remained stable (1.4/1000 admissions in both time periods). Over the same time period, the incidence of GBS late-onset SBI increased from 0.8 to 1.1 per 1000 admissions, and incidence of *E. coli* late-onset SBI increased from 2.2 to 2.5 per 1000 admissions.

Conclusions.—In our cohort, the incidence of GBS early-onset SBI decreased, whereas the incidence of late-onset SBI for *E. coli* and GBS increased.

▶ This retrospective analysis of early and late onset neonatal infections preintrapartum and postintrapartum antibiotic prophylaxis yielded interesting although not surprising results. Since the 1940s, we have seen epochs in which the predominant perinatal pathogens have been altered by widespread antibiotic use. In the 1940s, group A *Streptococcus* was responsible for the majority of puerperal sepsis and neonatal disease until the advent of penicillin. This, in turn, led to the emergence of *Staphylococcus* in the 1950s, until its eradication and subsequent replacement by gram negatives, especially *Escherichia coli.* Use of aminoglycosides once again altered the balance and led to the group B *Streptococcus* era in the 1970s. The message has been loud and clear, "Don't mess with Mother Nature." Bacterial adaptation is faster than big pharmaceutical's.

This study, which used a huge database, may be further evidence of this. Widespread use of intrapartum antibiotics appears to have accomplished its short-term goal, the reduction of early-onset group B *Streptococcus*, but perhaps at a significant cost: a rise in the incidence of late-onset infections caused by both group B *Streptococcus* and *E coli.* As the authors indicate, it is unclear whether this represents a true epidemiologic shift in pathogenetic organisms or a selective vulnerability of very preterm infants. It would be difficult to distinguish these in a retrospective, historically controlled review, but the red flag has been raised. Even well-intentioned strategies with favorable short-term benefits can have adverse long-term consequences.

S. M. Donn, MD

The Investment Case for Preventing NICU-Associated Infections
Donovan EF, on behalf of the Ohio Perinatal Quality Collaborative (Cincinnati Children's Hosp Med Ctr, OH)
Am J Perinatol 30:179-184, 2013

Background.—Nosocomial [hospital-associated or neonatal intensive care unit (NICU)-associated] infections occur in as many as 10 to 36% of very low-birth-weight infants cared for in NICUs.

Objective.—To determine the potentially avoidable, incremental costs of care associated with NICU-associated bloodstream infections.

Study Design.—This retrospective study included all NICU admissions of infants weighing 401 to 1500 g at birth in the greater Cincinnati region from January 1, 2005, through December 31, 2007. Nonphysician costs of care were compared between infants who developed at least one bacterial bloodstream infection prior to NICU discharge or death and infants who did not. Costs were adjusted for clinical and demographic characteristics that are present in the first 3 days of life and are known associates of infection.

Results.—Among 900 study infants with no congenital anomaly and no major surgery, 82 (9.1%) developed at least one bacterial bloodstream infection. On average, the cost of NICU care was $16,800 greater per infant who experienced NICU-associated bloodstream infection.

Conclusion.—Potentially avoidable costs of care associated with bloodstream infection can be used to justify investments in the reliable implementation of evidence-based interventions designed to prevent these infections.

▶ It is not the money, it is the amount. In this interesting article, the authors estimate the costs associated with nosocomial infections in the neonatal intensive care setting. Retrospective data from a 3-year period (2005 to 2007) were analyzed from infants sustaining at least 1 episode of bacterial sepsis prior to death or discharge. Nonphysician costs were increased by nearly $17 000 in 82 of the 900 infants studied.

Although one could quibble about the methodology and the assigned dollar values, the generalizable conclusions are valid: There is a relatively high incidence of hospital-acquired infections in the neonatal intensive care unit, and there is a significant incremental cost to treat them.

This article should be required reading for the neonatal world. It is nice that a group of investigators put some science behind the, "Yeah, I knew that."

S. M. Donn, MD

Central Line—Associated Bloodstream Infections in Neonatal Intensive care: Changing the Mental Model from Inevitability to Preventability
Suresh GK, Edwards WH (Dartmouth Med School, Lebanon, NH)
Am J Perinatol 29:57-64, 2012

Previously considered unavoidable complications of hospital care (reflecting an entitlement mental model), health care—associated infections are now considered as medical errors and cause significant preventable morbidity and mortality in neonates. Prevention of such infections, particularly central line—associated bloodstream infections (CLABSI), should be an important patient safety priority for all neonatal intensive care units (NICUs). An important first step is to promote a mental model of CLABSIs as preventable complications of care. Other general strategies are (1) promoting an organizational culture of safety and empowerment of staff; (2) hand hygiene; (3) avoiding overcrowding and understaffing;

(4) using breast milk for enteral feedings; and (5) involving families in infection prevention efforts. Specific strategies to prevent CLABSI are (1) insertion practices: insertion of all central vascular catheters under strict sterile conditions with the aid of a checklist; (2) maintenance practices: ensuring that entries into the lumen of the vascular catheter always occur under aseptic conditions, minimizing catheter disconnections, and replacement of intravenous infusion sets at recommended intervals; (3) removal of all central lines as soon as possible. Participation in national or statewide quality improvement collaboratives is an emerging trend in neonatology that can enhance CLABSI prevention efforts by NICUs.

▶ This review article contextualizes central line associated bloodstream infections (CLABSIs) in neonatal intensive care units (NICUs). Drawing on data from the Centers from Disease Control and Prevention, the National Healthcare Safety Network, and the Vermont Oxford Network, the authors outline the clinical and operational strategies for CLABSI reduction.

CLABSIs are the most common pediatric nosocomial infection and carry significant attributable morbidity and mortality for our patients and waste health care resources and dollars.[1] In 2008, the Centers for Medicare and Medicaid Services added CLABSI to the list of nonremunerable "never events," and it is striking to note that 2010 neonatal CLABSI rates are a fifth of what they were a decade prior.[1] This falling, highly variable CLABSI rate emphasizes the ongoing opportunity for eliminating residual, preventable harm.

The authors describe several important improvement strategies that may not be readily apparent to providers. To help distinguish signal from noise among events that are relatively infrequent in any single NICU, the authors introduce statistical process control as a complement to conventional biostatistics. Control charts empower local clinician leaders to bring statistical rigor to their small-scale quality improvement (QI) operations, enabling teams to collect and act on data simultaneously and continuously. QI collaboratives take this local data to the next level, employing data aggregation and cooperative benchmarking to accelerate learning, properly scale tests of change, and identify effective implementation strategies. Finally, the authors emphasize the impact of context on patient care, namely safe staffing and safety culture. The attitudes, beliefs, and availability of clinical care providers contribute to nosocomial infection rates much as technique and technology do.

This article does perpetuate some of the adult-centric and physician-centric CLABSI preconceptions. Adult intensive care units have enjoyed dramatic reductions in bloodstream infection rates by focusing on insertion practices, a focused task commonly performed by physicians. Yet, the preponderance of pediatric and neonatal CLABSIs occur weeks after insertion. Indeed, the long-term, daily maintenance practices are the main drivers of CLABSIs among children, and these diffuse activities fall predominantly within the nursing scope of practice.[2] Effective CLABSI reduction requires more than multidisciplinary collaboration; it demands effective application of implementation science. As the authors point out, there are already high grades of evidence for CLABSI prevention.

Yet, we commonly fail to build systems that enable providers to apply those evidence-based practices reliably.[3]

The traditional attitude that CLABSIs are inevitable and tolerable is clearly a barrier to more rigorous and widespread adoption of proven prevention methods, and the authors should be lauded for calling out the flawed mental model and proposing a better one. What we need most of all, however, are effective methods to actually get providers to change their mental models and behaviors. Ironically, this article suggests that NICUs with higher CLABSI rates should reduce them to levels seen in units with lower rates, implying an acceptably low rate above zero. It is a testament to how deeply rooted our flawed mental models are when we try to consciously update them, only to subconsciously fall back into our old ways of thinking.

M. Niedner, MD

References

1. National Healthcare Safety Network: NHSN Annual Reports. http://www.cdc.gov/nhsn/dataStat.htmls. Accessed July 31, 2012.
2. Miller MR, Niedner MF, Huskins WC, et al. Reducing PICU central line-associated bloodstream infections: 3-year results. *Pediatrics.* 2011;128:e1077-e1083.
3. Balas EA, Boren SA. Managing clinical knowledge for health care improvement. In: Bemmel J, McCray AT, eds. *Yearbook of Medical Informatics 2000: Patient-Centered Systems.* Stuttgart, Germany: Schattauer Verlagsgesellschaft mbH; 2000: 65-70.

Accuracy of Hospital Administrative Data in Reporting Central Line–Associated Bloodstream Infections in Newborns

Patrick SW, Davis MM, Sedman AB, et al (Univ of Michigan Health System, Ann Arbor; et al)
Pediatrics 131:S75-S80, 2013

Objectives.—Central line-associated bloodstream infections (CLABSIs) are a significant source of morbidity and mortality in the NICU. In 2010, Medicaid was mandated not to pay hospitals for treatment of CLABSI; however, the source of CLABSI data for this policy was not specified. Our objective was to evaluate the accuracy of hospital administrative data compared with CLABSI confirmed by an infection control service.

Methods.—We evaluated hospital administrative and infection control data for newborns admitted consecutively from January 1, 2008, to December 31, 2010. Clinical and demographic data were collected through chart review. We compared cases of CLABSI identified by administrative data (*International Classification of Diseases, Ninth Revision, Clinical Modification* 999.31) with infection control data that use national criteria from the Centers for Disease Control and Prevention as the gold standard. To ascertain the nature possible deficiencies in the administrative data, each patient's medical record was searched to determine if clinical phrases that commonly refer to CLABSI appeared.

TABLE 2.—Sensitivity, Specificity, Positive Predictive Value, Negative Predictive Value for Hospital Administrative Versus Infection Control Reporting

| | | CLABSI Cases Identified using CDC/NHSN Criteria Disease Present | | |
		Yes	No	Total
CLABSI in billing data	Yes	3	7	10
	No	42	2867	2909
	Total	45	2875	2920

Results.—Of 2920 infants admitted to the NICU during our study period, 52 were identified as having a CLABSI: 42 by infection control data only, 7 through hospital administrative data only, and 3 appearing in both. Against the gold standard, hospital administrative data were 6.7% sensitive and 99.7% specific, with a positive predictive value of 30.0% and a negative predictive value of 98.6%. Only 48% of medical records indicated a CLABSI.

Conclusions.—Our findings from a major children's hospital NICU indicate that *International Classification of Diseases, Ninth Revision, Clinical Modification* code 993.31 is presently not accurate and cannot be used reliably to compare CLABSI rates in NICUs (Table 2).

▶ Here we have a cautionary tale. Using data collected for 1 purpose for an entirely different end is fraught with hazard. In this instance, data collected to support hospital billing proved quite unreliable for identification of episodes of central line–associated bloodstream infections (CLABSIs): more than 90% of the actual CLABSI cases were not identified, and 70% of the putative cases were identified erroneously (Table 2). There may be many reasons for this discrepancy. Our system for payment of hospitals for care provided was not designed to capture comprehensive data about every patient's hospital course, only sufficient information to ensure correct compensation. Accordingly, many secondary diagnoses (such as CLABSI) are predictably underrepresented in those data. In addition, diagnostic criteria may differ when diagnoses are used for different purposes (eg, reimbursement vs quality benchmarking) and may not be applied consistently as physicians and other providers document their care. If providers are not aware of formal diagnostic criteria, as is very often the case, their documentation will not accurately reflect the clinical circumstances. Because administrative discharge data can only be drawn from provider documentation, to the exclusion of considering other data sources such as laboratory reports, provider documentation may deviate either way from strict data definitions. As this article demonstrates, the result is, not surprisingly, a very weak correlation between diagnostic classification based on chart abstraction for payment vs chart abstraction for quality oversight or clinical research. In addition, all such retroactive analyses very likely are much less accurate than real-time, prospective data collection. The analysis presented in this article demonstrates that such errors are, in fact, very substantial and may make administrative databases drawn from hospital reimbursement files virtually useless for other purposes, including quality- or outcomes-based modification of that reimbursement. Although the ready availability of such datasets makes them attractive resources for a variety of clinical, epidemiologic, and economic investigations, the results of these studies should be viewed with considerable skepticism, particularly if they are used to guide changes in practice or policy.

W. E. Benitz, MD

Prophylactic Probiotics to Prevent Death and Nosocomial Infection in Preterm Infants

Rojas MA, Lozano JM, Rojas MX, et al (Wake Forest School of Medicine, Winston-Salem, NC; Florida International Univ, Miami, FL; Pontificia Universidad Javeriana, Bogotá, Colombia; et al)
Pediatrics 130:e1113-e1120, 2012

Background and Objective.—It has been suggested that probiotics may decrease infant mortality and nosocomial infections because of their ability to suppress colonization and translocation of bacterial pathogens in the gastrointestinal tract. We designed a large double-blinded placebo-controlled trial using *Lactobacillus reuteri* to test this hypothesis in preterm infants.

Methods.—Eligible infants were randomly assigned during the first 48 hours of life to either daily probiotic administration or placebo. Infants in the intervention group were administered enterally 5 drops of a probiotic preparation containing 10^8 colony-forming units of *L reuteri* DSM 17938 until death or discharge from the NICU.

Results.—A total of 750 infants ≤2000 g were enrolled. The frequency of the primary outcome, death, or nosocomial infection, was similar in the probiotic and placebo groups (relative risk 0.87; 95% confidence interval: 0.63–1.19; $P = .376$). There was a trend toward a lower rate of nosocomial pneumonia in the probiotic group (2.4% vs 5.0%; $P = .06$) and a nonsignificant 40% decrease in necrotizing enterocolitis (2.4% vs 4.0%; $P = .23$). Episodes of feeding intolerance and duration of hospitalization were lower in infants ≤1500 g (9.6% vs 16.8% [$P = .04$]; 32.5 days vs 37 days [$P = .03$]).

Conclusions.—Although *L reuteri* did not appear to decrease the rate of the composite outcome, the trends suggest a protective role consistent with what has been observed in the literature. Feeding intolerance and duration of hospitalization were decreased in premature infants ≤1500 g (Table 2).

▶ Data regarding effects of probiotic use in preterm infants continues to accumulate, but evidence to guide incorporation into practice remains elusive. Results of clinical trials are inconsistent, and their implications remain controversial. These investigators deserve commendation for carrying out this carefully designed multicenter trial to illuminate this matter. It is unfortunate that this great effort has not brought resolution to the controversy, as the trial found neither safety

TABLE 2.—Nosocomial Infection—Related Outcomes of the Study Population

Primary Outcomes	Probiotic, $n = 372$	Placebo, $n = 378$	RR	95% CI	P
Death or NI, n (%)	57 (15.3)	67 (17.7)	0.87	0.63—1.19	.38
Death, n (%)	22 (5.9)	28 (7.4)	0.80	0.47—1.37	.41
NI, n (%)	47 (12.6)	57 (15.1)	0.88	0.61—1.28	.33
BSI, n (%)	24 (6.5)	17 (4.5)	1.44	0.78—2.63	.24
Positive culture, n (%)	34 (9.1)	40 (10.6)	0.86	0.56—1.33	.51
Nosocomial pneumonia, n (%)	9 (2.4)	19 (5.0)	0.48	0.22—1.05	.06
Nosocomial UTI, n (%)	7 (1.9)	3 (0.8)	2.37	0.62—9.10	.19
Nosocomial meningitis, n (%)	1 (0.3)	1(0.3)	1.02	0.06—16.20	.99
Necrotizing enterocolitis, n (%)	9 (2.4)	15 (4.0)	0.61	0.27—1.38	.23
Elevated C-reactive protein, n (%)	37 (10.0)	48 (12.7)	0.78	0.52—1.17	.24
Leukocytosis, n (%)	54 (14.5)	71 (18.8)	0.77	0.56—1.07	.12

BSI, bloodstream infection; UTI, urinary tract infection.

nor efficacy of administration of this probiotic. The optimistic tone of the abstract notwithstanding, none of the primary outcomes differed between treatment groups (Table 2). The abstract comments on a trend toward reduction in nosocomial pneumonia and a nonsignificant decrease in necrotizing enterocolitis but overlooks similar (nonsignificant) increases in rates of bloodstream and urinary tract infections. Of 27 outcome comparisons reported, only 2 (rates of feeding intolerance and duration of hospitalization in the subgroup of infants with birth weights < 1500 g) achieved statistical significance and only if no correction was made for multiple comparisons. There may be several potential explanations for these ambiguous results. Perhaps the choice of this particular probiotic strain was not propitious, or efficacy may require use of 2 or more complementary strains. Effects may have been masked by low rates of breast milk feeding (20%) in both groups. The number of subjects may have been insufficient to power detection of modest but potentially import differences. Or it may be that probiotic treatment is simply ineffective. Widespread adoption of this strategy should await standardization of agents and demonstration of efficacy and safety by ongoing clinical trials.

W. E. Benitz, MD

Unrecognized Viral Respiratory Tract Infections in Premature Infants during their Birth Hospitalization: A Prospective Surveillance Study in Two Neonatal Intensive Care Units
Bennett NJ, Tabarani CM, Bartholoma NM, et al (Upstate Golisano Children's Hosp, Syracuse, NY, et al)
J Pediatr 161:814-818.e3, 2012

Objective.—To determine the frequency and effects of nosocomial respiratory viral infections (RVIs) in premature neonates, including those who may be asymptomatic.

Study Design.—We performed a year-long surveillance for RVIs in infants <33 weeks gestational age admitted to 2 Syracuse neonatal intensive care units. Infants were enrolled within 3 days of neonatal intensive care unit admission and were sampled for RVIs until discharge using a multiplex polymerase chain reaction assay capable of detecting 17 different respiratory viruses or subtypes.

Results.—Twenty-six of 50 prematurely born infants (52%) tested positive for a respiratory virus at least once during their birth hospitalization. Testing positive for a respiratory virus was significantly associated with longer length of stay (70 days vs 35 days, $P = .002$) and prolonged ventilatory support (51 vs 13 days, $P = .002$). Infants who tested positive for a respiratory virus during their birth hospitalization had more than twice the rate of developing bronchopulmonary dysplasia ($P < .05$).

Conclusion.—Nosocomial RVIs were frequent in our study population, despite the absence of clinical indicators of illness. Length of hospital stay was significantly longer and a diagnosis of bronchopulmonary dysplasia was more common in infants who had respiratory viruses detected.

▶ Most neonates less than 33 weeks' gestation require some form of respiratory support, although the intensity and length of support vary considerably. This article demonstrates a previously underappreciated contributor to that variation: asymptomatic presence of respiratory viruses. Although previous studies have demonstrated the presence of asymptomatic respiratory viral infections following specific viral outbreaks,[1] this is the first study of widespread screening, demonstrating positive tests in 52% of study participants at some point between birth and discharge home. It is unclear whether the presence of respiratory viruses represented true infection vs transient carriage, although the serial detection of virus in multiple patients and the clinical correlations suggest true infection. Infected infants and noninfected infants were similar in terms of gestational age and birth weight; however, infected infants demonstrated significantly longer length of stay ($P = .002$), increased ventilator days ($P = .002$), increased duration of supplemental oxygen ($P = .022$), increased rate of developing bronchopulmonary dysplasia ($P < .05$), and more clinical deterioration ($P = .0001$), 71% of which were associated with positive respiratory viral infection studies. However, the authors do not report how many infants were asymptomatic at the time of positive virus detection.

This study brings forth the question of whether routine surveillance should be part of the standard of care for all neonates. These authors used multiplex polymerase chain reaction (PCR) testing, which allowed detection of 17 different viruses. Many centers still rely on direct fluorescent antibody testing, which is less expensive but also less sensitive; it remains unclear whether the cost of PCR testing is outweighed by benefits of the results from surveillance testing. Positive tests would not lead to treatment changes but may result in decreased antibiotic use, therefore decreasing the occurrence of antibiotic-related illnesses (such as necrotizing enterocolitis) and decreased antibiotic resistance. In addition, unit-wide surveillance may improve infection control measures, including improved hand hygiene practices, increased use of gowns and gloves during patient interactions, and stricter rules around visits from parents and siblings, especially during peak respiratory viral season.

Further studies are indicated to address appropriate timing for surveillance and whether clinical predictors can be linked to positive respiratory viral tests in asymptomatic patients.

S. S. Stone, MD, MBA

Reference

1. Cunney RJ, Bialachowski A, Thornley D, Smaill FM, Pennie RA. An outbreak of influenza A in a neonatal intensive care unit. *Infect Control Hosp Epidemiol.* 2000;21:449-454.

Risk of Fetal Death after Pandemic Influenza Virus Infection or Vaccination

Håberg SE, Trogstad L, Gunnes N, et al (Univ of Oslo, Norway; et al)
N Engl J Med 368:333-340, 2013

Background.—During the 2009 influenza A (H1N1) pandemic, pregnant women were at risk for severe influenza illness. This concern was complicated by questions about vaccine safety in pregnant women that were raised by anecdotal reports of fetal deaths after vaccination.

Methods.—We explored the safety of influenza vaccination of pregnant women by linking Norwegian national registries and medical consultation data to determine influenza diagnosis, vaccination status, birth outcomes, and background information for pregnant women before, during, and after the pandemic. We used Cox regression models to estimate hazard ratios for fetal death, with the gestational day as the time metric and vaccination and pandemic exposure as time-dependent exposure variables.

Results.—There were 117,347 eligible pregnancies in Norway from 2009 through 2010. Fetal mortality was 4.9 deaths per 1000 births. During the pandemic, 54% of pregnant women in their second or third trimester were vaccinated. Vaccination during pregnancy substantially reduced the risk of an influenza diagnosis (adjusted hazard ratio, 0.30; 95% confidence interval [CI], 0.25 to 0.34). Among pregnant women with a clinical diagnosis of influenza, the risk of fetal death was increased (adjusted hazard ratio, 1.91; 95% CI, 1.07 to 3.41). The risk of fetal death was reduced with vaccination during pregnancy, although this reduction was not significant (adjusted hazard ratio, 0.88; 95% CI, 0.66 to 1.17).

Conclusions.—Pandemic influenza virus infection in pregnancy was associated with an increased risk of fetal death. Vaccination during pregnancy reduced the risk of an influenza diagnosis. Vaccination itself was not associated with increased fetal mortality and may have reduced the risk of influenza-related fetal death during the pandemic. (Funded by the Norwegian Institute of Public Health.)

▶ During the influenza H1N1 pandemic of 2009, it was readily evident that infection was very bad for pregnant women, who all too often developed fulminant disease. The impacts on the fetus were not so clear. Transplacental infections appeared to be very rare, and only a very few isolated case reports have emerged over the intervening 4 years. This population-based report from Norway provides compelling evidence that H1N1 infection did have substantial effects on fetal viability. In an unadjusted comparison with women whose pregnancies did not coincide with the pandemic, the risk of fetal death among women who were pregnant during the pandemic was increased by 20% if they were not immunized (hazard ratio, 1.21; 95% confidence interval [CI], 1.00—1.48) and doubled if influenza was diagnosed (hazard ratio, 2.00; 95% CI, 1.20—3.32). The risk of fetal death was not increased among pregnant women during the pandemic if influenza was not diagnosed (hazard ratio, 1.11; 95% CI, 0.93—1.33) or if they were immunized (hazard ratio, 1.02; 95% CI, 0.79—1.32). Thus, H1N1 was bad for fetuses, too, and immunization was an effective (and safe) tool for prevention of excess fetal losses. Those national data are complemented by data from both Canada[1] and the United States,[2] showing that H1N1 immunization reduced rates of prematurity (birth before 32 and 36 weeks, respectively), low birth weight (< 2500 g), and intrauterine growth restriction as well. The latter report estimated that one preterm birth was prevented by every 24 maternal H1N1 immunizations, arguing that this intervention is highly cost effective. These studies add to the growing body of evidence that immunization of pregnant women during influenza epidemics should be a public health priority, both to protect them from severe effects of infection, to which they are exceptionally vulnerable, and to protect their fetuses. The decision to prioritize H1N1 immunization of pregnant women during the 2009 pandemic has been amply validated by these data.

W. E. Benitz, MD

References

1. Fell DB, Sprague AE, Liu N, et al. H1N1 influenza vaccination during pregnancy and fetal and neonatal outcomes. *Am J Public Health*. 2012;102:e33-e40.
2. Richards JL, Hansen C, Bredfeldt C, et al. Neonatal outcomes after antenatal influenza immunization during the 2009 H1N1 influenza pandemic: impact on preterm birth, birth weight, and small for gestational age birth. *Clin Infect Dis*. 2013;56:1216-1222.

Empiric Antifungal Therapy and Outcomes in Extremely Low Birth Weight Infants with Invasive Candidiasis

Greenberg RG, for the Eunice Kennedy Shriver National Institute of Child Health and Human Development Neonatal Research Network (Duke Univ, Durham, NC; et al)

J Pediatr 161:264-269.e2, 2012

Objective.—To assess the impact of empiric antifungal therapy for invasive candidiasis on subsequent outcomes in premature infants.

Study Design.—This was a cohort study of infants with a birth weight ≤1000 g receiving care at Neonatal Research Network sites. All infants had at least one positive culture for *Candida*. Empiric antifungal therapy was defined as receipt of a systemic antifungal on the day of or the day before the first positive culture for *Candida* was drawn. We created Cox proportional hazards and logistic regression models stratified on propensity score quartiles to determine the effect of empiric antifungal therapy on survival, time to clearance of infection, retinopathy of prematurity, bronchopulmonary dysplasia, end-organ damage, and neurodevelopmental impairment (NDI).

Results.—A total of 136 infants developed invasive candidiasis. The incidence of death or NDI was lower in infants who received empiric antifungal therapy (19 of 38; 50%) compared with those who had not (55 of 86; 64%; OR, 0.27; 95% CI, 0.08-0.86). There was no significant difference between the groups for any single outcome or other combined outcomes.

Conclusion.—Empiric antifungal therapy was associated with increased survival without NDI. A prospective randomized trial of this strategy is warranted.

▶ This report from the National Institute of Child Health and Human Development Neonatal Research Network provides evidence supporting one of our widely held suppositions—that, in general, earlier treatment leads to better outcomes. Using sophisticated statistical tools to analyze data collected on 136 infants with birth weight less than 1000 g from whom *Candida* was recovered in nonpermissive cultures, the consortium was able to detect a faint signal that was not apparent using more conventional tools. The lower incidence of death or neurodevelopmental impairment (NDI) among infants with proven *Candida* infection who received treatment on the day of or day before the diagnostic culture was obtained (50%) compared with those for whom treatment was initiated later (64%), was associated with an unadjusted odds ratio of 0.56 (95% confidence interval [CI], 0.26–1.21), but logistic regression modeling yielded a statistically significant adjusted odds ratio of 0.27 (95% CI, 0.08–0.86). This observation supports the conclusion that guidelines for empiric antifungal therapy of at-risk preterm infants are urgently needed.

The 136 cases described in this report were drawn from a sample of 1515 infants who underwent evaluations for suspected late-onset sepsis.[1] More than one-third (518) of those infants received empiric early antifungal therapy, yet more than two-thirds of those with *Candida* infection did not, indicating that clinician judgment is a very poor predictor of this infection. Based on this experience, however, some estimates of number needed to treat (NNT) can be made. Had none of the 137 infected babies received early empiric treatment, we might expect 49 to have survived without NDI; if they all had, we would expect approximately 69 survivors without NDI. If the criterion for empiric treatment is simply suspected sepsis (ie, eligibility for study enrollment), as these authors suggest, the NNT to prevent one case of death or NDI would be 75. This large NNT makes this universal empiric treatment strategy infeasible, so the challenge lies in identification of factors that reliably predict invasive *Candida* infection with a reasonably low false-positive rate. Application of the predictive model developed in the primary study from which this work is drawn, which has a receiver-operator curve optimum at a sensitivity of about 70% and specificity of approximately 75%, might reduce the NNT to a potentially more manageable 33. Yet, the need remains for better tools for selection of preterm infants who are good candidates for empiric antifungal therapy.

An alternative is to identify and adopt practices that help avoid the necessity for empiric antifungal therapy by reducing the incidence of invasive candidiasis, which ranged from 2% to 28% across the centers that participated in this study. Although the reasons for this variation are not fully understood, strategies might include minimizing use of broad-spectrum antibiotics (particularly cephalosporins) and corticosteroids, early removal of central venous catheters (which may be contingent on successful early initiation of enteric feedings), and shortening duration of parenteral nutrition and endotracheal intubation. Antifungal prophylaxis may be helpful in units with high attack rates. Surely, an ounce of prevention is worth a pound of cure.

W. E. Benitz, MD

Reference

1. Benjamin DK Jr, Stoll BJ, Gantz MG, et al. Neonatal candidiasis: epidemiology, risk factors, and clinical judgment. *Pediatrics*. 2010;126:e865-e873.

6 Cardiovascular System

Outcome of Extremely Preterm Infants (<1,000 g) With Congenital Heart Defects From the National Institute of Child Health and Human Development Neonatal Research Network
Pappas A, Shankaran S, Hansen NI, et al (Wayne State Univ, Detroit, MI; RTI International, Research Triangle Park, NC; et al)
Pediatr Cardiol 33:1415-1426, 2012

Little is known about the outcomes of extremely low birth weight (ELBW) preterm infants with congenital heart defects (CHDs). The aim of this study was to assess the mortality, morbidity, and early childhood outcomes of ELBW infants with isolated CHD compared with infants with no congenital defects. Participants were 401−1,000 g infants cared for at National Institute of Child Health and Human Development Neonatal Research Network centers between January 1, 1998, and December 31, 2005. Neonatal morbidities and 18−22 months' corrected age outcomes were assessed. Neurodevelopmental impairment (NDI) was defined as moderate to severe cerebral palsy, Bayley II mental or psychomotor developmental index <70, bilateral blindness, or hearing impairment requiring aids. Poisson regression models were used to estimate relative risks for outcomes while adjusting for gestational age, small-for-gestational-age status, and other variables. Of 14,457 ELBW infants, 110 (0.8 %) had isolated CHD, and 13,887 (96 %) had no major birth defect. The most common CHD were septal defects, tetralogy of Fallot, pulmonary valve stenosis, and coarctation of the aorta. Infants with CHD experienced increased mortality (48 % compared with 35 % for infants with no birth defect) and poorer growth. Surprisingly, the adjusted risks of other short-term neonatal morbidities associated with prematurity were not significantly different. Fifty-seven (52 %) infants with CHD survived to 18−22 months' corrected age, and 49 (86 %) infants completed follow-up. A higher proportion of surviving infants with CHD were impaired compared with those without birth defects (57 vs. 38 %, $p = 0.004$). Risk of death or NDI was greater for ELBW infants with CHD, although 20 % of infants survived without NDI.

▶ The information in this article includes the spectrum of congenital heart defects (CHD). If extremely-low-birth-weight (ELBW) infants with relatively uncomplicated lesions (ie, isolated atrial septal defect, isolated ventricular defect, pulmonary valve stenosis) and those with more complicated lesions are considered separately, a different picture emerges. The overall survival rate of ELBW infants with uncomplicated CHD was 85% compared with a rate of 65% for the ELBW cohort without CHD. This difference in mortality rate favoring the ELBW cohort with uncomplicated CHD most likely can be attributed to the higher rate of intrauterine growth retardation and older gestational age of the uncomplicated CHD cohort. In contrast, the overall survival rate for ELBW infants with complicated CHD was 27%. For specific complicated cardiac lesions, the mortality rates were 100% (truncus arteriosus, pulmonary atresia, single ventricle physiology, and tricuspid atresia), 80% (transposition of the great vessels), 66% (tetralogy of Fallot, pulmonary atresia, total anomalous pulmonary venous return, complete atrioventricular canal), 60% (double outlet right ventricle), and 56% (coarctation of the aorta). Although the rate of neurodevelopmental impairment among the 16 surviving ELBW infants with complicated CHD who were followed is not reported, it is implied from the discussion that greater than 80% of these infants had poor neurodevelopmental outcomes, approximately double the rate noted in the ELBW cohort without CHD.

Among term infants with CHD requiring open heart surgery, the reported rate of moderate-to-severe disability is approximately 43%, and there is mounting evidence suggesting that complicated CHD is associated with brain injury in utero.[1] The 2-fold increase in neurodevelopmental impairment reported in the article supports this supposition.

L. A. Papile, MD

Reference

1. Majnemer A, Limperopoulos C, Shevell MI, Rohlicek C, Rosenblatt B, Tchervenkov C. A new look at outcomes of infants with congenital heart disease. *Pediatr Neurol.* 2009;40:197-204.

Hemodynamic Effects of Fluid Restriction in Preterm Infants with Significant Patent Ductus Arteriosus

De Buyst J, Rakza T, Pennaforte T, et al (Hôpital Universitaire des Enfants Reine Fabiola, Brussels, Belgium; Hôpital Jeanne De Flandre, Lille, France)
J Pediatr 161:404-408, 2012

Objective.—To determine the hemodynamic impact of fluid restriction in preterm newborns with significant patent ductus arteriosus.

Study Design.—Newborns ≥ 24 and < 32 weeks' gestational age with significant patent ductus arteriosus were eligible for this prospective multicenter observational study. We recorded hemodynamic and Doppler echocardiographic variables before and 24 hours after fluid restriction.

Results.—Eighteen newborns were included (gestational age 24.8 ± 1.1 weeks, birth weight 850 ± 180 g). Fluid intake was decreased from 145 ± 15 to 108 ± 10 mL/kg/d. Respiratory variables, fraction of inspired oxygen, blood gas values, ductus arteriosus diameter, blood flow-velocities in ductus arteriosus, in the left pulmonary artery and in the ascending aorta, and the left atrial/aortic root ratio were unchanged after fluid restriction. Although systemic blood pressure did not change, blood flow in the superior vena cava decreased from 105 ± 40 to 61 ± 25 mL/kg/min ($P < .001$). The mean blood flow-velocity in the superior mesenteric artery was lower 24 hours after starting fluid restriction.

Conclusions.—Our results do not support the hypothesis that fluid restriction has beneficial effects on pulmonary or systemic hemodynamics in preterm newborns.

▶ Pointing out that numerous randomized trials have failed to demonstrate benefits from treatment to close a persistent patent ductus arteriosus (PDA) in preterm infants, recent systematic reviews have raised doubts about the utility of such measures. Most of those trials, as well as studies of factors that may predispose to delayed ductal closure, were conducted 20 or more years ago, so their relevance to care of extremely low-birthweight infants in the current era may be questioned. Studies such as this one, which reevaluate strategies for management of PDA, are therefore necessary and welcome. Several studies conducted before echocardiographic measurements of regional blood flow and cardiac output were readily available suggested that fluid intakes in excess of about 160 mL/kg/day are associated with prolongation of ductal patency, so fluid restriction has become a common component of PDA management. This report examines the short-term hemodynamic effects of fluid restriction in 18 infants representative of those whose patent ductus require management in current practice. Newborns eligible for inclusion were at least 10 days old, had at least clinical signs attributable to PDA, had echocardiographic confirmation of a significant left-to-right ductal shunt, and had failed to respond to 2 courses of treatment with intravenous ibuprofen. Clinical and physiologic variables were recorded and Doppler echocardiographic measurements were obtained before and 24 hours after reduction of fluid intakes from baseline rates between 140 and 160 mL/kg/day to 100 to 120 mL/kg/day. No significant changes in respiratory function, as reflected in fraction of inspired oxygen concentration, pH, partial pressure of carbon dioxide in arterial blood, or base excess, were observed. Most hemodynamic measurements, including heart rate, blood pressure, left atrial/aortic root ratio, ductal diameter and blood flow velocities, and left pulmonary artery and ascending aorta flow velocities, did not change following fluid restriction. However, there were significant reductions in superior vena cava and superior mesenteric artery flows (both by approximately 40%), and urine output fell by 60% following fluid restriction. In short, fluid restriction did not seem to ameliorate excessive pulmonary perfusion, but it may have compromised perfusion of brain, bowel, and kidneys. Although the immediate implications of these short-term observations for clinical practice remain uncertain, this study design may provide a template for much-needed clinical trials to define optimal management of preterm infants with persistent PDA.

W. E. Benitz, MD

Treatment of Patent Ductus Arteriosus and Neonatal Mortality/Morbidities: Adjustment for Treatment Selection Bias

Mirea L, on behalf of the Canadian Neonatal Network (Mount Sinai Hosp, Toronto, Ontario, Canada; et al)
J Pediatr 161:689-694.e1, 2012

Objective.—To examine the association between treatment for patent ductus arteriosus (PDA) and neonatal outcomes in preterm infants, after adjustment for treatment selection bias.

Study Design.—Secondary analyses were conducted using data collected by the Canadian Neonatal Network for neonates born at a gestational age ≤32 weeks and admitted to neonatal intensive care units in Canada between 2004 and 2008. Infants who had PDA and survived beyond 72 hours were included in multivariable logistic regression analyses that compared mortality or any severe neonatal morbidity (intraventricular hemorrhage grades ≥3, retinopathy of prematurity stages ≥3, bronchopulmonary dysplasia, or necrotizing enterocolitis stages ≥2) between treatment groups (conservative management, indomethacin only, surgical ligation only, or both indomethacin and ligation). Propensity scores (PS) were estimated for each pair of treatment comparisons, and used in PS-adjusted and PS-matched analyses.

Results.—Among 3556 eligible infants with a diagnosis of PDA, 577 (16%) were conservatively managed, 2026 (57%) received indomethacin only, 327 (9%) underwent ligation only, and 626 (18%) were treated with both indomethacin and ligation. All multivariable and PS-based analyses detected significantly higher mortality/morbidities for surgically ligated infants, irrespective of prior indomethacin treatment (OR ranged from 1.25-2.35) compared with infants managed conservatively or those who received only indomethacin. No significant differences were detected between infants treated with only indomethacin and those managed conservatively.

Conclusions.—Surgical ligation of PDA in preterm neonates was associated with increased neonatal mortality/morbidity in all analyses adjusted for measured confounders that attempt to account for treatment selection bias.

▶ To treat or not to treat is the ongoing controversy in the care of the infant with patent ductus arteriosus. Mirea et al take this debate a step further in this analysis of observational data from the Canadian Neonatal Network in which propensity score (PS)—adjusted outcomes are compared among infants with patent ductus arteriosus (PDA) receiving 1 of 4 approaches to PDA treatment: conservative management, indomethacin only, surgery only, or indomethacin and surgery. Through PS-adjusted and matched analyses, the authors attempted to adjust for confounding by indication or selection bias. Although outcomes were similar between infants with PDA managed conservatively or with indomethacin, infants who underwent surgery, with or without indomethacin treatment, were at greater risk of mortality and morbidities, including bronchopulmonary dysplasia, necrotizing enterocolitis, and severe retinopathy of prematurity. A randomized, controlled clinical trial is needed but likely will prove infeasible, especially given several biologically plausible explanations for increased risk associated with surgical PDA closure, including impaired cerebral autoregulation[1] and potential adverse effects of anesthesia on the developing brain.[2,3]

L. J. Van Marter, MD, MPH

References

1. Chock VY, Ramamoorthy C, Van Meurs KP. Cerebral autoregulation in neonates with a hemodynamically significant patent ductus arteriosus. *J Pediatr.* 2012;160: 936-942.
2. Davidson AJ. Anesthesia and neurotoxicity to the developing brain: the clinical relevance. *Paediatr Anaesth.* 2011;21:716-721.
3. Loepke AW, Soriano SG. An assessment of the effects of general anesthetics on developing brain structure and neurocognitive function. *Anesth Analg.* 2008;106: 1681-1707.

Treatment of Patent Ductus Arteriosus and Neonatal Mortality/ Morbidities: Adjustment for Treatment Selection Bias
Mirea L, on behalf of the Canadian Neonatal Network (Mount Sinai Hosp, Toronto, Ontario, Canada; et al)
J Pediatr 161:689-694.e1, 2012

Objective.—To examine the association between treatment for patent ductus arteriosus (PDA) and neonatal outcomes in preterm infants, after adjustment for treatment selection bias.

Study Design.—Secondary analyses were conducted using data collected by the Canadian Neonatal Network for neonates born at a gestational age ≤32 weeks and admitted to neonatal intensive care units in Canada between 2004 and 2008. Infants who had PDA and survived beyond 72 hours were included in multivariable logistic regression analyses that compared mortality or any severe neonatal morbidity (intraventricular hemorrhage grades ≥3, retinopathy of prematurity stages ≥3, bronchopulmonary dysplasia, or necrotizing enterocolitis stages ≥2) between treatment groups (conservative management, indomethacin only, surgical ligation only, or both indomethacin and ligation). Propensity scores (PS) were estimated for each pair of treatment comparisons, and used in PS-adjusted and PS-matched analyses.

Results.—Among 3556 eligible infants with a diagnosis of PDA, 577 (16%) were conservatively managed, 2026 (57%) received indomethacin only, 327 (9%) underwent ligation only, and 626 (18%) were treated with both indomethacin and ligation. All multivariable and PS-based analyses detected significantly higher mortality/morbidities for surgically ligated infants, irrespective of prior indomethacin treatment (OR ranged from 1.25-2.35) compared with infants managed conservatively or those who received only indomethacin. No significant differences were detected between infants treated with only indomethacin and those managed conservatively.

TABLE 3.—Multivariable Logistic Regression, PS-adjusted, and PS-matched Analyses of the Composite Outcome

OR (95% CIs)

Analyses	Indomethacin only vs Conservative Treatment*	Ligation only vs Conservative Treatment†	Both Indomethacin and Ligation vs Conservative Treatment‡	Any Ligation vs no Ligation§	Ligation Only vs Indomethacin Only¶
Univariate logistic regression‖	1.68 (1.4, 2.03)	4.58 (3.34, 6.29)	6.77 (5.13, 8.93)	3.91 (3.24, 4.73)	2.72 (2.05, 3.63)
Multivariable logistic regression‖	1.09 (0.86, 1.39)	1.77 (1.15, 2.73)	2.35 (1.66, 3.33)	2.0 (1.57, 2.54)	1.62 (1.09, 2.41)
PS-adjusted**	1.01 (0.78, 1.32)	1.93 (1.08, 3.45)	2.2 (1.43, 3.4)	1.99 (1.56, 2.54)	1.76 (1.13, 2.74)
PS-matched††	1.01 (0.74, 1.39)	1.69 (1.22, 2.36)	1.25 (1.03, 1.51)	2.1 (1.56, 2.83)	1.91 (1.14, 3.22)
[N matches]	[429 matches]	[117 matches]	[187 matches]	[700 matches]	[204 matches]

*PS was adjusted for: year of birth, site, GA, SGA, inborn/outborn, SNAPII score >20, cesarean delivery, chorioamnionitis, gestational diabetes, maternal hypertension, prenatal care, and the interactions SNAPII >20*SGA, SNAPII >20*cesarean delivery, GA*maternal hypertension, SGA*maternal hypertension, and cesarean*maternal hypertension.

†PS was adjusted for: year of birth, site, GA, SGA, inborn/outborn, 5-min Apgar ≤5, antenatal corticosteroids, gestational diabetes and the interactions GA*SGA, inborn/outborn*SGA, and 5-min Apgar ≤5*SGA.

‡PS was adjusted for: year of birth, site, GA, SGA, gestational diabetes, antenatal corticosteroids, chorioamnionitis, prenatal care, and the interactions GA*SGA, and chorioamnionitis*SGA.

§PS was adjusted for: year of birth, site, sex, GA, SGA, inborn/outborn, gestational diabetes, antenatal corticosteroids, and the interaction GA*SGA.

¶PS was adjusted for: year of birth, site, GA, SGA, inborn/outborn, SNAPII >20, 5-min Apgar ≤5, gestational diabetes, antenatal corticosteroids, chorioamnionitis and the interactions inborn/outborn* 5 min Apgar ≤5, inborn/outborn*year of birth, and inborn/outborn*antenatal corticosteroids.

‖Multivariable analyses were adjusted for: year of birth, site, sex, GA, SGA, inborn/outborn, SNAPII >20, maternal hypertension, and antenatal corticosteroids.

**All PS-adjusted analyses were also adjusted for: year of birth, site, sex, GA, SGA, inborn/outborn, SNAPII >20. Analyses comparing indomethacin only vs conservative treatment, any ligation vs no ligation, and ligation only vs indomethacin only were further adjusted for maternal hypertension.

††All PS-matched analyses were adjusted for: year of birth, site, GA, and SGA. Analyses of indomethacin only vs conservative treatment were also adjusted for gender, inborn/outborn, and SNAPII >20. Analyses of ligation only vs conservative treatment were also adjusted for: SNAPII >20 and cesarean delivery. Analyses of both indomethacin and ligation vs conservative treatment were also adjusted for gender, inborn/outborn, and SNAPII >20. Analyses of any ligation vs no ligation were also adjusted for gender, inborn/outborn, SNAPII >20, antenatal corticosteroids, and maternal hypertension. Analyses of ligation only vs indomethacin only were also adjusted for gender, antenatal corticosteroids, and chorioamnionitis.

Conclusions.—Surgical ligation of PDA in preterm neonates was associated with increased neonatal mortality/morbidity in all analyses adjusted for measured confounders that attempt to account for treatment selection bias (Table 3).

▶ Gleaning knowledge from retrospective analyses of past experience is an imperfect but constantly improving art, to which we must often resort in the absence of randomized, controlled trials addressing the question at hand. Because such analyses are fraught with potential biases and opportunities for erroneous conclusions, biostatisticians have developed tools—multivariate regression and adjustment for or matching by propensity scores (PS, a method for reducing all potential covariates to a single number)—that allow adjustment for baseline prognostic factors, including treatment selection bias. Using those methods, these investigators drew on data from a multicenter consortium to ask if treatment of patent ductus arteriosus in preterm infants, using indomethacin or surgical ligation, affected outcomes. The results (Table 3) are remarkable. First, the estimates of effect size (odds ratio) after risk adjustment are much smaller than those obtained with univariate regression for all intergroup comparisons, with the largest reductions seen when the most aggressive treatments (ligation or both indomethacin and ligation) are compared with the least aggressive (conservative management). This is consistent with the expectation that the most aggressive treatments were used in the sickest infants and suggests that the statistical adjustments are able to at least partially correct for that treatment selection bias. Second, the lack of a statistically significant effect of indomethacin, for either better or worse (odds ratio, 1.01 in both PS-adjusted and PS-matched models), is consistent with prior observations; this intervention is effective in closing the ductus in many babies but does not change the overall outcome. Third, worse outcomes among infants treated with surgical ligation, even after statistical adjustments, reinforces the need for concern about resorting to this measure if there is any possibility of avoiding it. The authors conclude with a note of caution: "Neither the multivariable nor the PS methods applied here can adjust for hidden bias due to...unmeasured confounders, and it is possible that our study results include residual bias and, therefore, should be interpreted with caution." Nonetheless, these results should give pause to the idea that indomethacin and ligation are beneficial, so we should proceed with caution in deciding how to treat babies who have persistent ductal patency as well, at least until there is strong evidence from clinical trials to guide our practices.

W. E. Benitz, MD

Timing of Patent Ductus Arteriosus Treatment and Respiratory Outcome in Premature Infants: A Double-Blind Randomized Controlled Trial

Sosenko IRS, Fajardo MF, Claure N, et al (Univ of Miami/Miller School of Medicine, FL)

J Pediatr 160:929-935.e1, 2012

Objective.—To determine whether "early" ibuprofen treatment, at the onset of subtle patent ductus arteriosus (PDA) symptoms, would improve respiratory outcome in premature infants compared with "expectant" management, with ibuprofen treatment only when the PDA becomes hemodynamically significant (HS).

Study Design.—We conducted a randomized double-blind controlled trial of infants with gestational ages 23 to 32 weeks and birth weights 500 to 1250 g who had echocardiography for subtle PDA symptoms (metabolic acidosis, murmur, bounding pulses). Infants were then randomized to "early" treatment (blinded ibuprofen; n = 54) or "expectant management" (blinded placebo, n = 51). If the PDA became HS (pulmonary hemorrhage, hypotension, respiratory deterioration), infants received open label ibuprofen. Infants with HS PDA at enrollment were excluded from the study. Respiratory outcomes and mortality and major morbidities were determined.

Results.—"Early" treatment infants received ibuprofen at median age of 3 days; infants in the "expectant group" in whom HS symptoms developed (20%) received ibuprofen at median of 11 days. A total of 49% of "expectant" infants never required ibuprofen or ligation. No significant differences were found in the primary outcome (days on oxygen [O_2] during the first 28 days), death, O_2 at 36 weeks, death or O_2 at 36 weeks, intestinal

TABLE 3.—Respiratory Outcomes Assessed From Birth Until Day 28, 36 Weeks PMA, and Discharge or Death

	All Infants		Birth Weight 500-800 g		Birth Weight 801-1250 g	
	Early (n = 54)	Expectant (n = 51)	Early (n = 24)	Expectant (n = 24)	Early (n = 30)	Expectant (n = 27)
Days on O_2 first 28 days	21 (7-27)	19 (5—26)	25 (14-27)	23 (14-27)	18 (6-26)	14 (2-24)
Total days on O_2	39 (9-133)	37 (10-97)	85 (17-146)	57 (26-119)	31 (7-62)	23 (4-59)
Days on MV first 28 days	10 (1-28)	8 (1-28)	24 (7-28)	23 (7-28)	3 (0-12)	4 (0-15)
Today days on MV	12 (1-68)	13 (1-59)	45 (5-76)	35 (7-68)	5 (1-18)	6 (0-21)
On O_2 at 36 weeks PMA	17 (33)	16 (33)	13 (59)	10 (46)	4 (13)	6 (22)
Death or O_2 at 36 weeks PMA	19 (35)	18 (35)	15 (63)	12 (50)	4 (13)	6 (22)
On O_2 >30% at 36 weeks PMA*	9 (17)	2 (4)	7 (32)	2 (9)	2 (7)	0 (0)
Death or O_2 >30% at 36 weeks PMA†	11 (20)	4 (8)	9 (38)	4 (17)	2 (7)	0 (0)

PMA, postmenstrual age.
Results expressed as median (10th-90th percentile) or number (%).
Variables O_2 at 36 weeks PMA and O_2 >30% at 36 weeks PMA as percent of all infants alive at assessment age.
*0.17 (0.03-0.88) expectant compared with early group, Mantel-Haenszel common OR estimate.
†0.27 (0.07-0.99) expectant compared with early group, Mantel-Haenszel common OR estimate.

perforation, surgical necrotizing enterocolitis, grades III and IV intracranial hemorrhage, periventricular leukomalacia, sepsis or retinopathy of prematurity.

Conclusion.—Infants with mild signs of PDA do not benefit from early PDA treatment compared with delayed treatment (Table 3).

▶ Evidence of the absence of utility of treatment to close the persistently patent ductus arteriosus (PDA) in preterm infants continues to accrue. Despite some limitations, this report is a significant addition to that literature. These authors set out to determine whether an aggressive approach to early closure of PDA (using intravenous ibuprofen) as soon as it could be recognized and documented by echocardiography produced better outcomes than a permissive expectant strategy (in which treatment consisted of placebo). Infants with hemodynamically significant PDA at enrollment were excluded. In both groups, open-label treatment was used if the PDA was deemed to be hemodynamically significant, as reflected by either pulmonary hemorrhage or cardiomegaly and pulmonary edema on chest radiographs accompanied by hypotension or respiratory failure (using well-specified criteria). The median age at first exposure to ibuprofen was 3 days in the "early" group and 11 days in the "expectant" group. Because of these features of the trial design, these data do not allow any conclusions regarding management of infants with hemodynamically significant PDA. Nonetheless, there was no apparent benefit from treatment with ibuprofen in infants with PDA associated with only mild clinical signs. Half of the infants in the permissive group never received treatment to close the PDA, but outcomes were not worse as a result. One might argue that the study was underpowered, because the study had to be stopped at two thirds of the planned enrollment when the study drug became unavailable. However, no trends toward differences in outcomes are evident from inspection of the data (Table 3), which actually suggest that some adverse outcomes (requirement for > 30% supplemental oxygen at 36 weeks or the combined outcome of that requirement or death) were actually significantly more likely in the early treatment group. This report, therefore, provides substantial reassurance that deferral of intervention to close the ductus into the second postnatal week is not harmful in this narrowly defined subgroup of preterm infants. More work is needed to determine how to manage infants with more severe hemodynamic consequences of ductal patency, whether they become apparent in the first week after birth or later in the course. The assumption that ductal closure in those instances is beneficial and, therefore, necessary is still not supported by empiric evidence.

W. E. Benitz, MD

Could ADMA levels in young adults born preterm predict an early endothelial dysfunction?

Bassareo PP, Puddu M, Flore G, et al (Univ of Cagliari, Italy)
Int J Cardiol 159:217-219, 2012

Background.—Sporadic data present in literature report how preterm birth and low birth weight are risk factors for the development of cardiovascular diseases in later life. High levels of asymmetric dimethylarginine (ADMA), a strong inhibitor of nitric oxide synthesis, are associated with the future development of adverse cardiovascular events and cardiac death.

Aims.—1) to verify the presence of a statistically significant difference between ADMA levels in young adults born preterm at extremely low birth weight (< 1000 g; ex-ELBW) and those of a control group of healthy adults born at term (C) and 2) to seek correlations between ADMA levels in ex-ELBW and anthropometric and clinical parameters (gender, chronological age, gestational age, birth weight, and duration of stay in Neonatal Intensive Care Unit).

Methods.—Thirty-two ex-ELBW subjects (11 males [M] and 21 females [F], aged 17–29 years, mean age 22.2 ± 2.3 years) were compared with 25 C (7M and 18F). ADMA levels were assessed by high-performance liquid chromatography with highly sensitive laser fluorescent detection.

Results.—ADMA levels were reduced in ex-ELBW subjects compared to C (0.606 + 0.095 vs 0.562 + 0.101 μmol/L, $p < 0.05$), and significantly correlated inversely with gestational age (r = −0.61, $p < 0.00001$) and birth weight (r = −0.57, $p < 0.0002$).

Conclusions.—Our findings reveal a significant decrease in ADMA levels of ex-ELBW subjects compared to C, underlining a probable correlation with preterm birth and low birth weight. Taken together, these

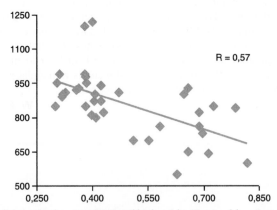

FIGURE 1.—Relationship between ADMA and birth weight. (Reprinted from Bassareo PP, Puddu M, Flore G, et al. Could ADMA levels in young adults born preterm predict an early endothelial dysfunction? *Int J Cardiol.* 2012;159:217-219, with permission from Elsevier Ireland.)

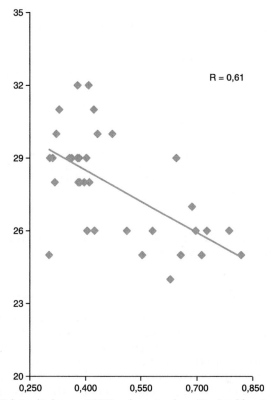

FIGURE 2.—Relationship between ADMA and gestational age. (Reprinted from International Journal of Cardiology. Bassareo PP, Puddu M, Flore G, et al. Could ADMA levels in young adults born preterm predict an early endothelial dysfunction? *Int J Cardiol*. 2012;159:217-219, Copyright 2012, with permission from International Society for Adult Congenital Heart Disease.)

results may underlie the onset of early circulatory dysfunction predictive of increased cardiovascular risk (Figs 1 and 2).

▶ Elevated levels of asymmetric dimethylarginine (ADMA), a methylated product of protein metabolism, interferes with L-arginine in the production of nitric oxide. Elevated levels are thought to be associated with adverse human health consequences, especially cardiovascular disease. Figs 1 and 2 in this study illustrate the relationship between plasma ADMA concentrations in young adults who were either born at term or preterm. The lower the birth weight or gestational age, the higher the concentration of plasma ADMA in young adulthood. Although these findings are preliminary, they suggest a partial mechanism for increased cardiovascular disease during adulthood in children who were born preterm. Whether the nitric oxide production in these individuals with higher ADMA concentrations actually differs is not tested in this study but would be an interesting topic of further investigation. The mechanism of why the ADMA is higher in those who were born preterm is not clear, but the authors propose this might be caused by altered renal function with poor clearance of ADMA. Low concentrations of arginine and high concentrations of ADMA have been measured in infants with pulmonary hypertension and have been associated with the development of chronic diseases in preterm infants.[1] The most important aspect of this finding appears to be its potential use as a marker for the increased potential for development of cardiovascular disease and the potential for early intervention.

J. Neu, MD

Reference

1. Vida G, Sulyok E, Lakatos O, Ertl T, Martens-Lobenhoffer J, Bode-Böger SM. Plasma levels of asymmetric dimethylarginine in premature neonates: its possible involvement in developmental programming of chronic diseases. *Acta Paediatr.* 2009;98:437-441.

Outcome and Resource Utilization of Infants Born with Hypoplastic Left Heart Syndrome in the Intermountain West

Menon SC, Keenan HT, Weng H-YC, et al (Univ of Utah, Salt Lake City)
Am J Cardiol 110:720-727, 2012

The objective of the present study was to characterize the outcomes and resource utilization of all infants born with hypoplastic left heart syndrome (HLHS) in the Intermountain West. This was a retrospective cohort study of all infants born with HLHS in the Intermountain West from January 1995 and January 2010. The cohort was divided into 3 eras: era 1, 1995 to 1999; era 2, 2000 to 2004; and era 3, 2005 to 2010. Cox proportional hazards regression analysis was performed to assess mortality. The lifetime hospitalization days and charges were also determined. Of the 245 infants identified, 65% were male infants and 172 (70%) underwent Stage 1 palliation. The transplant-free survival rate for the entire cohort was 33% at 14 years. The 1-year transplant-free survival rate for the surgical cohort was 60% in era 3. The infants whose initial presentation included shock, restrictive or intact atrial septum, chromosomal defects, or multiorgan dysfunction had an increased risk of death. A recent era of birth, greater birthweight, and older gestational age were associated with improved survival. The factors associated with mortality after stage 1 included surgical procedure type (Blalock-Taussig vs Sano shunt, hazard ratio 2.1), requirement for postoperative extracorporeal membrane oxygenation (hazard ratio 4.2), postoperative renal dysfunction (hazard ratio 3.0), anomalous pulmonary venous return (hazard ratio 2.9), and moderate or greater tricuspid valve regurgitation at any point (hazard ratio 2.0). For patients who had undergone stage 1, 2, or 3 palliation, the median cumulative lifetime hospitalization was 32, 48, and 65 days, and the median cumulative lifetime charges for hospitalization were $201,812, $253,183, and $296,213, respectively. In conclusion, although hospital-based studies of HLHS have shown significantly improved survival after surgical palliation,

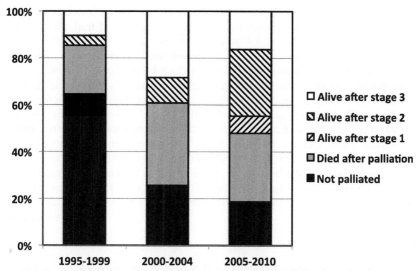

FIGURE.—Outcomes for infants with hypoplastic left heart syndrome in the Intermountain West, 1995-2010, based on. (Reprinted from the American Journal of Cardiology. Menon SC, Keenan HT, Weng H-YC, et al. Outcome and resource utilization of infants born with hypoplastic left heart syndrome in the Intermountain West. *Am J Cardiol.* 2012;110:720-7277, Copyright 2012, with permission from Elsevier.)

population-based studies have shown that HLHS continues to have a high mortality and high resource utilization (Fig).

▶ Given the prevalence and severity of the condition, it is surprising how difficult it is to find information on outcomes of serial surgeries for hypoplastic left heart syndrome (HLHS). The perioperative mortality rates posted online appear to exclude interstage mortalities, thereby giving the impression that outcomes are better than they actually are. This population-based report goes a long ways toward remediating this difficulty. Taking advantage of the ability to capture data for all diagnosed cases in a defined geographic area over more than 15 years, these authors report outcomes for 245 infants with HLHS, including 172 who had palliative surgery; follow-up information was available for nearly all (167) of the surgical cohort. They describe the changing patterns of care and outcomes across 3 eras of approximately 5 years each, beginning in 1995. Not surprisingly, the proportion of infants who underwent palliative surgery increased significantly, from 35% to 81% (Fig). Correspondingly, the number of perioperative and interstage deaths also increased, but the survival rate increased from 14% to 51%; however, only 16% of the infants in the final cohort achieved survival after stage 3 palliation (more than a third had not yet reached that stage), so the later rate constitutes an upper bound on the ultimate survival rate. Survival among surgical patients increased from 41% to 64%, but this change was not statistically significant. Actuarial estimates of survival rates provided by these authors, which are similar to reports from multicenter data collectives, suggest that 5-year transplant-free survival rates among infants who undergo stage 1 Norwood surgery still are only slightly in excess of 50%.

Reports of long-term neurodevelopmental findings in these infants are similarly worrisome. A recent nationwide report from Finland[1] found that survivors of surgery for HLHS had lower full-scale IQ (97 vs 121 in controls, $P < .001$) and were at risk for both major neurodevelopmental impairment (26% of patients) and minor neurologic dysfunction (43%). Magnetic resonance imaging abnormalities (mostly ischemic changes) were found in 82% of the patients with HLHS. Collectively, these data suggest that the probability of neurologically intact survival after surgical palliation for HLHS may be less than 15%, with an almost equal chance of survival with major neurodevelopmental impairment. These data show that the great advances in surgical technique and medical management of these complicated infants have fallen short of our aspirations. As we await further progress toward those goals, it is important for parents of babies with HLHS to be fully apprised of the prospects as they contemplate options for palliation end-of-life comfort care vs multistage surgical palliation.

W. E. Benitz, MD

Reference

1. Sarajuuri A, Jokinen E, Mildh L, et al. Neurodevelopmental burden at age 5 years in patients with univentricular heart. *Pediatrics*. 2012;130:e1636-e1646.

7 Respiratory Disorders

Randomized Trial of Early Bubble Continuous Positive Airway Pressure for Very Low Birth Weight Infants
Tapia JL, for the South American Neocosur Network (Pontificia Universidad Catolica de Chile, Santiago; et al)
J Pediatr 161:75-80.e1, 2012

Objective.—To determine whether very low birth weight infants (VLBWIs), initially supported with continuous positive airway pressure (CPAP) and then selectively treated with the INSURE (intubation, surfactant, and extubation to CPAP; CPAP/INSURE) protocol, need less mechanical ventilation than those supported with supplemental oxygen, surfactant, and mechanical ventilation if required (Oxygen/mechanical ventilation [MV]).

Study Design.—In a multicenter randomized controlled trial, spontaneously breathing VLBWIs weighing 800-1500 g were allocated to receive either therapy. In the CPAP/INSURE group, if respiratory distress syndrome (RDS) did not occur, CPAP was discontinued after 3-6 hours. If RDS developed and the fraction of inspired oxygen (FiO$_2$) was >0.35, the INSURE protocol was indicated. Failure criteria included FiO$_2$ >0.60, severe apnea or respiratory acidosis, and receipt of more than 2 doses of surfactant. In the Oxygen/MV group, in the presence of RDS, supplemental oxygen without CPAP was given, and if FiO$_2$ was >0.35, surfactant and mechanical ventilation were provided.

Results.—A total of 256 patients were randomized to either the CPAP/INSURE group (n = 131) or the Oxygen/MV group (n = 125). The need for mechanical ventilation was lower in the CPAP/INSURE group (29.8% vs 50.4%; P =.001), as was the use of surfactant (27.5% vs 46.4%; P =.002). There were no differences in death, pneumothorax, bronchopulmonary dysplasia, and other complications of prematurity between the 2 groups.

Conclusion.—CPAP and early selective INSURE reduced the need for mechanical ventilation and surfactant in VLBWIs without increasing morbidity and death. These results may be particularly relevant for resource-limited regions.

▶ This randomized, controlled trial was performed by the South American Neocosur Network, comprising investigators from Argentina, Chile, Peru, and Uruguay. The primary objective was to determine if selective use of the INSURE (intubation, surfactant, and extubation) technique could reduce the need for surfactant, mechanical ventilation, and supplemental oxygen without increasing the incidence of complications, including morbidity and mortality. A modest population of 256 infants (birth weights 600 to 1500 g) was studied. The groups were demographically similar. Infants were randomized to either continuous positive airway pressure (CPAP) or mechanical ventilation, and specific criteria dictated the use of surfactant, including redosing. The group assigned to the CPAP/INSURE arm required less mechanical ventilation and less surfactant than the group assigned to mechanical ventilation, and both differences were highly statistically significant. No differences in the rates of bronchopulmonary dysplasia, death, air leak, or other complications were found between groups.

This was a well-conducted clinical trial that used a reasonable and practical protocol to test the hypothesis that less is more. Not surprisingly, they were able to decrease costly treatments without increasing morbidity. However, the big question they now face is the generalizability of this trial to clinical practice in the rest of South America. There are likely to be population differences, obstetrical practices (about 90% of mothers of babies in this trial received antenatal corticosteroids), and the Hawthorne effect. One cost-saving thought, however, is to revise the surfactant redosing schedule from 6 to 12 hours to 12 to 24 hours.

It is gratifying, nonetheless, to see the evolution of research networks in resource-limited areas and how they ask questions pertinent to their own situation. I commend the authors on this superb study.

S. M. Donn, MD

Randomized Trial of Early Bubble Continuous Positive Airway Pressure for Very Low Birth Weight Infants

Tapia JL, for the South American Neocosur Network (Pontificia Universidad Catolica de Chile, Santiago; et al)
J Pediatr 161:75-80.e1, 2012

Objective.—To determine whether very low birth weight infants (VLBWIs), initially supported with continuous positive airway pressure (CPAP) and then selectively treated with the INSURE (intubation, surfactant, and extubation to CPAP; CPAP/INSURE) protocol, need less mechanical ventilation than those supported with supplemental oxygen, surfactant, and mechanical ventilation if required (Oxygen/mechanical ventilation [MV]).

Study Design.—In a multicenter randomized controlled trial, spontaneously breathing VLBWIs weighing 800-1500 g were allocated to receive either therapy. In the CPAP/INSURE group, if respiratory distress syndrome (RDS) did not occur, CPAP was discontinued after 3-6 hours. If RDS developed and the fraction of inspired oxygen (FiO_2) was >0.35, the INSURE protocol was indicated. Failure criteria included FiO_2 >0.60, severe apnea or respiratory acidosis, and receipt of more than 2 doses of surfactant. In the Oxygen/MV group, in the presence of RDS, supplemental oxygen without CPAP was given, and if FiO_2 was >0.35, surfactant and mechanical ventilation were provided.

Results.—A total of 256 patients were randomized to either the CPAP/ INSURE group (n = 131) or the Oxygen/MV group (n = 125). The need for mechanical ventilation was lower in the CPAP/INSURE group (29.8% vs 50.4%; *P* = .001), as was the use of surfactant (27.5% vs 46.4%; *P* = .002). There were no differences in death, pneumothorax, bronchopulmonary dysplasia, and other complications of prematurity between the 2 groups.

Conclusion.—CPAP and early selective INSURE reduced the need for mechanical ventilation and surfactant in VLBWIs without increasing morbidity and death. These results may be particularly relevant for resource-limited regions.

▶ More than 40 years after Gregory et al described use of continuous positive airway pressure (CPAP) as a treatment for respiratory distress syndrome in preterm infants,[1] we are still triangulating its optimal use. A handful of randomized, controlled trials reported in the past 5 years are shedding light on this matter, but the best approaches to management of these infants remain only partially defined. We know from the Surfactant Positive Airway Pressure and Pulse Oximetry Randomized Trial (SUPPORT), for example, that early initiation of CPAP in the delivery room results in rates of survival and bronchopulmonary dysplasia equivalent to those achieved with early intubation, surfactant administration, and mechanical ventilation, along with less use of epinephrine in the delivery room, less treatment with postpartum steroids, and fewer days of mechanical ventilation.[2] Others have proposed that a best of both approach consisting of early CPAP with selective use of surfactant followed by immediate extubation to CPAP (the INSURE strategy) might be better than either SUPPORT strategy. However, evidence from at least 2 trials has failed to demonstrate an advantage of routine early surfactant over selective use of surfactant among babies for whom support with CPAP was initiated soon after birth.[3,4]

A cursory reading of only the results section of the abstract of this article might lead one to believe that it provides evidence supporting use of routine early intubation and prophylactic surfactant, resulting in less need for mechanical ventilation and less surfactant use. However, closer examination of study design reveals that early INSURE was not one of the treatment strategies studied. The study compared early CPAP with early supplemental oxygen with different rescue strategies: INSURE (in the early CPAP group) and mechanical ventilation and surfactant (in the supplemental oxygen group). Because the initial treatment differed substantially between the 2 arms, no conclusions regarding the relative merits of INSURE can be drawn from these data. One major outcome difference between groups—less use of mechanical ventilation in the early CPAP group— may be tautological, because a trial of CPAP was not an available rescue option in the supplemental oxygen arm. Nonetheless, the authors' primary conclusion that early initiation of bubble CPAP—an easy and inexpensive intervention— significantly reduces subsequent resource consumption is probably sound. An important secondary lesson is that clinical application of this evolving literature requires very careful attention to the particulars of trial designs as well as the clinical outcomes.

W. E. Benitz, MD

References

1. Gregory GA, Kitterman JA, Phibbs RH, Tooley WH, Hamilton WK. Treatment of the idiopathic respiratory-distress syndrome with continuous positive airway pressure. *N Engl J Med.* 1971;284:1333-1340.
2. Finer NN, Carlo WA, Walsh MC, et al. Early CPAP versus surfactant in extremely preterm infants. *N Engl J Med.* 2010;362:1970-1979.
3. Rojas MA, Lozano JM, Rojas MX, et al. Very early surfactant without mandatory ventilation in premature infants treated with early continuous positive airway pressure: a randomized, controlled trial. *Pediatrics.* 2009;123:137-142.
4. Dunn MS, Kaempf J, de Klerk A, et al. Randomized trial comparing 3 approaches to the initial respiratory management of preterm neonates. *Pediatrics.* 2011;128: e1069-e1076.

Randomized Trial of Prongs or Mask for Nasal Continuous Positive Airway Pressure in Preterm Infants

Kieran EA, Twomey AR, Molloy EJ, et al (The Natl Maternity Hosp, Dublin, Ireland)
Pediatrics 130:e1170-e1176, 2012

Objective.—To determine whether nasal continuous positive airway pressure (NCPAP) given with nasal prongs compared with nasal mask reduces the rate of intubation and mechanical ventilation in preterm infants within 72 hours of starting therapy.

Methods.—Infants <31 weeks' gestation treated with NCPAP were randomly assigned to receive it via either prongs or mask. Randomization was stratified by gestational age (<28 weeks, 28—30 weeks) and according to whether NCPAP was started as a primary treatment for respiratory distress or postextubation. Infants were intubated and ventilated if they fulfilled 2 or more of 5 failure criteria (worsening signs of respiratory distress; recurrent apnea treated with mask positive pressure ventilation; fraction of inspired oxygen >0.4 to keep oxygen saturation >88% sustained for 30 minutes; pH <7.2 on 2 blood gases ≥30 minutes apart; Pco_2 >9 kPa [68 mm Hg] on 2 blood gases ≥30 minutes apart) within 72 hours of starting therapy. The groups were treated the same in all other respects. We recorded relevant secondary outcomes and analyzed data by using the intention-to-treat principle.

Results.—We enrolled 120 infants. Thirty-two of 62 (52%) infants randomly assigned to prongs were intubated within 72 hours, compared with 16/58 (28%) of those randomly assigned to mask ($P = .007$). There were no statistically significant differences between the groups in any secondary outcomes.

Conclusions.—In premature infants, NCPAP was more effective at preventing intubation and ventilation within 72 hours of starting therapy when given via nasal masks compared with nasal prongs.

▶ As this study demonstrates, details matter. We often use shorthand descriptions of treatment strategies, such as CPAP for continuous positive airway pressure, as though they fully define the intervention, and assume that small differences in the particulars are inconsequential. Confronted with gradual adoption of nasal masks for delivery of CPAP in their unit, however, these authors asked the crucial question of whether the outcomes achieved using those devices differed from those resulting from use of the nasal prongs, which had been the previous standard. Contrary to their expectations, they found that infants managed with nasal masks were significantly ($P = .007$) less likely to require intubation within 72 hours after initiation of CPAP, estimating a number needed to treat of 4 to prevent reintubation of 1 infant. These results have 2 important implications. First, this trial provides an important proof of concept that the small but crucial choices made every day in our nurseries can be successfully evaluated in well-designed, randomized trials. Selection of the outcome to test is a critical element, as the sample size required to demonstrate significant impacts on long-term outcomes such as mortality rates will certainly be prohibitive. We should all aspire to conduct our process improvement activities with similar rigor. Second, the rest of us should consider following the advice of these authors by standardizing our method of CPAP administration on use of masks, at least for the first 72 hours, while exploring the mechanisms that mediate the differential efficacy of these interface devices. Whether the difference relates to larger leaks around prongs, more frequent episodes, device displacement resulting in suboptimal pressure delivery, larger pressure drops across the small, high resistance orifice of prongs, or to some other mechanism, this knowledge may guide further enhancement of our ability to provide effective, noninvasive respiratory support for preterm infants. The authors circumspectly note that they studied only a single type of device for delivery of CPAP, the Viasys Infant Flow System, for which nasal prongs and masks are interchangeable, so their observations may not be applicable to other CPAP-generating devices. Those details deserve similar systematic evaluation.

W. E. Benitz, MD

Randomised weaning trial comparing assist control to pressure support ventilation
Shefali-Patel D, Murthy V, Hannam S, et al (King's College London, UK)
Arch Dis Child Fetal Neonatal Ed 97:F429-F433, 2012

Objectives.—To determine if the work of breathing was lower, respiratory muscle strength greater, but the degree of asynchrony higher during weaning by assist control ventilation (ACV) rather than pressure support ventilation (PSV) and if any differences were associated with a shorter duration of weaning.

Design.—Randomised trial.

Setting.—Tertiary neonatal unit.

Patients.—Thirty-six infants, median gestational age 29 (range 24 to 39) weeks.

Intervention.—Weaning by either ACV or PSV.

Main Outcome Measures.—At baseline, 24 hours after entering the study and immediately prior to extubation, the work of breathing (PTPdi), thoracoabdominal asynchrony (TAA) and respiratory muscle strength (Pimax) were assessed and weaning duration recorded.

Results.—There were no significant differences in the median PTPdi, TAA and Pimax results at any time point. The inflation times during ACV and PSV were similar. The median duration of weaning was 34 (range 7–100) hours in the ACV group and 27 (range 10–169) hours in the PSV group ($p = 0.88$).

Conclusion.—No significant differences were found between weaning by PSV and ACV when similar inflation times were used.

▶ This trial aimed to determine differences in the work of breathing and duration of weaning in infants randomly assigned to either assist/control ventilation or pressure support ventilation while receiving a modest degree of respiratory support. This is an important clinical question to answer, as weaning practices are among the most heterogenous aspects of neonatal respiratory care. This was a relatively small, single-center study. As such, it would have been better to have concentrated on a more homogeneous group of babies, such as preterm infants with respiratory distress syndrome, and not added babies with congenital diaphragmatic hernia or other surgical conditions. Entry criteria were stratified by gestational age, but results were not. Furthermore, extubation was not done according to protocol but according to clinical practice. Although pre-extubation caffeine was part of the protocol, 5 of the 36 babies (14%) failed to receive it.

The investigators found no differences in the outcomes of interest. However, before we dismiss pressure support as no better than assist/control, we need to examine the design of this study. In both groups, the ventilator rate was set at 40 breaths per minute (control and synchronized intermittent mandatory ventilation [SIMV] rates). How much spontaneous breathing should we expect in SIMV/pressure support if the baby receives 40 mandatory breaths per minute? Setting the pressure support properly is also a key element. The investigators attempted to use a termination sensitivity (expiratory trigger) of 5% to 10% but did not provide information about the inspiratory time limit. To know that the baby is terminating breaths by flow rather than by time, the inspiratory time limit needs to be set long enough to observe that inspiration ends by flow termination rather than by time. Presumably, the infants in the assist/control arm were treated with time-cycling, but it is not clear whether they received constant flow, pressure-limited ventilation, or pressure control ventilation with an accelerating/decelerating inspiratory flow. This could have had a significant effect on study results. Finally, it has been my experience that permissive hypercapnia (used in this trial after day 7) cannot be achieved in patient-triggered ventilation without severely perturbing ventilator settings (eg, delivering a suboptimal tidal volume) or heavily sedating the infant.

Given these limitations, I would accept that pressure support is no worse than assist/control. But the question remains—could it be better?

S. M. Donn, MD, FAAP

Surfactant Administration via Thin Catheter During Spontaneous Breathing: Randomized Controlled Trial
Kanmaz HG, Erdeve O, Canpolat FE, et al (Ankara Univ School of Medicine, Turkey)
Pediatrics 131:e502-e509, 2013

Background.—The primary aim of this randomized study was to describe the feasibility of early administration of surfactant via a thin catheter during spontaneous breathing (Take Care) and compare early mechanical ventilation (MV) requirement with the InSurE (Intubate, Surfactant, Extubate) procedure.

Methods.—Preterm infants, who were <32 weeks and stabilized with nasal continuous positive airway pressure (nCPAP) in the delivery room, were randomized to receive early surfactant treatment either by the Take Care or InSurE technique. Tracheal instillation of 100 mg/kg poractant α via 5-F catheter during spontaneous breathing under nCPAP was performed in the intervention group. In the InSurE procedure, infants were intubated, received positive pressure ventilation for 30 seconds after surfactant instillation, and placed on nCPAP immediately.

Results.—One hundred infants in each group were analyzed. The MV requirement in the first 72 hours of life was significantly lower in the Take Care group when compared with the InSurE group (30% vs 45%, $P = .02$, odds ratio -0.52, 95% confidence interval -0.94 to -0.29). Mean duration of both nCPAP and MV were significantly shorter in the Take Care group (P values .006 and .002, respectively). Bronchopulmonary dysplasia rate was significantly lower among the infants treated with the Take Care technique (relative risk -0.27, 95% confidence interval -0.1 to -0.72).

Conclusions.—The Take Care technique is feasible for the treatment of respiratory distress syndrome in infants with very low birth weight. It significantly reduces both the need and duration of MV, and thus the bronchopulmonary dysplasia rate in preterm infants.

▶ The recognition that mechanical ventilation (MV) is a major risk factor for bronchopulmonary dysplasia (BPD) and that simply replacing MV with continuous positive airway pressure (CPAP) does not reduce the risk of BPD, has led to a search for optimal ways to combine surfactant administration with noninvasive respiratory support. In this study of infants with moderately severe respiratory distress syndrome born before 32 weeks of gestation who were hospitalized at Zekai Tahir Burak Maternity Teaching Hospital in Turkey, Kanmaz et al join others[1-4] in leading the effort to discover the optimal approach to minimally inva-sive surfactant administration. In this study, 200 infants on CPAP at fraction of inspired oxygen 0.40 or greater were randomly assigned to receive surfactant by one of 2 methods: InSurE (intubation, surfactant administration, brief manual ventilation, and extubation to CPAP) or Take Care (intratracheal administration of surfactant via a modified nasogastric under direct laryngoscopy without the use of Magill forceps, while on CPAP). Although both techniques resulted in lower inspired oxygen over the first 24 hours after treatment, the Take Care approach was found to be superior and was associated with reductions in MV in the first 72 postnatal hours (30% vs 45%; $P = .02$), duration of CPAP and MV (if needed), and the composite outcome of death or BPD (22% vs 32%; $P = .15$). Let's hope this approach or a modification of it provides a much needed key to optimal respiratory support and BPD prevention among preterm infants.

L. J. Van Marter, MD, MPH

References

1. Verder H, Robertson B, Greisen G, et al. Surfactant therapy and nasal continuous positive airway pressure for newborns with respiratory distress syndrome. Danish-Swedish Multicenter Study Group. *N Engl J Med.* 1994;331:1051-1055.
2. Kribs A, Härtel C, Kattner E, et al. Surfactant without intubation in preterm infants with respiratory distress: first multi-center data. *Klin Padiatr.* 2010;222:13-17.
3. Gopel W, Kribs A, Ziegler A, et al; German Neonatal Network. Avoidance of mechanical ventilation by surfactant treatment of spontaneously breathing preterm infants (AMV): an open-label randomised, controlled trial. *Lancet.* 2011;378: 1627-1634.
4. Dargaville PA, Aiyappan A, De Paoli AG, et al. Minimally-invasive surfactant therapy in preterm infants on continuous positive airway pressure. *Arch Dis Child Fetal Neonatal Ed.* 2013;98:F122-F126.

Impaired surfactant protein B synthesis in infants with congenital diaphragmatic hernia

Cogo PE, Simonato M, Danhaive O, et al (Bambino Gesú Children's Hosp, Rome, Italy; Med Ctr and Univ of Padua, Italy; Univ of California San Francisco; et al)
Eur Respir J 41:677-682, 2013

Pulmonary hypoplasia and hypertension account for significant morbidity and mortality in neonates with congenital diaphragmatic hernia (CDH). Whether CDH is associated with surfactant dysfunction remains controversial. Therefore, we measured disaturated phosphatidylcholine (DSPC) and surfactant protein (SP)-B concentration in tracheal aspirates and their synthesis rate in infants with CDH compared to infants without lung disease.

^2H_2O as a precursor of DSPC and $1\text{-}^{13}C$-leucine as a precursor of SP-B were administered to 13 infants with CDH and eight controls matched for gestational age. DSPC and SP-B were isolated from tracheal aspirates, and their fractional synthesis rate was derived from ^2H and ^{13}C enrichment curves obtained by mass spectrometry. DSPC and SP-B amounts in tracheal aspirates were also measured.

In infants with CDH, SP-B fractional synthesis rate and amount were $62 \pm 27\%$ and $57 \pm 22\%$ lower, respectively, than the value found in infants without lung disease ($p < 0.01$ and $p < 0.05$, respectively). There were no significant group differences in DSPC fractional synthesis rate and amount.

Infants with CDH have a lower rate of synthesis of SP-B and less SP-B in tracheal aspirates. In these infants, partial SP-B deficiency could contribute to the severity of respiratory failure and its correction might represent a therapeutic goal.

▶ It is always reassuring when a nice piece of science reinforces clinical impressions. This group of investigators applied stable isotope technology to show that infants with congenital diaphragmatic hernias have lower rates of synthesis of surfactant protein B as well as a decreased concentration of surfactant protein B in tracheal aspirates. This is not a surprising finding, as the pulmonary hypoplasia that accompanies congenital diaphragmatic hernia results in fewer type II alveolar cells to explain diminished surfactant production.

Surfactant dosing has, until recently, been rather arbitrary, with many flawed assumptions about surfactant pharmacokinetics. Carnielli's group has been instrumental in enhancing our understanding about surfactant synthesis and turnover using the stable isotope methodology. This most recent study from Carnielli's group provides some evidence that surfactant repletion in infants with congenital diaphragmatic hernia has a biological basis and seems to be a reasonable therapeutic consideration.

S. M. Donn, MD

Automated Closed Loop Control of Inspired Oxygen Concentration
Claure N, Bancalari E (Univ of Miami Miller School of Medicine, FL)
Respir Care 58:151-161, 2013

Oxygen therapy is extensively used in premature infants and adults with respiratory insufficiency. In the premature infant the goal during manual control of the F_{IO_2} is to maintain adequate oxygenation and to minimize the exposure to hypoxemia, hyperoxemia, and oxygen. However, this is frequently not achieved during routine care, which increases the risks of associated side effects affecting the eye, lungs, and central nervous system. In the adult the primary goal is to avoid hypoxemia, but conventional methods of oxygen supplementation may fall short during periods of increased demand. On the other hand, there are growing concerns related to unnecessarily high F_{IO_2} levels that increase the exposure to hyperoxemia and excessive oxygen use in settings where resources are limited. Systems for automated closed loop control of F_{IO_2} have been developed for use in neonates and adults. This paper will give an overview of the rationale for the development of these systems, present the evidence, and discuss important advantages and limitations.

▶ The ability to tightly limit the excursions of arterial oxygen saturation has been one of neonatology's holy grails. Multiple studies, as well as everyone's personal experiences, have found that preterm infants spend little time within the intended target range, and the consequences of both hypoxia and hyperoxia do not need to be elaborated here. In this article, Claure and Bancalari nicely review the concepts of closed loop control of oxygen concentration, where the pulse oximetry—derived saturation value is used to regulate the oxygen blender. In both the original pilot trial in their center and in a follow-up multicenter trial (in which I participated), infants displayed much tighter control of inspired oxygen and fewer severe fluctuations while on automated control compared with manual. There were strikingly fewer manual interventions required to adjust fraction of inspired oxygen while on automated control as well. Currently, the automated system has been tested only in mechanically ventilated infants, and trials of using the system during noninvasive ventilation are in the planning stages.

After the clinical trials, the automated device was approved for use in Europe by the European Medicines Agency, the equivalent of the US Food and Drug Administration (FDA) in Europe. It was immediately accepted by the neonatal community and is in widespread use. In the United States, the FDA has yet to approve the device despite reasonable clinical evidence of both efficacy and safety. As the authors rightly indicated, the optimal range of saturation has yet to be identified. Yet, although the device may or may not help to define the limits, it can certainly ameliorate wide swings in oxygen saturation, which appear to be potentially dangerous. Reduction of pulse oximetry alarms, while maintaining the baby in a desirable range, would certainly be a laudable goal. Ask any neonatal nurse!

S. M. Donn, MD, FAAP

Does the ex utero intrapartum treatment to extracorporeal membrane oxygenation procedure change outcomes for high-risk patients with congenital diaphragmatic hernia?
Stoffan AP, Wilson JM, Jennings RW, et al (Harvard Med School, Boston, MA)
J Pediatr Surg 47:1053-1057, 2012

Purpose.—In the most severe cases of congenital diaphragmatic hernia (CDH), significant barotrauma or death can occur before advanced therapies such as extracorporeal membrane oxygenation (ECMO) can be initiated. We have previously examined the use of the ex utero intrapartum treatment (EXIT) to ECMO procedure (EXIT with placement on ECMO) in high-risk infants and reported a survival advantage. We report our experience with EXIT to ECMO in a more recent cohort of our patients with most severe CDH.

Methods.—Every patient with less than 15% predicted lung volume during January 2005 to December 2010 was included. We obtained data on prenatal imaging, size and location of the defect, and survival.

Results.—Seventeen high-risk infants were identified. All 17 (100%) received ECMO and required a patch. Six children were delivered by EXIT to ECMO, and only 2 (33%) survived. An additional patient was delivered by EXIT to intubation with ECMO on standby and died. Of the 10 children who did not receive EXIT, 5 (50%) survived.

Conclusions.—No clear survival benefit with the use of the EXIT to ECMO procedure was demonstrated in this updated report of our high-risk CDH population. The general application of EXIT to ECMO for CDH is not supported by our results.

▶ The ex utero intrapartum treatment (EXIT) to extracorporeal membrane oxygenation (ECMO) procedure is a glamorous, labor-intense, and highly technical procedure, usually performed when there has been a prenatally diagnosed, life-threatening anomaly of the airway or lung not likely to respond to conventional therapy. I have been involved in this, with upward of 2 dozen of my closest colleagues present in the operating room.

This article reviewed a 6-year experience of 1 center with the intrapartum management of 17 ECMO-treated babies with prenatally diagnosed diaphragmatic hernia, where predicted lung volume was less than 15% of normal. Ten of these babies were delivered by standard methods (3 vaginal, 7 cesarean) and 5 survived. One baby was delivered by EXIT and was intubated with ECMO on standby (and used later) and died. Six babies underwent EXIT to ECMO and 4 died. The authors concluded that in this high-risk population, EXIT to ECMO offers no apparent survival advantage.

Although the numbers are very small, they come from an institution with considerable experience in both EXIT and ECMO and should be heeded. It appears that we may be subjecting a large number of infants to a costly, painful, high-risk procedure with a high degree of futility. Since it is not likely that a large, randomized trial is feasible, careful consideration needs to be given when this is being contemplated.

It begs the question, "Just because we can, should we?"

S. M. Donn, MD

C reactive protein: impact on peripheral tissue oxygenation and perfusion in neonates
Pichler G, Pocivalnik M, Riedl R, et al (Med Univ Graz, Austria)
Arch Dis Child Fetal Neonatal Ed 97:F444-F448, 2012

Objective.—C reactive protein (CRP) is a sensitive marker of acute inflammation of infectious and non-infectious origin. Aim was to use near-infrared spectroscopy (NIRS) to analyse peripheral oxygenation and perfusion in term and preterm neonates with elevated CRP levels, at a time when routine haemodynamic variables are still normal.

Design.—Prospective observational study.

Settings.—Peripheral-muscle NIRS was performed in the first week of life. Tissue-oxygenation index (TOI), mixed venous oxygenation (SvO$_2$), fractional oxygen extraction (FOE), haemoglobin flow (Hbflow), oxygen delivery (DO$_2$) and oxygen consumption (VO$_2$) were assessed. Blood samples were taken within 3 h of the NIRS measurements.

Patients.—Cardiocirculatory stable term and preterm neonates with infection-related and infection-unrelated CRP elevations > 10 mg/l were compared with neonates without CRP elevation. The two groups were matched for gestational and postnatal age.

Results.—33 neonates with CRP elevation (gestational age 37.7 ± 2.9 weeks) were compared with 33 controls (gestational age 37.3 ± 2.9 weeks). In neonates with CRP elevation, TOI (68.9 ± 6.6%), SvO$_2$ (66.9 ± 7.3%) DO$_2$ (39.2 ± 16.1 μmol/100 ml/min) and VO$_2$ (10.9 ± 3.4 μmol/100 ml/min) were significantly lower compared with controls (TOI 72.9 ± 3.8%, SvO$_2$ 70.2 ± 4.7%, DO$_2$ 48.8 ± 18.4 μmol/ 100 ml/min, VO$_2$ 12.3 ± 3.8 μmol/100 ml/min). There was no significant difference in any other NIRS or routine haemodynamic parameter between the two groups.

Conclusion.—Inflammatory processes with CRP elevation cause impaired peripheral oxygenation and perfusion in neonates even when routine haemodynamic variables are still normal. NIRS might offer a new non-invasive tool for the early recognition and diagnosis of infectious and non-infectious inflammatory processes.

▶ Inflammation has been linked with a host of neonatal morbidities, including but not limited to, intracranial white matter injury, bronchopulmonary dysplasia, and persistent pulmonary hypertension of the newborn. In this study, Pichler et al studied the association between C reactive protein (CRP), a powerful indicator of inflammation, and tissue perfusion, as assessed by near infrared spectroscopy (NIRS). The investigators found an elevated CRP level to be associated with impaired peripheral tissue perfusion and oxygenation even when hemodynamic parameters were normal. It is unclear whether CRP acts directly on peripheral tissues or simply serves as a marker for tissue effects of inflammation and related processes, possibly warranting further study. This study also provides evidence favoring broader consideration and evaluation of potential new applications of NIRS in noninvasive assessment of tissue perfusion and oxygenation.

L. J. Van Marter, MD, MPH

Spectrum of chronic lung disease in a population of newborns with extremely low gestational age

Hjalmarson O, Brynjarsson H, Nilsson S, et al (The Sahlgrenska Academy at Univ of Gothenburg, Sweden; Chalmers Univ of Technology, Gothenburg, Sweden)

Acta Paediatr 101:912-918, 2012

Aims.—To determine how the ability to oxygenate the blood develops after birth in infants of extremely low gestational age (ELGANs) and to find risk factors for chronic lung disease.

Method.—A prospective, population-based, cohort study was under- taken in one tertiary-care centre. The alveolar—arterial oxygen pressure difference ($AaDO_2$) was monitored.

Results.—Of 41 survivors, 21 had a period of normal lung function in the first week of life, after which oxygenation deteriorated. Low gestational age and low Apgar score at 5 min were found to be strong and independent predictors of $AaDO_2$ in the first month of life. Mechanical ventilation did not appear as a risk factor. Lung function at 36 weeks of gestation and duration of oxygen treatment could be better predicted by the severity of lung disease in the first month than by gestational age at birth.

Conclusions.—Difficulty in oxygenation was a general observation in ELGANs and not only a particular subset. Gestational age and Apgar score were independent predictors of the degree of difficulty over the first month of life. As oxygenation failure often developed after a few days, the process may be possible to treat or prevent once the pathogenesis is known.

▶ Very premature birth is frequently associated with chronic respiratory morbidity, particularly in infants who developed bronchopulmonary dysplasia (BPD). There are many risk factors for BPD; infants may have a genetic predis- position and there is an inverse relationship of BPD occurrence with gestational age. Male[1] and small-for-gestational-age[2] infants have an increased risk of BPD and chronic respiratory morbidity. BPD is more common in infants who had severe respiratory failure, but very prematurely born infants may develop BPD having initially had minimal or no respiratory distress after birth.[3]

Hjalmarson et al[4] report serial measurements of the alveolar arterial oxygen difference ($AaDO_2$) in 41 extremely low gestational age survivors. Transcuta- neous measurements, which were used in the calculation of the $AaDO_2$, had been shown in a previous study to correlate well with results of arterial PaO_2 measurements.[5] Others, however, have not had such success[6] and limited clinical applicability of transcutaneous measurements has been reported resulting from burns. The majority of the measurements were performed in the prone position, this is important as even at 36 weeks' postmenstrual age (PMA)[7] and in older infants[8] prone vs sleeping position is associated with better oxygenation. In Hjalmarson's study, septicemia and chorioamnionitis were diagnosed clinically. It had been reported that chorioamnionitis was a significant risk factor for BPD,[9] although others[10] highlighted that chorioamnionitis was only significantly associated with BPD if infants subsequently developed postnatal sepsis or required prolonged ventilation.[10] Subsequently, only 6 of 18 studies demonstrated an association of BPD with chorioamnionitis,[11] and in the studies in which gestational age was taken into account, chorioamnionitis was no longer a risk factor for BPD. In addition, lung function results at 36 weeks' PMA did not differ significantly between very prematurely born infants exposed or unexposed to chorioamnionitis.[12]

A strength of Hjalmarson's study is the longitudinal data. Their analysis further emphasizes that a period of normal lung function in the first week after birth does not preclude BPD development. In addition, they highlight that low gestational age and low Apgar score at 5 minutes were independent predictors of increased $AaDO_2$ levels in the first month after birth, emphasizing the importance of reducing very premature delivery and having more effective resuscitation strategies. Respiratory function monitoring in the labor suite has demonstrated that, despite completing appropriate training, pediatricians frequently do not follow international resuscitation guidelines,[13] in particular much shorter inflation times were used than those recommended. In addition, tidal volumes and exhaled carbon dioxide levels significantly increased only when the infant took their first breath during resuscitation.[14] Further studies incorporating long-term outcomes are required to optimize resuscitation of extremely low gestational age infants.

A. Greenough, MD

References

1. Peacock J, Marston L, Marlow N, et al. Neonatal and infant outcome in boys and girls born very prematurely. *Ped Res.* 2012;71:305-310.
2. Peacock JL, Lo J, D'Costa W, Calvert S, Marlow N, Greenough A. Respiratory morbidity at follow up of small for gestational age infants born very prematurely. *Pediatr Res.* 2013;73:457-463.
3. Rojas MA, Gonzalez A, Bancalari E, et al. Changing trends in the epidemiology and pathogenesis of chronic lung disease. *J Pediatr.* 1995;126:605-610.
4. Hjalmarson O, Brynjarsson H, Nilsson S, et al. Spectrum of chronic lung disease in a population of newborns with extremely low gestational age. *Acta Paediatr.* 2012;101:912-918.
5. Sandberg KL, Brynjarsson H, Hjalmarson O. Transcutaneous blood gas monitoring during neonatal intensive care. *Acta Paediatr.* 2011;100:676-679.
6. Coalson JJ. Pathology of bronchopulmonary dysplasia. *Semin Perinatol.* 2006;30:179-184.
7. Bhat RY, Leipala JA, Singh NR, et al. Effect of posture on oxygenation, lung volume, and respiratory mechanics in premature infants studied before discharge. *Pediatrics.* 2003;112:29-32.
8. Saiki T, Rao H, Landolfo F, et al. Sleeping position, oxygenation and lung function in prematurely born infants studied post term. *Arch Dis Child.* 2009;94:F133-F137.
9. Watterberg KL, Demers LM, Scott SM, et al. Chorioamnionitis and early lung inflammation in infants in whom bronchopulmonary dysplasia develops. *Pediatrics.* 1996;97:210-215.
10. Van Marter LJ, Ammann O, Allred EN, et al. Chorioamnionitis, mechanical ventilation and postnatal sepsis as modulators of chronic lung disease in preterm infants. *J Pediatr.* 2002;140:171-176.
11. Been JV, Zimmerman LJI. Histological chorioamnionitis and respiratory outcome in preterm infants. *Arch Dis Child Fetal Neonatal Ed.* 2009;94:F218-F225.

12. Prendergast M, May C, Broughton S, et al. Chorioamnionitis, lung function and bronchopulmonary dysplasia in prematurely born infants. *Arch Dis Child Fetal Neonatal Ed.* 2011;96:F270-F274.
13. Murthy V, Dattani N, Fox G, et al. The first five inflations during resuscitation of prematurely born Infants. *Arch Dis Child.* 2012;97:F249-F253.
14. Murthy V, O'Rourke-Potocki A, Dattani N, et al. End tidal carbon dioxide levels during the resuscitation of prematurely born infants. *Early Hum Dev.* 2012;88: 783-787.

Long-term reparative effects of mesenchymal stem cell therapy following neonatal hyperoxia-induced lung injury

Sutsko RP, Young KC, Ribeiro A, et al (Univ of Miami Miller School of Medicine, FL)
Pediatr Res 73:46-53, 2013

Background.—Mesenchymal stem cell (MSC) therapy may prevent neonatal hyperoxia-induced lung injury (HILI). There are, however, no clear data on the therapeutic efficacy of MSC therapy in established HILI, the duration of the reparative effects, and the exact mechanisms of repair. The main objective of this study was to evaluate whether the long-term reparative effects of a single intratracheal (IT) dose of MSCs or MSC-conditioned medium (CM) are comparable in established HILI.

Methods.—Newborn rats exposed to normoxia or hyperoxia from post-natal day (P)2—P16 were randomized to receive IT MSCs, IT CM, or IT placebo (PL) on P9. Alveolarization and angiogenesis were evaluated at P16, P30, and P100.

Results.—At all time periods, there were marked improvements in alveolar and vascular development in hyperoxic pups treated with MSCs or CM as compared with PL. This was associated with decreased expression of inflammatory mediators and an upregulation of angiogenic factors. Of note, at P100, the improvements were more substantial with MSCs as compared with CM.

Conclusion.—These data suggest that acute effects of MSC therapy in HILI are mainly paracrine mediated; however, optimum long-term improvement following HILI requires treatment with the MSCs themselves or potentially repetitive administration of CM.

▶ This report, and similar results from the laboratory of Dr Bernard Thebaud in Canada,[1] provide a glimpse into the future of neonatal medicine. Working in rat models of oxygen toxicity in developing lungs, both groups have found remarkable attenuation of the alveolar and vascular developmental arrest that characterizes the new bronchopulmonary dysplasia. Intratracheal administration of stem cells, or even just medium conditioned by those cells in culture, markedly reduced increases in mean linear intercept and average alveolar area, reflecting preservation of alveolar septation. Similar but smaller effects were found on lung vascular density and right ventricular systolic pressures. These results are obtained with both syngenic and xenogenic cells, derived from bone marrow of adult rats (Sutsko et al) or from human umbilical cord blood or vessels,[1] respectively, providing proof of concept that the donor stem cells need not be closely matched to the recipient or derived from the recipients themselves. A great deal of work remains before such treatments enter clinical practice. Criteria for selection of infants likely to benefit from such treatments need to be established. Optimal timing, frequency, and dosing and whether stem cells themselves, conditioned medium, or some cocktail containing the critical elements of condition medium are the best agents remain to be determined. The possibility that the more modest effects of stem cell therapy on vascular (compared with alveolar septal) development may be insufficient to substantially alter outcomes for extremely-low-birth-weight babies needs to be explored, and strategies to address this may have to be developed. Anatomically remote and long-term effects, including potential adverse effects not recognized to date, need to be delineated. Logistics of production and distribution of live therapeutic agents will have to be worked out and standards for good manufacturing practices established. Attitudinal barriers to treatment of newborn infants with living cells—although already widely accepted when used in the form of bone marrow transplantation—will have to be understood and overcome. These are surmountable challenges, and the potential benefits are very likely to recompense the effort required. We should follow further developments in this work closely, as we may soon need to be ready to apply this new technology in our neonatal intensive care units.

W. E. Benitz, MD

Reference

1. Pierro M, Ionescu L, Montemurro T, et al. Short-term, long-term and paracrine effect of human umbilical cord-derived stem cells in lung injury prevention and repair in experimental bronchopulmonary dysplasia. *Thorax.* 2013;68:475-484.

Adapted ECMO criteria for newborns with persistent pulmonary hypertension after inhaled nitric oxide and/or high-frequency oscillatory ventilation
van Berkel S, Binkhorst M, van Heijst AFJ, et al (Radboud Univ Nijmegen Med Centre, The Netherlands)
Intensive Care Med 39:1113-1120, 2013

Purpose.—Early prediction of extracorporeal membrane oxygenation (ECMO) requirement in term newborns with persistent pulmonary hypertension (PPHN), partially responding to inhaled nitric oxide (iNO) and/or high-frequency oscillatory ventilation (HFOV), based on oxygenation parameters.

Methods.—This was a retrospective cohort study in 53 partial responders from among 133 term newborns with PPHN born between 2002 and 2007. Alveolar-to-arterial oxygen gradient ($AaDO_2$) values were determined in these 53 partial responders during the initial 72 h of iNO and/or HFOV treatment and compared between newborns who ultimately did ($n = 11$) and did not ($n = 42$) need ECMO.

Results.—Over 72 h, partial responders not requiring ECMO showed a more profound $AaDO_2$ decrease than those who needed ECMO (median decline 242.5 mm Hg, IQR 144 to 353 mm Hg, vs. 35 mm Hg, IQR −15 to 123 mm Hg; $p = 0.0007$). A decline of <123 mm Hg over 72 h predicted the need for ECMO (sensitivity 82%, specificity 79%). At 72 h, $AaDO_2$ was significantly lower in partial responders without the need for ECMO than in those who did need ECMO (median 369 mm Hg, IQR 258 to 478 mm Hg, vs. 570 mm Hg IQR 455 to 590 mm Hg; $p = 0.0008$). An $AaDO_2$ >561 mm Hg at 72 h predicted the need for ECMO (sensitivity 64%, specificity 95%, positive predictive value 78%).

Conclusions.—In term newborns with PPHN partially responding to iNO and/or HFOV, oxygenation-based prediction of the need for ECMO appears to be possible after 72 h. ECMO centers are encouraged to develop their own prediction model in order to prevent both lung damage and unnecessary ECMO runs.

▶ As part of an original center offering neonatal extracorporeal membrane oxygenation (ECMO) for intractable respiratory failure, I was always troubled by the selection criteria for use in persistent pulmonary hypertension of the newborn. The 2 most prominent of these were the oxygenation index and the alveolar-arterial oxygen difference ($A\text{-}aDO_2$). The former was flawed because once optimal lung inflation was achieved, further increases in peak airway pressure or end-expiratory pressure would only lead to hyperinflation and increases in pulmonary vascular resistance and, thus, a reduction in oxygenation. To meet ECMO criteria and justify cannulation only required the clinician to go up on the pressure. This became further complicated by the introduction of high-frequency application into clinical practice, where the mean airway pressure is not equivalent to that produced during tidal ventilation. The $A\text{-}aDO_2$ was utilized at a time when the primary management strategy included deliberate hypocapnia. If the clinician was successful in achieving hypocapnia, the $A\text{-}aDO_2$ increased as a consequence of simple arithmetic. Thus, successful treatment moved a baby closer to the need for ECMO. There was little to no validation of these indices, and they differed from one center to another.

This study re-examined the utility of serial $A\text{-}aDO_2$ measurements as predictive indices for ECMO in the era of inhaled nitric oxide (iNO). Using a retrospective cohort study, they determined that ECMO was likely if the $A\text{-}aDO_2$ was greater than 561 torr after 72 hours of nitric oxide therapy. They also advised the need for developing institution-specific criteria, something we learned early in the course of ECMO. Nevertheless, their work is important in giving us a new framework to gauge the success of iNO. Prospective validation would certainly be useful in deciding which patients might require (or escape from) our most invasive respiratory intervention.

S. M. Donn, MD

ECMO hospital volume and survival in congenital diaphragmatic hernia repair

Davis JS, Ryan ML, Perez EA, et al (Univ of Miami Miller School of Medicine, FL)
J Surg Res 178:791-796, 2012

Purpose.—This study examined survival in newborn patients after congenital diaphragmatic hernia (CDH) repair.

Methods.—We analyzed the Kids' Inpatient Database Years 2000, 2003, and 2006 for patients admitted at fewer than 8 d of age undergoing CDH repair. We analyzed patient demographics, clinical characteristics, socio-economic measures, hospital type, operative case volume, and survival using Fisher's exact test and a multivariate binary logistic regression model.

Results.—Of 847 patients identified, most were male (61%) and white (57%), were treated at urban (99.8%) and teaching (96%) hospitals, and had private insurance (57%). Survival to discharge was 95% in non-extracorporeal membrane oxygenation (ECMO) patients versus 51% for those requiring ECMO ($P < 0.0001$). Univariate analysis revealed significantly lower survival rates in blacks, Medicaid patients, and patients undergoing repair after 7 d of life. Among ECMO patients, we noted higher survival rates at hospitals conducting four or more ECMO cases per year (66% versus 47%; $P = 0.03$). Multivariate analysis identified ECMO (hazards ratio [HR] 16.23, $P < 0.001$), CDH repair at >7 d of age (HR 2.70, $P = 0.004$), and ECMO patients repaired at hospitals performing <4 CDH ECMO cases per year (HR 3.59, $P = 0.03$) as independent predictors of mortality.

Conclusions.—We conclude that ECMO hospital volume is associated with survival in patients requiring ECMO for CDH repair.

▶ This report attempts to further explore the potential contribution of center experience with outcomes in infants born with congenital diaphragmatic hernia (CDH) using the Kids' Inpatient Database (KID). Several prior studies using different databases have found a positive association between volume of CDH cases and survival.[1-3] Bucher et al[3] also examined overall extracorporeal membrane oxygenation (ECMO) volume and did not find an association with survival in infants with CDH, but none has specifically examined the potential relationship between volume of CDH patients requiring ECMO and outcome. The KID is attractive in that it includes all payers and information from all public hospitals, academic medical centers, and pediatric hospitals. It does, however, capture only a random sample of cases (80% of complicated in-hospital births and other pediatric cases), and, as with all large databases, there is potential for coding errors. The authors analyzed demographic data, socioeconomic data, clinical characteristics, hospital type, operative case volume (including need for ECMO), and survival data for all newborns in the database in 2000, 2003, and 2006 who were less than 8 days of age and who underwent a CDH repair. Overall survival rate to discharge was 95% in those infants who did not require ECMO, and 57% in those who required ECMO. Survival was lower in blacks,

Medicaid patients, patients undergoing repair after 7 days, and patients requiring ECMO who were cared for at centers caring for fewer than 4 CDH patients requiring ECMO per year (univariate analysis). Requirement for ECMO, repair at less than 7 days of age, and repair at hospitals performing less than 4 CDH ECMO cases per year remained significant predictors of mortality on multivariate analysis.

Although these findings are of interest and certainly justify further investigation, their significant limitations should be taken into consideration. The inclusion of only infants who underwent CDH repair eliminates any infant who did not survive to undergo repair, which may include patients who received ECMO as well as those who died before receiving ECMO and could potentially skew the data in either direction. In addition, the presence or absence of other congenital anomalies, genetic syndromes, or prematurity, all previously identified risk factors for mortality, were not examined in this data set. In addition, information on overall neonatal ECMO volume would have been helpful in further exploring the association. The authors do make a valid argument that ECMO in the setting of CDH is potentially more complicated, and a higher-risk procedure, such as the association with ECMO-CDH volume, even if there is not a clear association with overall ECMO volume, is plausible and warrants further investigation.

S. M. Donn, MD

References

1. Javid PJ, Jaksic T, Skarsgard ED, Lee S. Survival rate in congenital diaphragmatic hernia: the experience of the Canadian Neonatal Network. *J Pediatr Surg.* 2004; 39:657-660.
2. Grushka JR, Laberge JM, Puligandla P, Skarsgard ED. Effect of hospital case volume on outcome in congenital diaphragmatic hernia: the experience of the Canadian Pediatric Surgery Network. *J Pediatr Surg.* 2009;44:873-876.
3. Bucher BT, Guth RM, Saito JM, Najaf T, Warner BW. Impact of hospital volume on in-hospital mortality of infants undergoing repair of congenital diaphragmatic hernia. *Ann Surg.* 2010;252:635-642.

Respiratory morbidity at follow-up of small-for-gestational-age infants born very prematurely

Peacock JL, Lo JW, D'Costa W, et al (King's College London, UK; et al)
Pediatr Res 73:457-463, 2013

Background.—The aim of this study was to determine whether small-for-gestational-age (SGA) infants born very prematurely had increased respiratory morbidity in the neonatal period and at follow-up.

Methods.—Data were examined from infants recruited into the United Kingdom Oscillation Study (UKOS). Of the 797 infants who were born at <29 wk of gestational age, 174 infants were SGA. Overall, 92% were exposed to antenatal corticosteroids and 97% received surfactant; follow-up data at 22—28 mo were available for 367 infants.

Results.—After adjustment for gestational age and sex, SGA infants had higher rates of supplementary oxygen dependency at 36 wk postmenstrual age (odds ratio (OR): 3.23; 95% confidence interval: 2.03, 5.13), pulmonary hemorrhage (OR: 3.07; 95% CI: 1.82, 5.18), death (OR: 3.32; 95% CI: 2.13, 5.17), and postnatal corticosteroid requirement (OR: 2.09; 95% CI: 1.35, 3.23). After adjustment for infant and respiratory morbidity risk factors, a lower mean birth weight z-score was associated with a higher prevalence of respiratory admissions (OR: 1.40; 95% CI: 1.03, 1.88 for 1 SD change in z-score), cough (OR: 1.28; 95% CI: 1.00, 1.65), and use of chest medicines (OR: 1.32; 95% CI: 1.01, 1.73).

Conclusion.—SGA infants who were born very prematurely, despite routine use of antenatal corticosteroids and postnatal surfactant, had increased respiratory morbidity at follow-up, which was not due to poor neonatal outcome.

▶ This report is a spinoff of the United Kingdom Oscillation Study trial, which compared the use of high-frequency oscillation with conventional tidal volume in a population of extremely low-birth-weight infants. It attempted to address whether small-for-gestational age infants had long-term respiratory morbidity, even if treated with antenatal corticosteroids and surfactant. It is not clear whether this was planned a priori or if it represents data dredging after the fact. The authors conclude that infants with intrauterine growth restriction had both short- and long-term problems related to growth restriction, which distinguished them from their normally grown counterparts.

Data were analyzed both by small-for-gestational-age vs appropriate-for-gestational-age status and by birth weight Z-score status. The latter appears to have more significance, but given the large number of comparisons, the *P* values should have been subjected to a Bonferroni correction, which would have diminished the statistical significance. Most of the difference appears to be related to rehospitalization for respiratory illnesses, which were not specified. Information about palivizumab treatment would have been helpful. In addition, examining differences related to the assigned modality of ventilation might have been meaningful.

Finally, despite using sophisticated statistical manipulations, let's remember that the Apgar score is a discontinuous variable and cannot be averaged.

S. M. Donn, MD

8 Central Nervous System and Special Senses

Neurodevelopmental Outcomes of Extremely Low-Gestational-Age Neonates With Low-Grade Periventricular-Intraventricular Hemorrhage
Payne AH, for the Eunice Kennedy Shriver National Institute of Child Health and Human Development Neonatal Research Network (Case Western Reserve Univ, Cleveland, OH; et al)
JAMA Pediatr 167:451-459, 2013

Importance.—Low-grade periventricular-intraventricular hemorrhage is a common neurologic morbidity among extremely low-gestational-age neonates, yet the outcomes associated with this morbidity are not fully understood. In a contemporary multicenter cohort, we evaluated the impact of such hemorrhages on early (18-22 month) neurodevelopmental outcomes of extremely premature infants.

Objective.—To compare neurodevelopmental outcomes at 18 to 22 months' corrected age for extremely low-gestational-age infants with low-grade (grade 1 or 2) periventricular-intraventricular hemorrhage with those of infants with either no hemorrhage or severe (grade 3 or 4) hemorrhage demonstrated on cranial ultrasonography.

Design.—Longitudinal observational study.

Setting.—Sixteen centers of the Eunice Kennedy Shriver National Institute of Child Health and Human Development Neonatal Research Network.

Participants.—A total of 1472 infants born at less than 27 weeks' gestational age between January 1, 2006, and December 31, 2008, with ultrasonography results within the first 28 days of life and surviving to 18 to 22 months with complete follow-up assessments were eligible.

Main Exposure.—Low-grade periventricular-intraventricular hemorrhage.

Main Outcome Measures.—Outcomes included cerebral palsy; gross motor functional limitation; cognitive and language scores according to the Bayley Scales of Infant Development, 3rd Edition; and composite measures of neurodevelopmental impairment. Regression modeling evaluated the association of hemorrhage severity with adverse outcomes while controlling for potentially confounding variables and center differences.

Results.—Low-grade hemorrhage was not associated with significant differences in unadjusted or adjusted risk of any adverse neurodevelopmental outcome compared with infants without hemorrhage. Compared with low-grade hemorrhage, severe hemorrhage was associated with decreased adjusted continuous cognitive (β, -3.91 [95% CI, -6.41 to -1.42]) and language (β, -3.19 [-6.19 to -0.19]) scores as well as increased odds of each adjusted categorical outcome except severe cognitive impairment (odds ratio [OR], 1.46 [0.74 to 2.88]) and mild language impairment (OR, 1.35 [0.88 to 2.06]).

Conclusions and Relevance.—At 18 to 22 months, the neurodevelopmental outcomes of extremely low-gestational-age infants with low-grade periventricular-intraventricular hemorrhage are not significantly different from those without hemorrhage. Additional study at school age and beyond would be informative.

▶ Intraventricular hemorrhages (IVH) leading to ventricular dilatation (grade 3) or intraparenchymal hemorrhages (grade 4) in extremely low-birth-weight infants are clearly associated with higher incidences of cerebral palsy and worse cognitive outcomes compared with no hemorrhages. However, the significance of isolated germinal matrix hemorrhages (grade 1) or of IVH without ventricular dilatation (grade 2) has been less clearly established. In this study, Dr Payne and investigators from the Eunice Kennedy Shriver National Institute of Child Health and Human Development Neonatal Research Network evaluated 1472 infants born at less than 27 weeks of gestation and admitted to 16 centers between 2006 and 2008 who survived 18 to 22 months (87% follow-up rate). Contrary to the authors' initial hypothesis, the study found that, after adjusting for potential confounders in a multivariate regression mode, infants with grade 1 to 2 IVH did not have an increased incidence of poor neurodevelopmental outcome at 18 to 22 months compared with infants without IVH. These findings were somewhat surprising because they were in disagreement with the most recent prior studies reporting neurodevelopmental outcomes in infants with grade 1 or 2 IVH, which pointed toward a greater negative effect.[1-3] The reasons for the discrepancies between those reports and the Payne study are likely multifactorial and include differences in the populations of preterm infants studied (the Payne study only included infants born at < 27 weeks of gestation) and changes over time in medical practice, particularly the use of prenatal and postnatal steroids (which were included in the analysis of the Payne study but not the previous studies). Overall, this new study provides us with welcome data from a large, contemporary cohort of extremely preterm infants indicating that, in current times, the neurodevelopmental outcome of high-risk preterm infants in whom grade 1 or 2 IVH develops is no different from that of infants with no hemorrhage, at least at 18 to 20 months.

M. Sola-Visner, MD

References

1. Ancel PY, Livinec F, Larroque B, et al. Cerebral palsy among very preterm children in relation to gestational age and neonatal ultrasound abnormalities: the EPIPAGE cohort study. *Pediatrics.* 2006;117:828-835.
2. Sherlock RL, Anderson PJ, Doyle LW. Neurodevelopmental sequelae of intraventricular haemorrhage at 8 years of age in a regional cohort of ELBW/very preterm infants. *Early Hum Dev.* 2005;81:909-916.
3. Patra K, Wilson-Costello D, Taylor HG, Mercuri-Minich N, Hack M. Grades I-II intraventricular hemorrhage in extremely low birth weight infants: effects on neurodevelopment. *J Pediatr.* 2006;149:169-173.

Impact of low-grade intraventricular hemorrhage on long-term neurodevelopmental outcome in preterm infants

Klebermass-Schrehof K, Czaba C, Olischar M, et al (Med Univ of Vienna, Austria)

Childs Nerv Syst 28:2085-2092, 2012

Purpose.—Despite a decreasing incidence, intraventricular hemorrhage (IVH) remains a point of major concern in neonatology due to its association to adverse neurodevelopmental outcome (NDO). Aim of this study was to compare outcome of preterm infants with different grades of IVH born below 32 weeks of gestational age (GA) with outcome of controls without IVH and to especially evaluate the influence of low grade IVH on NDO.

Methods.—Four hundred seventy-one preterm infants with a GA below 32 weeks were admitted to our neonatal intensive care unit between 1994 and 2005 and included into analysis.

Results.—IVH patients showed significantly lower mean psychomotor and mental developmental indices and a significantly higher percentage of cerebral palsy and visual impairment. Results of IVH patients born below 28 weeks of GA were significantly worse than results of IVH patients born at or above 28 weeks of GA. In all parameters, an increase of abnormal results with increasing grade of IVH could be observed; even patients with low-grade IVH (grades I and II) showed higher percentages of impairment compared to controls without any IVH.

Conclusion.—Even low-grade IVH has an significant impact on neurodevelopmental outcome of preterm patients and gestational age influences the impact of intraventricular hemorrhage on neurodevelopmental outcome (Fig).

▶ Observations made soon after in vivo neuroimaging techniques came into clinical use suggested that lower grades (I or II) of intraventricular hemorrhage (IVH) in preterm infants had minimal, if any, effects on long-term neurodevelopment. Those correlations predominantly came from infants who would now be considered relatively mature, so their relevance to the very immature infants who now populate our neonatal intensive care units is, at best, uncertain. The

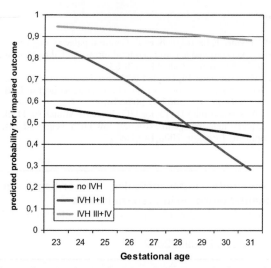

FIGURE.—Influence of gestational age on the impact of IVH on neurodevelopmental outcome. Predicted probabiliy of impaired outcome (=1) for infants with no IVH (*blue line*), infant with low-grade IVH (grades I and II) and infants with high-grade IVH (grades III and IV); gestational age is given in weeks. For interpretation of the references to color in this figure legend, the reader is referred to web version of this article. (With kind permission from Springer Science+Business Media. Klebermass-Schrehof K, Czaba C, Olischar M, et al. Impact of low-grade intraventricular hemorrhage on long-term neurodevelopmental outcome in preterm infants. *Childs Nerv Syst.* 2012;28:2085-2092, Copyright 2012.)

belief that lower grades of IVH are inconsequential has been slow to disappear, however. Drawing upon a single-center experience over a 12-year period (1994—2005), this report provides valuable data to remedy any remaining ambiguity. These authors identified 471 infants born before 32 weeks of gestation who had cerebral ultrasound scans performed on days 1, 3, 5, 7, and 10 after birth and then weekly until discharge, and who were assessed in the neonatal follow-up clinic at 1, 2, 3.5, and 5.5 years of age. (The total number of potentially eligible subjects is not specified.) No IVH was seen in 287 infants, grade I IVH was found in 37, grade II in 84, grade III in 18, and grade IV in 12; 33 infants who had additional neuroimaging abnormalities (periventricular leucomalacia or cerebellar injuries) were excluded from the analysis. Much information about outcomes is presented in the Tables of the report, for each grade of IVH and for the cohorts of infants born before or after 28 weeks of gestation (interested readers should consult the full publication for details). Neurodevelopmental outcomes were dependent on both gestational age at birth and grade of IVH. Impaired neurologic function was more likely or more severe in less mature infants overall and for each grade of IVH except grade IV (for which outcomes were poor in both age groups). Increasing IVH grade was associated with worse developmental outcome, especially among infants greater than 28 weeks of gestation. Even grade I or II IVH increased the risk of neurodevelopmental impairment (Fig). For example, among infants born before 28 weeks of gestation, the prevalence of cerebral palsy at age 5.5 years increased from 14.3% for infants without IVH to 34.8%, 55.0%, 63.6%, and 90.9%, respectively, with grade I, II, III, or IV IVH; for infants born at or after 28 weeks, those rates were 8.5%, 12.5%, 23.5%, 60.0%, and 100.0%, respectively (all differences from subjects with no IVH are statistically significant). Although it remains true that the implications of grade III and IV IVH may be grave, we cannot be entirely sanguine about the prognosis for infants with less severe IVH. To be sure, even multiple normal cerebral sonograms do not guarantee intact neurodevelopment. The results presented in this report will be useful in informing thought about this important subject.

W. E. Benitz, MD

An overlooked aspect on metabolic acidosis at birth: blood gas analyzers calculate base deficit differently

Mokarami P, Wiberg N, Olofsson P (Lund Univ, Malmö, Sweden)
Acta Obstet Gynecol Scand 91:574-579, 2012

Objective.—Metabolic acidosis (MA) at birth is commonly defined as umbilical cord arterial pH < 7.0 plus base deficit (BD) $\geq$ 12.0 mmol/L. Base deficit is not a measured entity but is calculated from pH and P_{CO_2} values, with the hemoglobin (Hb) concentration [Hb] included in the calculation algorithm as a fixed or measured value. Various blood gas analyzers use different algorithms, indicating variations in the MA diagnosis. The objective was therefore to calculate the prevalence of MA in blood and extracellular fluid with algorithms from three blood gas analyzer brands relative to the Clinical and Laboratory Standards Institute (CLSI) algorithm.
Design.—Comparative study.
Setting.—University hospital.
Sample.—Arterial cord blood from 15 354 newborns.
Main outcome measure.—Prevalence of MA.
Methods.—Blood was analyzed in a Radiometer ABL 735 analyzer. Base deficit was calculated post hoc with algorithms from CLSI and Corning and Roche blood gas analyzers, and with measured and fixed (9.3 mmol/L) values of [Hb].
Results.—The prevalence of BD $\geq$ 12.0 mmol/L in blood was with the CLSI algorithm 1.97%, Radiometer 5.18%, Corning 3.84% and Roche 3.29% (CLSI vs. other; McNemar test, $p < 0.000001$). Likewise, MA prevalences were 0.58, 0.66, 0.64 and 0.64%, respectively ($p \leq 0.02$). Base deficit $\geq$ 12.0 mmol/L and MA rates were lower in extracellular fluid than in blood ($p \leq 0.002$). Algorithms with measured or fixed Hb concentration made no differences to MA rates ($p \geq 0.1$).
Conclusions.—The neonatal metabolic acidosis rate varied significantly with blood gas analyzer brand and fetal fluid compartment for calculation of BD.

▶ Base excess (or deficit) is an important component of the American Academy of Pediatrics/American College of Obstetricians and Gynecologists and

International Consensus criteria for recognition of intrapartum hypoxic-ischemic injury and for determining eligibility for neuroprotective cooling. This report highlights technical inconsistencies in the formulas used to calculate that value among 3 commercial blood gas analyzers, which all differ from the standard promulgated by the Clinical Laboratory Standards Institute (CLSI). One analyzer not included in this analysis (i-Stat®, Abbott) uses equations consistent with CLSI guidelines, so at least 4 different sets of values may result from analysis of any specimen. To complicate matters further, base excess values come in 2 flavors: blood base excess and extracellular fluid base excess, which differ from each other and among analyzers; either result may be chosen for posting by each hospital's clinical laboratory. These ambiguities are not inconsequential. Recalculating values for base excess estimates from data accrued from nearly 16 000 cord blood specimens, these authors show substantial differences in the proportion of newborn infants who would be categorized as having a significantly elevated extracellular fluid base deficit ($BD_{ECF} \geq 12.0$ mmol/L), ranging from 0.73% using algorithms from the Corning 178 analyzer (Ciba Corning Diagnostics) to 2.26% with those from the Roche cobas b 221 analyzer (Hoffmann-La Roche); rates of elevated BD_{ECF} for all 3 analyzers differed significantly from that determined using CLSI standards. Similar discrepancies were found for rates of significant metabolic acidosis (pH < 7.0 and $BD_{ECF} \geq 12.0$ mmol/L). These observations have 2 important implications. First, because analyses of relationships between cord blood or initial postnatal base deficit values and neurologic injury and clinical trials of neuroprotective interventions typically do not specify (and may not have standardized) the algorithm used for calculation of those values, it is difficult or impossible to know whether a particular patient is comparable to the subjects enrolled in those studies. The external validity of those studies, therefore, may be compromised. Second, standardization of laboratory measurements that serve as surrogates for the severity of intrapartum asphyxia injury is essential. Rather than persisting in use of calculated values for base deficits, it may be better to adopt lactate levels, as these authors suggest. Lactate levels in blood are directly measured (not derived), are readily available at a reasonable cost, and directly reflect anaerobic metabolism resulting from hypoxic-ischemic conditions. Addition of lactate measurements as a standard component of the laboratory evaluation of neonates with possible hypoxic-ischemic injury may be an idea whose time has come. Accrual of those data over time will help ascertain the utility of that surrogate of severity of anoxic insults in identification of infants at risk and estimate the potential benefit from hypothermia or other treatments.

W. E. Benitz, MD

Neonatal Encephalopathy: An Inadequate Term for Hypoxic–Ischemic Encephalopathy

Volpe JJ (Harvard Med School, Boston, MA)
Ann Neurol 72:156-166, 2012

This Point of View article addresses neonatal encephalopathy (NE) presumably caused by hypoxia-ischemia and the terminology currently in wide use for this disorder. The nonspecific term NE is commonly utilized for those infants with the clinical and imaging characteristics of neonatal hypoxic—ischemic encephalopathy (HIE). Multiple magnetic resonance imaging studies of term infants with the clinical setting of presumed hypoxia—ischemia near the time of delivery have delineated a topography of lesions highly correlated with that defined by human neuropathology and by animal models, including primate models, of hypoxia—ischemia. These imaging findings, coupled with clinical features consistent with perinatal hypoxic—ischemic insult(s), warrant the specific designation of neonatal HIE.

▶ This article is a superb review of hypoxic encephalopathy, including the neuropathology, pathophysiology, neuroimaging, and clinical features succinctly compressed into 8 pages of text, but referencing 125 articles. I would recommend this to all neonatologists.

At the end of the article, Dr Volpe acknowledges the medico-legal conundrum of ascribing the proper terminology to a newborn infant's condition. He is dissatisfied that so many affected babies are coded as "neonatal encephalopathy" rather than "hypoxic-ischemic encephalopathy." I think this really is a matter of what information is available at the time. An analogy is sepsis. At the time of an admission history and physical examination, we may only have enough information to list "suspected sepsis" or "sepsis syndrome" as our admitting diagnosis. It is not "strep B sepsis" until the cultures are positive.

An encephalopathic newborn could have any number of underlying conditions. It would not be improper to use the "neonatal encephalopathy" diagnosis until there are sufficient data to ascribe the cause as hypoxia-ischemia. One of the problems of using "hypoxic—ischemic encephalopathy" is that it is unclear as to when the brain injuring event occurred, and unfortunately, there is generally a presumption that it was an intrapartum event. I do concur that we need to be precise in all phases of medical record documentation.

S. M. Donn, MD

Biomarkers of Brain Injury in Neonatal Encephalopathy Treated With Hypothermia

Massaro AN, Chang T, Kadom N, et al (Children's Natl Med Ctr, Washington, DC)
J Pediatr 161:434-440, 2012

Objective.—To determine if early serum S100B and neuron-specific enolase (NSE) levels are associated with neuroradiographic and clinical evidence of brain injury in newborns with encephalopathy.

Study Design.—Patients who received therapeutic whole-body hypothermia were prospectively enrolled in this observational study. Serum specimens were collected at 0, 12, 24, and 72 hours of cooling. S100B and NSE levels were measured by enzyme linked immunosorbent assay. Magnetic resonance imaging was performed in surviving infants at 7-10 days of life. Standardized neurologic examination was performed by a child neurologist at 14 days of life. Multiple linear regression analyses were performed to evaluate the association between S100B and NSE levels and unfavorable outcome (death or severe magnetic resonance imaging injury/significant neurologic deficit). Cutoff values were determined by receiver operating curve analysis.

Results.—Newborns with moderate to severe encephalopathy were enrolled (n = 75). Median pH at presentation was 6.9 (range, 6.5-7.35), and median Apgar scores of 1 at 1 minute, 3 at 5 minutes, and 5 at 10 minutes. NSE and S100B levels were higher in patients with unfavorable outcomes across all time points. These results remained statistically significant after controlling for covariables, including encephalopathy grade at presentation, Apgar score at 5 minutes of life, initial pH, and clinical seizures.

Conclusion.—Elevated serum S100B and NSE levels measured during hypothermia were associated with neuroradiographic and clinical evidence of brain injury in encephalopathic newborns. These brain-specific proteins may be useful immediate biomarkers of cerebral injury severity.

▶ This was an interesting observational study that correlated the changes in 2 biomarkers specific to brain injury (serum S100B and neuron-specific enolase) during therapeutic hypothermia with short-term neurologic outcome, assessed by magnetic resonance imaging (MRI) and neurologic examination. The investigators found a positive correlation, with statistically significant differences at all time points between those with unfavorable vs favorable outcomes. This was a well-done study, and it will be interesting to see how clinicians use these data. It is hard to imagine discontinuing hypothermia in light of elevated neuron-specific enolase or S100B. In the study, both were found to have reasonable specificity but less than stellar sensitivity. Might it be useful in discriminating infants who could be spared the expense of an MRI?

Perhaps a more important application will be incorporating these measurements into ongoing clinical cooling trials, which are examining depth and duration of cooling, where they may give important information about neuronal injury and recovery.

The relationship of elevated biomarkers to long-term outcome is unknown. This study is yet another reminder of the value of the neurological examination at discharge. When all else fails, look at the baby.

S. M. Donn, MD

Biomarkers of Brain Injury in Neonatal Encephalopathy Treated with Hypothermia

Massaro AN, Chang T, Kadom N, et al (Children's Natl Med Ctr, Washington, DC)

J Pediatr 161:434-440, 2012

Objective.—To determine if early serum S100B and neuron-specific enolase (NSE) levels are associated with neuroradiographic and clinical evidence of brain injury in newborns with encephalopathy.

Study Design.—Patients who received therapeutic whole-body hypothermia were prospectively enrolled in this observational study. Serum specimens were collected at 0, 12, 24, and 72 hours of cooling. S100B and NSE levels were measured by enzyme linked immunosorbent assay. Magnetic resonance imaging was performed in surviving infants at 7-10 days of life. Standardized neurologic examination was performed by a child neurologist at 14 days of life. Multiple linear regression analyses were performed to evaluate the association between S100B and NSE levels and unfavorable outcome (death or severe magnetic resonance imaging injury/significant neurologic deficit). Cutoff values were determined by receiver operating curve analysis.

Results.—Newborns with moderate to severe encephalopathy were enrolled (n = 75). Median pH at presentation was 6.9 (range, 6.5-7.35), and median Apgar scores of 1 at 1 minute, 3 at 5 minutes, and 5 at 10 minutes. NSE and S100B levels were higher in patients with unfavorable outcomes across all time points. These results remained statistically significant after controlling for covariables, including encephalopathy grade at presentation, Apgar score at 5 minutes of life, initial pH, and clinical seizures.

Conclusion.—Elevated serum S100B and NSE levels measured during hypothermia were associated with neuroradiographic and clinical evidence of brain injury in encephalopathic newborns. These brain-specific proteins may be useful immediate biomarkers of cerebral injury severity.

▶ Sequelae of neonatal hypoxic—ischemic encephalopathy (HIE) cover a wide spectrum, ranging from no disability to severe disability or death. Therapeutic cooling improves outcomes and has become an accepted standard of care, but optimal effect requires initiation within 6 hours after the insult, so early iden-tification of infants who are most likely to benefit is essential. The best strategy for doing so remains elusive. Apgar scores and blood gas measurements are nonspecific. The Sarnat grading system of mild, moderate, and severe encephalopathy correlates better with neurologic outcome, but relies on clinical examination over days rather than hours. This has prompted efforts to identify serum biomarkers that might help predict severity of neurodevelopmental outcome within the first few hours after birth. Reliable serum biomarkers might allow stratification of infants into 2 classes: those with mild or severe injuries whose outcomes are unlikely to be altered by cooling, and an intermediate group most likely to benefit from cooling.

In this prospective observational study of 75 infants treated with whole-body hypothermia at a single institution, the investigators sought to determine if levels of neuron-specific enolase (NSE) or S100B obtained at 0, 12, 24, and 72 hours after birth are associated with poor outcomes. NSE is a marker of neuronal injury; S100B is released with astrocytic injury. Outcome measures were death or severe magnetic resonance imaging (MRI)-related injury at 7 to 10 days of age, or death or significant neurologic deficit by exam at 14 days of age. NSE and S100B levels were higher in patients with adverse outcomes at all time points, even after controlling for various potential confounders. Measurements at the initiation of cooling were better predictors of death or severe MRI injury, whereas levels at the end of cooling were more predictive of death or severe neurologic deficit. It is not clear which of these endpoints might correlate best with long-term outcomes because no late follow-up data were reported. Using cutpoints selected for maximal diagnostic accuracy, these measurements had only modest sensitivity and specificity (64% and 84%, respectively, for S100B at 0 hours, for example). Selection of cutpoints to optimize specificity (up to 91% and 93% for S100B and NSE, respectively, at 0 hours), and thereby minimize false-positive results, resulted in low sensitivities (40% and 30%, respectively, at 0 hours).

Nevertheless, this well-designed study is the first to evaluate early use of serum biomarkers to prognosticate neurodevelopmental outcome in neonates with HIE. The study did not address the utility of these tests for prediction of long-term neurodevelopmental outcome, focusing on the more immediate outcome measures noted previously, for which the specificity and sensitivity of these biomarkers are regrettably low. Although not sufficient to permit immediate incorporation of these tests into clinical practice, these data suggest potential roles for such measurements, perhaps in combination with clinical examination and ambulatory encephalogram, to identify infants most likely to benefit from cooling. An accurate prediction tool would be quite useful, allowing referring hospitals to determine whether to transfer a patient to initiate cooling and cooling centers to recognize infants for whom cooling is not indicated or ineffective, for example.

N. A. Shah, MD

Increased Inspired Oxygen in the First Hours of Life is Associated with Adverse Outcome in Newborns Treated for Perinatal Asphyxia with Therapeutic Hypothermia

Sabir H, Jary S, Tooley J, et al (Univ of Bristol, UK; Univ Hosps Bristol, UK)
J Pediatr 161:409-416, 2012

Objective.—To assess whether increased inspired oxygen and/or hypocarbia during the first 6 hours of life are associated with adverse outcome at 18 months in term neonates treated with therapeutic hypothermia.

Study Design.—Blood gas values and ventilatory settings were monitored hourly in 61 newborns for 6 hours after birth. We investigated if there was an association between increased inspired oxygen and/or hypocarbia and adverse outcome (death or disability by Bayley Scales of Newborn Development II examination at 18-20 months).

Results.—Hypothermia was started from 3 hours 45 minutes (10 minutes-10 hours) and median lowest Pco_2 level within the first 6 hours of life was 30 mm Hg (16.5-96 mm Hg). The median highest fraction of inspiratory oxygen within the first hour of life was 0.43 (0.21-1.00). The area under the curve fraction of inspiratory oxygen and Pao_2 for hours 1-6 of life was 0.23 (0.21-1.0) and 86 mm Hg (22-197 mm Hg), respectively. We did not find any association between any measures of hypocapnia and adverse outcome ($P > .05$), but increased inspired oxygen correlated with adverse outcome, even when excluding newborns with initial oxygenation failure ($P < .05$).

Conclusion.—Increased fraction of inspired oxygen within the first 6 hours of life was significantly associated with adverse outcome in newborns treated with therapeutic hypothermia following hypoxic ischemic encephalopathy.

▶ The effect of hypothermia is dependent on oxygenation in the first hours of life. Hypothermia for newborn hypoxic ischemic encephalopathy (HIE) has become standard therapy.[1] Guidelines also state that "it is best to start resuscitation of term or near term newborns with air rather than 100% oxygen." However, is the hypothermia effect dependent on the initial oxygen concentration before cooling is initiated? This is a relevant question because animal studies have found that hyperoxic resuscitation induces inflammation in the brain.[2] Sabir et al[3] tried to answer this question in a clinical setting by comparing outcomes of babies in need of hypothermia related to the oxygen load the child experienced from 1 to 6 hours of life. This is, therefore, not a strict analysis of the effect of delivery room oxygen concentration on later outcome in cooled babies. Because random selection of term babies in need of resuscitation to cooling or not, or to air or 100% oxygen, is no longer possible, Sabir et al chose to use a retrospective approach to shed light on this question.

Our own approach has been to study (1) oxygen-glucose—deprived (OGD) human neurons (NT2-N) in culture exposed to different oxygen concentrations and temperatures and (2) newborn animals in need of resuscitation. In studies of neuronal cells in culture after OGD; 20-minute exposure to 1%, 21%, or 100%

oxygen; followed by 20.5 hours of hypothermia (33.0°C) or normothermia (37.0°C), the oxygen level did not affect cell viability.[4] Hypoxic newborn pigs randomly assigned to resuscitation with air or 100% oxygen were further randomly assigned to normothermia (rectal temperature, 35.0°C) or moderate hypothermia (rectal temperature, 29°C) for 6.5 hours. Histologic damage to the striatum was reduced by cooling only in animals resuscitated with 100% O_2.[5] Further, gene expression of DNA glycosylases Neil 1, Neil 3, and Oggi 1 were reduced by hypothermia, indicating reduced protection against oxidative DNA damage.[6]

To penetrate this question further, in collaboration with Marianne Thoresen and her group, hypoxia-ischemia was induced in newborn rats followed by 30 minutes of reoxygenation in either 21% or 100% oxygen before the animals were randomly assigned to 5 hours of normothermia (37°C) or hypothermia (32°C). Hippocampal injury was lowest for 21% + hypothermia followed by 21% + normothermia. When hypothermia followed resuscitation with 100% oxygen, the cooling effect was strongly reduced.[7] This study indicates that hyperoxia before cooling more or less blocked the hypothermia effect. This is in accordance with the findings of Sabir et al. In cooled babies with HIE, these authors found a significant association between the area of FiO_2 in the first 6 hours of life and adverse effects. They also found that high FiO_2 (>0.4) the first hour after birth also was associated with poor outcome. This may indicate that the effect of hypothermia reported in randomized studies and meta-analyses[8,9] underestimated the cooling effect.

It is unfortunate that Sabir et al's study is retrospective. It also uses a mixture of venous, capillary, and arterial blood gas results. The next step, if possible, should be to correlate FiO_2 levels confined to the delivery room only to outcomes of babies needing cooling. Such data might, however, be difficult to obtain.

O. D. Saugstad, MD, PhD

References

1. Perlman JM, Wyllie J, Kattwinkel J, et al; Neonatal Resuscitation Chapter Collaborators. Part 11: Neonatal resuscitation: 2010 International Consensus on Cardiopulmonary Resuscitation and Emergency Cardiovascular Care Science With Treatment Recommendations. *Circulation.* 2010;122:S516-S538.
2. Munkeby BH, Børke WB, Bjørnland K, et al. Resuscitation with 100% O2 increases cerebral injury in hypoxemic piglets. *Pediatr Res.* 2004;56:783-790.
3. Sabir H, Jary S, Tooley J, Liu X, Thoresen M. Increased inspired oxygen in the first hours of life is associated with adverse outcome in newborns treated for perinatal asphyxia with therapeutic hypothermia. *J Pediatr.* 2012;161:409-416.
4. Dalen ML, Frøyland E, Saugstad OD, Mollnes TE, Rootwelt T. Post-hypoxic hypothermia is protective in human NT2-N neurons regardless of oxygen concentration during reoxygenation. *Brain Res.* 2009;1259:80-89.
5. Dalen ML, Alme TN, Munkeby BH, et al. Early protective effect of hypothermia in newborn pigs after hyperoxic, but not after normoxic, reoxygenation. *J Perinat Med.* 2010;38:545-556.
6. Dalen ML, Alme TN, Bjørås M, Munkeby BH, Rootwelt T, Saugstad OD. Reduced expression of DNA glycosylases in post-hypoxic newborn pigs undergoing therapeutic hypothermia. *Brain Res.* 2010;1363:198-205.
7. Dalen ML, Liu X, Elstad M, et al. Resuscitation with 100% oxygen increases injury and counteracts the neuroprotective effect of therapeutic hypothermia in the neonatal rat. *Pediatr Res.* 2012;71:247-252.

8. Jacobs S, Hunt R, Tarnow-Mordi W, Inder T, Davis P. Cooling for newborns with hypoxic ischaemic encephalopathy. *Cochrane Database Syst Rev.* 2007;(4): CD003311.

9. Edwards AD, Brocklehurst P, Gunn AJ, et al. Neurological outcomes at 18 months of age after moderate hypothermia for perinatal hypoxic ischaemic encephalopathy: synthesis and meta-analysis of trial data. *BMJ.* 2010;340:c363.

Association of nucleated red blood cells and severity of encephalopathy in normothermic and hypothermic infants
Walsh BH, Boylan GB, Dempsey EM, et al (Cork Univ Maternity Hosp, Wilton, Ireland)
Acta Paediatr 102:e64-e67, 2013

Aim.—To determine whether hypothermia alters the discriminative ability of postnatal nucleated red blood cells (NRBCs) to distinguish between mild and moderate/severely encephalopathic infants.

Methods.—A prospective cohort study recruited full-term neonates with hypoxic ischaemic encephalopathy (HIE) from 2003 to 2012 (prehypothermic and hypothermic eras). The NRBC count was analysed in the first 24 h in all infants and compared between normothermic and hypothermic cohorts. The severity of encephalopathy was categorized using both clinical Sarnat score and continuous multichannel EEG.

Results.—Eighty-six infants with HIE were included: in the normothermic group, 19 were clinically mild, 24 moderate/severe; in the hypothermic group, 22 were mild, 21 moderate/severe encephalopathy. NRBC count discriminated between mild and moderate/severe Sarnat scores in the normothermic group ($p = 0.03$) but not in the hypothermic group ($p = 0.9$). This change was due to a decrease in NRBCs among moderately encephalopathic infants in the hypothermic cohort.

Conclusion.—Postnatal NRBCs distinguished between mild and moderate/severe encephalopathy in normothermic infants but not in infants undergoing therapeutic hypothermia. We advise caution when using postnatal blood samples to study diagnostic biomarkers for HIE without first analysing the potential impact of hypothermia upon these markers.

▶ Use of blood or serum biomarkers to determine the nature, timing, severity, or presence of hypoxic-ischemic brain injury in the perinatal period is both important and difficult. Interpretation of such measurements requires careful attention to their context, timing, evolution, and potential confounding conditions. The circulating nucleated red blood cell count is one of the oldest and most thoroughly studied potential biomarkers for perinatal asphyxial injury. Unfortunately, the older literature (and some more recent work) on this topic is confounded by the anachronistic tradition of reporting nucleated red blood cells (NRBC) counts in terms of NRBC/100 white blood cells rather than as NRBC per cubic millimeters or microliter of blood. That notwithstanding, there is evidence that significant episodes of acute intrapartum asphyxia are typically followed by an early but transient elevation of the NRBC count in the first 6 to 8 hours after the event to levels typically between 4000 and 10 000/μL, returning to normal (< 2000/μL) within 24 hours. Counts obtained too early (from cord blood, for example) or too late (on the second day) often miss this transient phenomenon. Elevation of NRBC counts to substantially higher levels or for longer intervals are more likely caused by prolonged intrauterine hypoxia (and old, established injury before labor or birth) or to other conditions, such as infection or maternal diabetes. This report emphasizes the necessity to recognize that novel therapies—in this case, neuroprotective hypothermia—may significantly alter the NRBC response to an asphyxial episode. Although infants with severe neonatal encephalopathy who met criteria for hypoxic-ischemic injury (arterial pH < 7.1 in the first hour; 5-min Apgar score, 6; initial capillary or arterial lactate > 7 mmol/L; or resuscitation at delivery requiring intubation) had higher NRBC counts in both the prehypothermia and hypothermia eras (median, 3594/μL; range, 2695—8498 and median, 7420/μL; range, 4855—11 108, respectively), NRBC counts in infants with moderate encephalopathy were elevated only for the prehypothermia cohort (median, 2992/μL; range, 885—5940 vs median, 620/μL; range, 196—1834 in the hypothermia era). Some infants with mild encephalopathy had modest elevations in both eras (median, 1800/μL; range, 850—3365 and median, 1810/μL; range, 882-3315, respectively). Although these results indicate that high NRBC counts may still be consistently associated with severe encephalopathy, this finding is no longer a reliable marker of moderate injury in the hypothermia era. Therefore, this marker cannot be used as a prognostic indicator (infants with normal NRBC counts may have moderate encephalopathy and be at risk for permanent sequelae) or to exclude a hypoxic-ischemic mechanism of injury unless there are clinical signs of severe encephalopathy. In addition, the authors draw the more general and correct conclusion that use of biomarkers to diagnose, stage, or time hypoxic-ischemic insults or to prognosticate about affected infants must be independently validated in populations of infants treated with this new therapy.

W. E. Benitz, MD

Hypothermia for Neonatal Hypoxic Ischemic Encephalopathy: An Updated Systematic Review and Meta-analysis
Tagin MA, Woolcott CG, Vincer MJ, et al (Univ of Toronto, Ontario, Canada; Dalhousie Univ, Halifax, Nova Scotia, Canada)
Arch Pediatr Adolesc Med 166:558-566, 2012

Objective.—To establish the evidence of therapeutic hypothermia for newborns with hypoxic ischemic encephalopathy (HIE).

Data Sources.—Cochrane Central Register of Controlled Trials, Oxford Database of Perinatal Trials, MEDLINE, EMBASE, and previous reviews.

Study Selection.—Randomized controlled trials that compared therapeutic hypothermia to normothermia for newborns with HIE.

Intervention.—Therapeutic hypothermia.

Main Outcome Measures.—Death or major neurodevelopmental disability at 18 months.

Results.—Seven trials including 1214 newborns were identified. Therapeutic hypothermia resulted in a reduction in the risk of death or major neurodevelopmental disability (risk ratio [RR], 0.76; 95% CI, 0.69-0.84) and increase in the rate of survival with normal neurological function (1.63; 1.36-1.95) at age 18 months. Hypothermia reduced the risk of death or major neurodevelopmental disability at age 18 months in newborns with moderate HIE (RR, 0.67; 95% CI, 0.56-0.81) and in newborns with severe HIE (0.83; 0.74-0.92). Both total body cooling and selective head cooling resulted in reduction in the risk of death or major neurodevelopmental disability (RR, 0.75; 95% CI, 0.66-0.85 and 0.77; 0.65-0.93, respectively).

Conclusion.—Hypothermia improves survival and neurodevelopment in newborns with moderate to severe HIE. Total body cooling and selective head cooling are effective methods in treating newborns with HIE. Clinicians should consider offering therapeutic hypothermia as part of routine clinical care to these newborns.

▶ This is an important article because the updated meta-analysis includes the 3 most recent large, randomized, controlled trials performed in Europe, China, and Australia. This increases the number of infants to approximately 1200 participants. This is the first analysis to document that hypothermia is protective for term neonates who present with either moderate or severe encephalopathy when cooling is initiated within 6 hours of birth. Also, this analysis demonstrates that both whole-body cooling and selective head cooling are protective against death and disability at 18 months of age. However, this report includes the 1998 pilot study by Gunn, which was a sequential allocation to 3 different target temperatures and not a randomized trial. The 1998 study was a safety study and outcome data abstracted from subsequent reports. The randomized, controlled trial of safety and efficacy performed by Eicher, a large pilot study, could have been included in spite of only having a 12-month outcome report.

This meta-analysis raises some discussion: The authors have considered the clinical evaluation of encephalopathy and the amplitude integrated electroencephalogram as equivalent. This is not clear from the literature; in fact, it could be argued that an abnormal amplitude-integrated electroencephalogram used as eligibility criteria in the randomized, controlled trials might select a subset of infants among those with either moderate or severe encephalopathy. Although identifying early predictors of nonresponders to hypothermia would be clinically very useful, currently none are available for use within the therapeutic window of 6 hours of age. Data from this meta-analysis and the recommendation of the American Heart Association[1] and the International Consensus on Cardiopulmonary Resuscitation[2] adds to the evidence that initiation of therapy with hypothermia (after the infant has been stabilized at birth and moderate or severe encephalopathy is diagnosed within this window) should be standard practice. The 2 recent publications[3,4] on childhood outcome after neonatal hypothermia therapy have established that hypothermia is beneficial with neuroprotective effects noted at 18 months of age that continue to childhood. Information on clinical,[5] cerebral functioning,[6,7] and imaging[8,9] biomarkers of hypothermia therapy are now available; thus, clinicians are better equipped to offer prognosis to families. Although hypothermia is effective and safe in high- and middle-resource countries, hypothermia as neuroprotection needs to be examined in the low-resource countries. Other questions that remain unanswered or unproven are: cooling initiated beyond 6 hours of age, cooling for infants < 36 weeks' gestation or cooling outside the published protocol, initiating cooling in the delivery room, cooling for < 72 hours, or at a target temperature outside the 33–34°C range.

S. Shankaran, MD

References

1. Kattwinkel J, Perlman JM, Aziz K, et al. Neonatal resuscitation: 2010 American Heart Association Guidelines for Cardiopulmonary Resuscitation and Emergency Cardiovascular Care. *Pediatrics.* 2010;126:e1400-e1413.
2. Perlman JM, Wyllie J, Kattwinkel J, et al. Neonatal resuscitation: 2010 International Consensus on Cardiopulmonary Resuscitation and Emergency Cardiovascular Care Science with Treatment Recommendations. *Pediatrics.* 2010;126: e1319-e1344.
3. Guillet R, Edwards AD, Thoresen M, et al; CoolCap Trial Group. Seven- to eight-year follow-up of the CoolCap trial of head cooling for neonatal encephalopathy. *Pediatr Res.* 2012;71:205-209.
4. Shankaran S, Pappas A, McDonald SA, et al; Eunice Kennedy Shriver NICHD Neonatal Research Network. Childhood outcomes after hypothermia for neonatal encephalopathy. *N Engl J Med.* 2012;366:2085-2092.
5. Shankaran S, Laptook AR, Tyson JE, et al; Eunice Kennedy Shriver National Institute of Child Health and Human Development Neonatal Research Network. Evolution of encephalopathy during whole body hypothermia for neonatal hypoxic-ischemic encephalopathy. *J Pediatr.* 2012;160:567-572.e3.
6. Thoresen M, Hellström-Westas L, Liu X, de Vries LS. Effect of hypothermia on amplitude-integrated electroencephalogram in infants with asphyxia. *Pediatrics.* 2010;126:e131-e139.
7. Shankaran S, Pappas A, McDonald SA, et al; Eunice Kennedy Shriver National Institute of Child Health and Human Development Neonatal Research Network. Predictive value of an early amplitude integrated electroencephalogram and neurologic examination. *Pediatrics.* 2011;128:e112-e120.
8. Rutherford M, Ramenghi LA, Edwards AD, et al. Assessment of brain tissue injury after moderate hypothermia in neonates with hypoxic-ischaemic encephalopathy: a nested substudy of a randomised controlled trial. *Lancet Neurol.* 2010;9:39-45.
9. Shankaran S, Barnes PD, Hintz SR, et al; MD for the Eunice Kennedy Shriver National Institute of Child Health and Human Development Neonatal Research Network. Brain injury following trial of hypothermia for neonatal hypoxic-ischemic encephalopathy. *Arch Dis Child.* 2012 Jul 17 [Epub ahead of print].

Passive cooling during transport of asphyxiated term newborns
O'Reilly D, Labrecque M, O'Melia M, et al (Boston Children's Hosp, MA)
J Perinatol 33:435-440, 2013

Objective.—To evaluate the efficacy and safety of passive cooling during transport of asphyxiated newborns.

Study Design.—Retrospective medical record review of newborns with perinatal asphyxia transported for hypothermia between July 2007 and June 2010.

Result.—Of 43 newborns transported, 27 were passively cooled without significant adverse events. Twenty (74%) passively cooled newborns arrived with temperature between 32.5 and 34.5°C. One newborn arrived with a temperature <32.5, and 6 (22%) had temperatures >34.5°C. Time from birth to hypothermia was significantly shorter among passively cooled newborns compared with newborns not cooled (215 vs 327 min, $P < 0.01$), even though time from birth to admission to Boston Children's Hospital was similar (252 vs 259 min, $P = 0.77$). Time from birth to admission was the only significant predictor of increased time to reach target temperature ($P = 0.001$).

Conclusion.—Exclusive passive cooling achieves significantly earlier initiation of effective hypothermia for asphyxiated newborns but should not delay transport for active cooling.

▶ One of the challenges facing centers offering therapeutic hypothermia for the treatment of neonatal hypoxic-ischemic encephalopathy (HIE) is how to assure that infants born at referring centers are appropriately cooled in a timely manner. Several studies have evaluated cooling during transport of infants with HIE, in most cases with both passive and active cooling procedures, and there has been one previous report of exclusive passive cooling in which 11% of affected infants were noted to have temperatures less than the target range upon arrival at the treating center.[1]

In the above observational study, the authors analyzed data from 2 distinct epochs after the initiation of a therapeutic hypothermia protocol at a single center. During the first epoch, infant temperature was maintained in the normo-thermic range until arrival at the center whereas during the second epoch, passive cooling was started as soon as the referral was received. Passive cooling consisted of removing all external heat sources at the referring center and placing the infant in an isolette without active heating during transport.

Passive cooling was initiated 74 (mean) minutes after birth, and target temperature was reached 128 (mean) minutes after passive cooling was started. Even though transport distances were short and the time from birth to admission was similar for the 2 cohorts, infants who were passively cooled reached target temperature at least an hour sooner.

It should be noted that the target therapeutic temperature range in the above study is wider than that in other published reports (32.50°C to 34.50°C vs 33.0°C to 34.0°C) and that the site at which temperatures were measured during transport was the axilla. A comparison of simultaneously recorded axillary and esophageal temperatures before and after the initiation of active cooling showed a mean difference (esophageal-axillary) of 0.30°C (range, 0.1°C to 0.60°C). A previously reported study of passive cooling for neonatal HIE reported that axillary temperatures were also in good agreement with rectal temperatures (mean difference, 0.10°C).[1]

Cumulative observational data suggest that the strategy of passive cooling in the field is feasible and safe, although a certain percentage of babies will inadvertently be overcooled or not reach the target temperature. A recent pilot study from the United Kingdom demonstrated the feasibility of using a servo-control device for cooling during neonatal transport.[2] However, until equipment for the precise measurement of core temperature and the delivery of hypothermia during transport becomes widely available and affordable, it behooves centers offering hypothermia for neonatal HIE to develop detailed protocols for initiating cooling at the referring hospital and during transport to assure that affected infants receive therapy as soon as possible.

L. A. Papile, MD

References

1. Kendall GS, Kapetanakis A, Ratnavel N, Azzopardi D, Robertson NJ; On behalf of the Cooling on Retrieval Study G. Passive cooling for initiation of therapeutic hypothermia in neonatal encephalopathy. *Arch Dis Child Fetal Neonatal Ed.* 2010;95:F408-F412.
2. Johnston ED, Becher J-C, Mitchell AP, Stenson BJ. Provision of servo-controlled cooling during neonatal transport. *Arch Dis Child Fetal Neonatal Ed.* 2012;97: F365-F367.

The assessment of bulging fontanel and splitting of sutures in premature infants: an interrater reliability study by the Hydrocephalus Clinical Research Network

Wellons JC 3rd, Hydrocephalus Clinical Research Network (Univ of Alabama, Birmingham)
J Neurosurg Pediatr 11:12-14, 2013

Object.—Previous studies from the Hydrocephalus Clinical Research Network (HCRN) have shown a great degree of variation in surgical decision making for infants with posthemorrhagic hydrocephalus, such as when to temporize, when to shunt, or when to convert. Since much of this clinical decision making is dictated by clinical signs of increased intracranial pressure (including bulging fontanel and splitting of sutures), the authors investigated whether there was variability in how these signs were being assessed by neurosurgeons. They wanted to answer the following question: is there acceptable interrater reliability in the neurosurgical assessment of bulging fontanel and split sutures?

Methods.—Explicit written definitions of "bulging fontanel" and "split sutures" were agreed upon with consensus across the HCRN. At 5 HCRN centers, pairs of neurosurgeons independently assessed premature infants in the first 3 months of life for the presence of a split suture and/or bulging fontanel, according to the a priori definitions. Interrater reliability was then calculated between pairs of observers using the Cohen simple kappa coefficient. Institutional board review approval was obtained at each center and at the University of Utah Data Coordinating Center.

Results.—A total of 38 infants were assessed by 13 different raters (10 faculty, 2 fellows, and 1 resident). The kappa for bulging fontanel was 0.65 (95% CI 0.41-0.90), and the kappa for split sutures was 0.84 (95% CI 0.66-1.0). No complications from the study were encountered.

Conclusions.—The authors have found a high degree of interrater reliability among neurosurgeons in their assessment of bulging fontanel and split sutures. While decision making may vary, the clinical assessment of this cohort appears to be consistent among these physicians, which is crucial for prospective studies moving forward.

▶ The Hydrocephalus Clinical Research Network (HCRN) is a collaboration of neurosurgeons at 7 pediatric hospitals in North America whose goal is to improve hydrocephalus treatment by conducting multicenter clinical trials. One of the proposed HCRN studies is the management of intraventricular hemorrhage (IVH) in preterm infants. In the process of designing an intervention trial for IVH, the HCRN has developed treatment rubrics for the clinical assessment of increased intracranial pressure in preterm infants, which includes measuring head circumference, assessing the presence of a bulging fontanel, and splitting of the cranial sutures. Although there are data regarding the reliability of measuring head circumference, no such published data exist for evaluating either a bulging fontanel or splitting of the sutures in preterm infants. The intent of this article was to gather these data. The kappa coefficient of 0.84 for split sutures does indicate a high degree of interrater reliability, but the kappa coefficient of 0.65 for bulging fontanel, although acceptable, suggests that it is a less reliable measure. However, because the time interval between the 2 independent assessments could be as long as 6 hours, the lower reliability of a bulging fontanel may reflect a change in the infant's clinical condition (eg, body position, degree of irritability) rather than a true variability in the assessment. Nonetheless, it appears that both measures would be useful in identifying eligible preterm infants for a randomized, clinical trial comparing the timing of various interventions for IVH.

L. A. Papile, MD

Neonatal White Matter Abnormalities an Important Predictor of Neurocognitive Outcome for Very Preterm Children

Woodward LJ, Clark CAC, Bora S, et al (Univ of Canterbury, Christchurch, New Zealand; Univ of Oregon, Eugene; et al)
PLoS One 7:e51879, 2012

Background.—Cerebral white matter abnormalities on term MRI are a strong predictor of motor disability in children born very preterm. However, their contribution to cognitive impairment is less certain.

Objective.—Examine relationships between the presence and severity of cerebral white matter abnormalities on neonatal MRI and a range of neurocognitive outcomes assessed at ages 4 and 6 years.

Design/Methods.—The study sample consisted of a regionally representative cohort of 104 very preterm (≤32 weeks gestation) infants born from

1998–2000 and a comparison group of 107 full-term infants. At term equivalent, all preterm infants underwent a structural MRI scan that was analyzed qualitatively for the presence and severity of cerebral white matter abnormalities, including cysts, signal abnormalities, loss of white matter volume, ventriculomegaly, and corpus callosal thinning/ myelination. At corrected ages 4 and 6 years, all children underwent a comprehensive neurodevelopmental assessment that included measures of general intellectual ability, language development, and executive functioning.

Results.—At 4 and 6 years, very preterm children without cerebral white matter abnormalities showed no apparent neurocognitive impairments relative to their full-term peers on any of the domain specific measures of intelligence, language, and executive functioning. In contrast, children born very preterm with mild and moderate-to-severe white matter abnormalities were characterized by performance impairments across all measures and time points, with more severe cerebral abnormalities being associated with increased risks of cognitive impairment. These associations persisted after adjustment for gender, neonatal medical risk factors, and family social risk.

Conclusions.—Findings highlight the importance of cerebral white matter connectivity for later intact cognitive functioning amongst children born very preterm. Preterm born children without cerebral white matter abnormalities on their term MRI appear to be spared many of the cognitive impairments commonly associated with preterm birth. Further follow-up will be important to assess whether this finding persists into the school years.

▶ Efforts to identify early perinatal markers of later neurodevelopmental risk among very preterm infants have included screening with neuroimaging, particularly magnetic resonance imaging (MRI), at term equivalent. The presence of cerebral white matter abnormalities (WMA) on MRI at term has been shown to be predictive of later neurodevelopmental impairment, particularly cerebral palsy.[1,2] In this report, the authors suggest that very preterm born children who did not have WMA on MRI at term can be expected to have similar levels of preschool and early-school-age cognitive functioning as their full-term peers.

MRI was done between 39 and 41 weeks corrected age. Each MRI was graded using a qualitative scoring system consisting of five 3-point scales assessing the presence and severity of periventricular white matter volume loss, white matter signal abnormality, the presence of cystic abnormalities, ventricular dilation, and thinning of the corpus callosum and reduction of myelination. Of the 104 very preterm infants included in the study, 82% had evidence of WMA, 76% of whom were classified as mild.

At 6 years of age, children in the no-WMA and mild-WMA cohorts had similar rates of severe delay in intellectual ability (9.1% vs 11.7%), language development (4.5% vs 5.1%), and executive function (18.2% vs 20%). No significant differences were found between full-term comparison children (N = 107) and very preterm born children with no WMA (N = 25) on any of the outcome measures assessed. However, the relative risk (RR) for any or severe delay was 1.2 to 1.7 and 1.6 to 3.2, respectively. Children with mild WMA (N = 60) had a higher risk of any delay (RR, 1.7—3.0), but the risk for severe delay was similar to that of the no-WMA cohort (1.8—3.6). Thus, although very preterm born children with no WMA had similar outcomes relative to their full-term peers in each of the domain-specific measures, when overall neurocognitive outcome is considered, very preterm born children did not perform as well as their full-term peers.

L. A. Papile, MD

References

1. Skiold B, Vollmer B, Bohm B, et al. Neonatal magnetic resonance imaging and outcome at 30 months in very preterm infants. *J Pediatr.* 2012;160:559-566.e1.
2. Spittle AJ, Cheong J, Doyle LW, et al. Neonatal white matter abnormality predicts childhood motor impairment in very preterm children. *Dev Med Child Neurol.* 2011;53:1000-1006.

Effects of Endotracheal Intubation and Surfactant on a 3-Channel Neonatal Electroencephalogram

Shangle CE, Haas RH, Vaida F, et al (Univ of California San Diego Med Ctr, La Jolla; Univ of California San Diego)
J Pediatr 161:252-257, 2012

Objective.—To evaluate the effects of surfactant administration on the neonatal brain using 3-channel neonatal electroencephalography (EEG).

Study Design.—A prospective cohort of 30 infants had scalp electrodes placed to record brain waves using 3-channel EEG (Fp1-O1, C3-C4, and Fp2-O2). Sixty-second EEG epochs were collected from a 10-minute medication-free baseline, during premedication for endotracheal intubation, at surfactant administration, and at 10, 20, and 30 minutes after surfactant administration for amplitude comparisons. Oxygen saturation and heart rate were monitored continuously. Blood pressure and transcutaneous carbon dioxide were recorded every 5 minutes.

Results.—Eighteen of 29 infants (62%) exhibited brain wave suppression on EEG after surfactant administration ($P \leq .008$). Four of those 18 infants did not receive premedication. Nine infants exhibited evidence of EEG suppression during endotracheal intubation, all of whom received premedication before intubation. Five infants had EEG suppression during endotracheal suctioning. Oxygen saturation, heart rate, and blood pressure were not independent predictors of brain wave suppression.

Conclusion.—Eighteen of 29 intubated infants (62%) had evidence of brain wave suppression on raw EEG after surfactant administration. Nine patients had evidence of brief EEG suppression with endotracheal intubation alone, a finding not previously reported in neonates. Intubation and surfactant administration have the potential to alter cerebral function in neonates.

▶ Life in the neonatal intensive care unit (NICU) in no way resembles intra-uterine life, and no one knows this better than our tiny patients who must endure the light, noise, and tactile and painful stimuli associated with NICU care. Studies of the effects of NICU environmental stimuli on neurodevelopment have raised awareness of the potential long-term neurodevelopmental hazards of preterm birth, other neonatal conditions, and NICU environmental stimuli among the most fragile humans on the planet. However, we largely ignore the potential neurologic downsides of life-saving interventions such as intubation and surfactant administration. Shangle et al provide a wake-up call in the form of a study of amplitude-integrated electroencephalographic (aEEG) patterns among term and preterm infants undergoing NICU procedures. They found that laryngoscope insertion, intubation, and surfactant administration each were associated with significant suppression of aEEG activity. These effects were observed in both term and preterm infants. Interestingly, the common vital sign parameters we often use to assess physiologic well-being (ie, heart rate, blood pressure, and oxygen saturation) were not independent predictors of brain wave suppression. Further studies are needed to establish the long-term implications of these findings. These observations, however, might open the door to continuous brain monitoring by aEEG or near-infrared spectroscopy and real-time assessment of brain effects of physiologic states, such as hypogly-cemia and a host of delivery room and NICU interventions, including resuscita-tion, administration of inotropes, analgesics, sedatives, and other medications.

L. J. Van Marter, MD, MPH

Neonatal stroke
Rutherford MA, Ramenghi LA, Cowan FM (Hammersmith Hosp, London, UK; Fondazione Policlinico IRCCS Ospedale Cá Granda Neonatal Unit and NICU, Milan, Italy; Hammersmith/St Mary's Comprehensive Biomed Res Centre, London, UK)
Arch Dis Child Fetal Neonatal Ed 97:F377-F384, 2012

Neonatal stroke encompasses a range of focal and multifocal ischaemic and haemorrhagic tissue injuries. This review will concentrate on focal brain injury that occurs as a consequence of arterial infarction, most frequently the left middle cerebral artery, or more rarely as a consequence of cerebral sinus venous thrombosis (CSVT). Both conditions are multifac-torial in origin. The incidence of both acquired and genetic thrombophilic disorders in both mothers and infants is high although rarely causal in isolation. Neurodevelopmental morbidity occurs in over 50% of chil-dren. Specific therapy in the form of anticoagulation is currently only recommended in CSVT and needs to be carefully monitored in the presence of haemorrhage.

▶ In childhood, the incidence of stroke is highest in the neonatal period. Neuroimaging data have provided important insights about the broad range of cerebrovascular pathology (arterial and venous, ischemic and/or hemorrhagic) in preterm and term neonates. The authors of this review cite incidences of 1 in 2300-4000 deliveries for perinatal arterial ischemic stroke (AIS), and 1—2.69/ 100 000 newborns for cerebral sinus venous thrombosis (CSVT), and comment that these values may be underestimates.

This review highlights evidence of prothrombotic risk factors (maternal and infant) in published series and, equally important, that subsequent stroke risk beyond the neonatal period is very low. The authors emphasize that it is the combination of maternal and neonatal clinical factors that predominates over individual prothrombotic variants with respect to perinatal stroke risk. Thus, it is somewhat surprising that they recommend early testing for protein-based assays of coagulation function; they do not provide a strong rationale for this advice or explicitly address the clinical utility of thrombophilia testing (in terms of acute management of neonatal stroke). The authors justifiably recommend "placental assessment," but they do not address the practical challenges inherent in implementing this recommendation (given that the diagnosis of neonatal stroke is often established several days postpartum).

The illustrative magnetic resonance (MR) imaging represents a significant strength of this review and the figures provide an excellent teaching tool. The authors' recommendations for neurodiagnostic imaging reflect their own experience and practice in a highly specialized neonatal unit. They recommend inclusion of MR angiography in all cases; however, the likelihood that this study will provide incremental data that inform clinical management in most settings is very low.

One of the most challenging issues in the management of neonatal stroke is the role of anticoagulation. Available evidence to support implementation of antithrombotic therapy in neonates with AIS and CSVT is weak. The authors cite American College of Chest Physician treatment guidelines as the basis for their recommendation to use heparin to treat AIS in neonates with an identified cardioembolic source; the wording of the current guidelines,[1] published after this article, are more circumspect and suggest treatment with heparin (unfractionated [UFH] or low molecular weight [LMWH]), based on Grade 2C evidence. These guidelines include the same suggestion for treatment of neonates with CSVT without significant intracranial hemorrhage: "…anticoagulation, initially with UFH or LMWH and subsequently with LMWH, for a total therapy duration between 6 weeks and 3 months rather than shorter or longer treatment duration (Grade 2C)."

In the final sentence of this review, the authors speculate that acceptance of hypothermia as standard of care for neonatal hypoxic ischemic encephalopathy will prompt trials of cooling in neonatal AIS. Given the heterogeneity of mechanisms and severity of neonatal stroke, and the broad range of outcomes, summarized well by the authors, clinical trials to improve neurodevelopmental outcome will be very challenging to implement in this population. Because the diagnosis of neonatal stroke is often delayed for several days, it is unlikely that implementation of therapeutic hypothermia will be feasible within a pathophysiologically relevant time window. Treatments that promote neural repair and/or neuroplasticity could ultimately benefit affected infants.

F. S. Silverstein, MD

Reference

1. Monagle P, Chan AK, Goldenberg NA, et al. American College of Chest Physicians. Antithrombotic therapy in neonates and children: Antithrombotic Therapy and Prevention of Thrombosis, 9th ed: American College of Chest Physicians Evidence-Based Clinical Practice Guidelines. *Chest.* 2012;141:e737S-e801S.

Findings of perinatal ocular examination performed on 3573, healthy full-term newborns
Li L-H, Li N, Zhao J-Y, et al (Maternal and Children's Hosp, Kunming, Yunnan, China; Capital Univ of Med Sciences, Beijing, China; et al)
Br J Ophthalmol 97:588-591, 2013

Objective.—To document the findings of a newborn eye examination programme for detecting ocular pathology in the healthy full-term newborn.

Methods.—This is a cross-sectional study of the majority of newborns born in the Kunming Maternal and Child Healthcare Hospital, China, between May 2010 and June 2011. Infants underwent ocular examination within 42 days after birth using a flashlight, retinoscope, handheld slit lamp microscope and wide-angle digital retinal image acquisition system. The retinal fundus examination utilised the RetCam wide-field digital imaging system (Clarity Medical Systems, Pleasanton, California, USA). The external eye, pupillary light reflex, red reflex, opacity of refractive media, anterior chamber and posterior segments were also examined.

Results.—A total of 3573 healthy full-term newborns were enrolled and examined in the programme. There was detection of 871 abnormal cases (24.4%). The majority of abnormal exams were 769 (21.52%) retinal haemorrhages. Of these, there were 215 cases of significant retinal haemorrhage, possible sight threatening or amblyogenic, representing 6.02% of the total. In addition, 67 cases (1.88%) involved macular haemorrhage. The other 107 cases (2.99%) with abnormal ocular findings included subconjunctival haemorrhage, congenital microphthalmos, congenital corneal leukoma, posterior synechia, persistent pupillary membrane, congenital cataract, enlarged C/D ratio, retinal hamartoma versus retinoblastoma, optic nerve defects, macular pigment disorder and non-specific peripheral retinopathy.

Conclusion.—Ocular examination of healthy newborns leads to the detection of a significant number of ocular pathologies. The most commonly discovered ocular abnormality during examination of the newborns in this study is retinal haemorrhage. The long-term impact of these

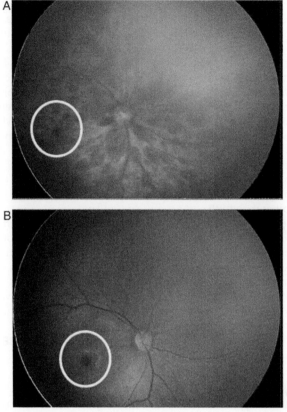

FIGURE 2.—(A) Above: oculus dexter (OD) with Grade 3 retinal and macular haemorrhage; (B) Bottom: Review after 3 weeks shows persistent macular haemorrhage OD; retinal haemorrhage OS completely absorbed. (Reprinted from Li L-H, Li N, Zhao J-Y, et al. Findings of perinatal ocular examination performed on 3573, healthy full-term newborns. *Br J Ophthalmol*. 2013;97:588-591, with permission from the BMJ Publishing Group Ltd.)

findings is unknown. Although presumed by some to benign, neonatal retinal haemorrhages due to birth trauma could be involved in altering visual development. Further work, including prospective examination of newborns with long-term follow-up, is needed and supported by our findings (Fig 2).

▶ Traditionally the initial eye examination has focused on ruling out conjunctivitis, glaucoma, and cataracts together with establishing the presence of red reflex. This article from China highlights the pathology that can be found with detailed examination of the eye in a large population. The RetCam, used in this study, not only facilitates examination of the retina but provides a permanent record of the examination, permitting verification of the pathology. As would be anticipated, retinal hemorrhage (RH) was the most common finding. Li et al do not know the long-term outcome of these infants with RH, particularly in the 2% with macula involvement. They also point out that it is impractical and not cost effective to perform this depth of screening on all eyes. But it was revealing to observe how much ocular pathology was detected in these healthy newborns.

Emerson et al[1] in 2001, using indirect ophthalmoscopy, studied 149 newborns to determine the prevalence, associated biometric factors, and rate of disappearance of neonatal RH. Newborns with RH (34%) were reexamined biweekly until hemorrhage resolved. The hemorrhage varied from a single dot hemorrhage in one eye to bilateral widespread hemorrhages, occasionally with white centers. Hemorrhage was more frequent after vacuum-assisted (75%) than for spontaneous vaginal deliveries (33%) and was least frequent for infants delivered by cesarean section (7%). By 2 weeks after birth, RH resolved in 86% of eyes, and at 4 weeks no intraretinal hemorrhage was present. They noted that RH in infants older than 1 month should heighten suspicion that the hemorrhage is associated with factors other than birth.

Some 12 years later, Watts et al[2] scoured the medical literature and databases and reported on 13 studies representing 1777 infants. The studies found that 1 in 4 newborns born via spontaneous vaginal deliveries had RH. In contrast, infants delivered by vacuum extraction had a 43% rate of RH, and infants delivered by double-instrument deliveries (forceps and vacuum) had a 52% rate of RH. Most RH (83%) resolved by 10 days, and few persisted beyond 6 weeks.

Awareness of RH after vacuum and forceps delivery should induce more detailed eye examinations in these infants.

A. A. Fanaroff, MBBCh, FRCPE

References

1. Emerson MV, Pieramici DJ, Stoessel KM, Berreen JP, Gariano RF. Incidence and rate of disappearance of retinal hemorrhage in newborns. *Ophthalmology.* 2001;108:36-39.
2. Watts P, Maguire S, Kwok T, et al. Newborn retinal hemorrhages: a systematic review. *J AAPOS.* 2013;17:70-78.

The relationship between patterns of intermittent hypoxia and retinopathy of prematurity in preterm infants
Di Fiore JM, Kaffashi F, Loparo K, et al (Case Western Reserve Univ, Cleveland, OH)
Pediatr Res 72:606-612, 2012

Background.—We have previously shown an increased incidence of intermittent hypoxemia (IH) events in preterm infants with severe retinopathy of prematurity (ROP). Animal models suggest that patterns of IH events may play a role in ROP severity as well. We hypothesize that specific IH event patterns are associated with ROP in preterm infants.

Methods.—Variability in IH event duration, severity, and the time interval between IH events ($\leq 80\%$ ≥ 10 s, and ≤ 3 min) along with the

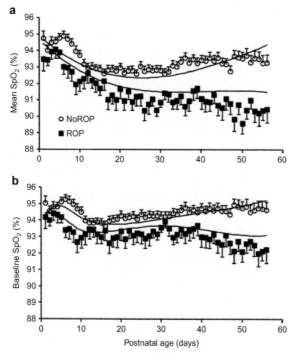

FIGURE 1.—Mean and baseline SpO_2 in infants with and without severe ROP. Both (a) mean SpO_2 and (b) baseline SpO_2, excluding IH events, were significantly lower in the severe ROP group ($P < 0.05$ and $P < 0.01$, respectively). Open circles, no or mild ROP; filled squares, severe ROP; solid line, covariate-adjusted models. Mean ± SEM. IH, intermittent hypoxemia; ROP, retinopathy of prematurity; SpO_2, oxygen saturation. (Reprinted from Di Fiore JM, Kaffashi F, Loparo K, et al. The relationship between patterns of intermittent hypoxia and retinopathy of prematurity in preterm infants. *Pediatr Res.* 2012;72:606-612, with permission from International Pediatric Research Foundation, Inc.)

frequency spectrum of the oxygen saturation (SpO_2) waveform were assessed.

Results.—Severe ROP was associated with (i) an increased mean and SD of the duration of IH event ($P < 0.005$), (ii) more variability (histogram entropy) of the time interval between IH events ($P < 0.005$), (iii) a higher IH nadir ($P < 0.05$), (iv) a time interval between IH events of 1–20 min ($P < 0.05$), and (v) increased spectral power in the range of 0.002–0.008 Hz ($P < 0.05$), corresponding to SpO_2 waveform oscillations of 2–8 min in duration. Spectral differences were detected as early as 14 d of life.

Conclusion.—Severe ROP was associated with more variable, longer, and less severe IH events. Identification of specific spectral components in the SpO_2 waveform may assist in early identification of infants at risk for severe ROP (Fig 1).

▶ The pivotal role of excessive oxygen in the pathogenesis of retinopathy of prematurity was established decades ago, but the optimal goals for oxygen therapy in preterm infants remain a subject of uncertainty and, too often, controversy. The SUPPORT trial showed that a lower oxygen saturation (SpO_2) target range (85% to 89%, rather than 91% to 95%) in infants born at less than 28 weeks of gestation, from the day of birth to 36 weeks postmenstrual age or weaning to room air, was associated with a lower rate of severe retinopathy of prematurity (ROP) but increased mortality. This elegant analysis of pulse oximetry data from a similar population of infants, comparing those who required laser therapy for severe ROP with those who had no or mild ROP, suggests a more complex relationship. First, infants with severe ROP had lower, rather than higher, mean and baseline SpO_2 levels, particularly after the second postnatal week (Fig). Second, severe ROP was associated with measures of increased variability and duration (but reduced severity) of intermittent hypoxemia episodes. In particular, severe ROP correlated with more numerous hypoxemia events 1 to 20 minutes in duration and with increased spectral power corresponding to oximetry oscillations 2 to 8 minutes in duration, both beginning at about 14 days of age. A related publication describes an increase in hypoxemic events in SUPPORT trial subjects assigned to the lower SpO_2 target range, but those differences were related to events less than 1 minute in duration and were evident only at less than 12 or greater than 57 days of age.[1] It is not clear how to reconcile these seemingly disparate observations. One possible explanation may lie in the hypothesis that the role of oxygen in retinal vasculogenesis is biphasic, with early hyperoxemia inducing vasoconstriction, retinal hypoxemia, and increased vascular endothelial growth factor (VEGF) production in the avascular retina, whereas later hypoxemia (or variability in oxygen levels) in the vascularizing retina prolongs or augments VEGF production and vasoproliferative disease. That hypothesis would lead to an expectation that severe ROP might be minimized by initial relative oxygen restriction followed by slightly higher SpO_2 targets later. Assuming that the relationships described in this report are causal and not merely correlative, they also suggest that measures to reduce periodic variability in SpO_2 between 2 and 6 weeks after birth will be beneficial. The analysis from the SUPPORT subjects[1] suggests that simply adjusting inspired oxygen supplementation to higher SpO_2 targets will not achieve that goal, implying that other strategies will have to be developed. Further application of the tools of signal analysis, as shown here, promises to identify patterns of oximetry measurements that correlate with, predict, and ultimately guide development of measures to prevent severe ROP.

W. E. Benitz, MD

Reference

1. Di Fiore JM, Walsh M, Wrage L, et al. Low oxygen saturation target range is associated with increased incidence of intermittent hypoxemia. *J Pediatr.* 2012;161:1047-1052.

Mechanisms and Management of Retinopathy of Prematurity

Hartnett ME, Penn JS (Univ of Utah, Salt Lake City; Vanderbilt Univ School of Medicine, Nashville, TN)
N Engl J Med 367:2515-2526, 2013

Background.—Along with the increased incidence of premature births worldwide is an increased incidence of retinopathy of prematurity in countries with the technology to save preterm infants. Retinopathy of prematurity is now a leading cause of childhood blindness. Its management is evolving, as is the understanding of its pathogenesis.

Pathogenesis.—Through clinical evaluation and research using relevant animal models, specifically the mouse and the rat, retinopathy of prematurity is now characterized as having two phases: phase 1, delayed physiologic retinal vascular development, and phase 2, vasoproliferation. Models of oxygen-induced retinopathy have revealed signaling pathways involved in the pathogenesis of these two phases. Pathways affected by oxygen stresses in cell culture and oxygen-induced retinopathy include those that involve hypoxia, oxidative signaling, inflammation, and poor postnatal growth or extrauterine growth restriction. These pathways interact and overlap, affecting angiogenesis and the occurrence of oxygen-induced retinopathy. Retinal hypoxia leads to stabilization and translocation of hypoxia-inducible factors (HIFs), resulting in the transcription of angiogenic genes, including those encoding vascular endothelial growth factor (VEGF), cyclooxygenase, erythropoietin, and angiopoietin 2. VEGF signaling can disorder endothelial cells and contribute to the tortuosity and dilation of retinal vessels. The endothelial cells then proliferate outside the retinal plane into the vitreous. Inhibiting VEGF may reorient the endothelial cells and aid physiologic retinal vascular development, but using the optimal dose is critical. The Janus-associated kinase-n-signal transducers and activators of transcription (JAK-STAT) signaling pathway reduces physiologic retinal vascular development, which improves vascularization, possibly positively affecting both phase 1 and phase 2 disease. Insulin-like growth factor 1 (IGF-1) is especially important in fetal growth during the third trimester, with premature infants having insufficient production of IGF-1. Extrauterine growth restriction is associated with a higher risk of severe retinopathy of prematurity, so IGF-1 administered to infants may have a role in reducing disease severity. Various other substances may also affect the development of retinopathy.

Clinical Implications.—Although oxidative stress is associated with retinopathy of prematurity, clinical trials indicate no clear support for the use of antioxidants or document unacceptable side effects. Very-low-birth-weight infants are at high risk for both retinopathy of prematurity and neurodevelopmental impairment, so erythropoietin has been proposed as a neuroprotective agent. The best time to administer erythropoietin to preterm infants remains to be seen. Anti-VEGF agents also have shown serious side effects; further studies are needed to determine drug dose and timing, type of agent to be used, and safety. The weight, IGF, neonatal retinopathy of prematurity (WINROP) algorithm is used to assess individual risk for severe retinopathy of prematurity. A simplified version is used to study poor postnatal weight gain as an indicator of high risk for severe retinopathy of prematurity. However, its sensitivity varies with different populations, so its usefulness needs to be explored further.

Conclusions.—Oxygen stress may lead to the development of retinopathy of prematurity through various signaling pathways. Treatment currently includes laser therapy and visual rehabilitation. Further study may add to this arsenal of weapons.

▶ The preservation of normal vision is a vitally important advantage to surviving premature infants in their quest for optimal development and quality of life. As the authors of this excellent review article make clear, we are in a phase of rapid evolution in the science of retinopathy of prematurity (RoP), both in the understanding of mechanisms of disease and pursuit of potential preventive therapies. Drs Hartnett and Penn provide a superb summary of the pathogenesis and laboratory models of RoP, describing signaling pathways involved in oxygen-induced retinopathy, the role of retinal hypoxia in pathogenesis, and potential role of insulinlike growth factor (IGF)-1 in protecting the developing retina. All of the major clinical trials to date are presented, and implications of current proposed or actual therapies, including antioxidants, erythropoietin, anti−vascular endothelial growth factor agents, and the WINROP (weight, IGF, neonatal RoP) are discussed.

L. J. Van Marter, MD, MPH

Children With Sensorineural Hearing Loss After Passing the Newborn Hearing Screen
Dedhia K, Kitsko D, Sabo D, et al (Univ of Pittsburgh Med Ctr (UPMC), PA; Children's Hosp of Pittsburgh of UPMC, PA)
JAMA Otolaryngol Head Neck Surg 139:119-123, 2013

Objectives.—To identify and describe the findings of children who passed their newborn hearing screen (NHS) and were subsequently found to have childhood hearing loss.

Setting.—Academic tertiary care center.

Design.—Retrospective medical chart review.

Methods.—With approval of the institutional review board, hospital records were reviewed for children diagnosed as having hearing loss. We identified 923 children with hearing loss from 2001 to 2011. Patients who passed the NHS with subsequent hearing loss were included.

Results.—Seventy-eight patients were included in our study. The suspicion of hearing loss in patients who passed the NHS was most often from parental concerns (n = 28 [36%]) and failed school hearing screens (n = 25 [32%]). Speech and language delay and failed primary care physician screens accounted for 17% and 12%, respectively. Configuration of the audiogram was bilateral symmetric (n = 42 [54%]), bilateral asymmetric (n = 16 [21%]), and unilateral (n = 20 [26%]) loss. Thirty-seven patients (47%) had severe or profound hearing loss. The etiology was unknown in 42 patients (54%); the remaining was attributed to genetics (n = 13 [17%]), anatomic abnormality (n = 11 [14%]), acquired perinatal (n = 9 [12%]), and auditory neuropathy (n = 3 [4%]).

Conclusions.—This is the largest study to characterize children with hearing loss who passed the NHS. In our review, parental concerns and school hearing screens were the most common method to diagnose hearing loss after passing the NHS. Families and primary care physicians may have a false sense of security when patients pass the NHS and overlook symptoms of hearing loss. This study raises the question whether further screens would identify hearing loss in children after passing the NHS.

▶ With the integration of universal newborn hearing screening (UNHS) into routine newborn care there has been a dramatic improvement of early identification of children with hearing loss, resulting in timely intervention and subsequent improvement in speech and language and cognitive development. However, as the above report points out, passing a newborn hearing screening test does not assure that a child will not have a severe or profound hearing loss. Among the 314 pediatric patients with hearing loss who had undergone UNHS, the authors noted that 25% had passed the screening test, as reported by the parent. One-third had a profound hearing loss and an additional 13% had a severe hearing loss. The mean age at diagnosis for profound and severe hearing loss was similar (4 years, 7 months).

The study highlights the importance of recognizing the possibility that children who pass the UNHS may have hearing loss. Although the American Academy of Pediatrics recommendations for preventive pediatric health care include hearing assessment at every well child visit,[1] only 15% of the children were referred for otolaryngology consultation by their primary care physician because of a failed hearing assessment. As the authors speculate, primary care physicians may be less diligent in identifying hearing loss when a young child has passed a newborn screening test.

L. A. Papile, MD

Reference

1. American Academy of Pediatrics. Recommendations for preventive pediatric health care. *Pediatrics.* 2000;105:645.

9 Behavior and Pain

A Randomized Placebo-Controlled Trial of Massage Therapy on the Immune System of Preterm Infants
Ang JY, Lua JL, Mathur A, et al (Children's Hosp of Michigan, Detroit; Wayne State Univ School of Medicine, Detroit, MI; et al)
Pediatrics 130:e1549-e1558, 2012

Objectives.—The aim of this study was to investigate the effects of massage therapy (MT) on the immune system of preterm infants. The primary hypothesis was that MT compared with sham therapy (control) will enhance the immune system of stable premature infants by increasing the proportion of their natural killer (NK) cell numbers.

Methods.—A randomized placebo-controlled trial of MT versus sham therapy (control) was conducted among stable premature infants in the NICU. Study intervention was provided 5 days per week until hospital discharge for a maximum of 4 weeks. Immunologic evaluations (absolute NK cells, T and B cells, T cell subsets, and NK cytotoxicity), weight, number of infections, and length of hospital stay were also evaluated.

Results.—The study enrolled 120 infants (58 massage; 62 control). At the end of the study, absolute NK cells were not different between the 2 groups; however, NK cytotoxicity was higher in the massage group, particularly among those who received ≥ 5 consecutive days of study intervention compared with control (13.79 vs 10 lytic units, respectively; $P = .04$). Infants in the massage group were heavier at end of study and had greater daily weight gain compared with those in the control group; other immunologic parameters, number of infections, and length of stay were not different between the 2 groups.

Conclusions.—In this study, MT administered to stable preterm infants was associated with higher NK cytotoxicity and more daily weight gain. MT may improve the overall outcome of these infants. Larger studies are needed.

▶ It is human nature to enjoy being comforted with tactile stimulation and stroking. Massage is listed among the nonpharmacologic approaches to relief of pain and discomfort in neonates. Massage is itself a huge industry; however, this is not the case regarding preterm infants, as Field et al[1] reported that preterm infant massage is only practiced in less than 40% of neonatal intensive care units. Moderate-pressure massage therapy has led to enhanced weight gain in preterm infants. This ultimately results in shorter hospital stays, which translates into significant hospital cost savings. The massage may be enhanced with the use

143

of oils, including coconut oil and safflower oil, which may increase vagal activity. The increases noted in vagal activity, gastric motility, and insulin and insulin-like growth factor—1 levels after moderate-pressure massage are potential underlying mechanisms of the increased weight gain. Furthermore, passive movement of the limbs in preterm infants results in both gained weight and an increase in bone density. Haley et al[2] reported that tactile kinesthetic stimulation improves bone strength in premature infants by attenuating the decrease that normally follows preterm birth. They observed that biomarkers of bone metabolism showed a modification in bone turnover in tactile/kinesthetic stimulation (TKS) infants in favor of bone accretion. Their interpretation was that TKS improves bone mineralization.

Rudnicki et al[3] in Poland observed that the amplitude of the amplitude-integrated electroencephalography trend during massage significantly increased. Massage also impacted the dominant frequency delta waves. Frequency significantly increased during the massage and returned to baseline after treatment. Oxygen saturation significantly decreased during massage. In 4 premature infants, massage was discontinued because of desaturation less than 85%. Pulse frequency during the massage decreased but remained within physiologic limits of greater than 100 beats per minute in all infants. Doppler flow values in the anterior cerebral artery measured before and after massage did not show statistically significant changes.

Ang et al confirm the weight gain benefit of systematic massage and also show enhanced natural killer (NK) cell function, implying a more robust immune mechanism accompanying the massage. Fewer NK cells showed more killing ability after massage.

These data suggest that massage is good for babies. One can anticipate better weight gain, stronger bones, and an enhanced immune system in addition to positive behavioral responses. The correct techniques are needed and pulse oximetry should be monitored.

A. A. Fanaroff, MBBCh, FRCPE

References

1. Field T, Diego M, Hernandez-Reif M. Preterm infant massage therapy research: a review. *Infant Behav Dev.* 2010;33:115-124.
2. Haley S, Beachy J, Ivaska KK, Slater H, Smith S, Moyer-Mileur LJ. Tactile/kinesthetic stimulation (TKS) increases tibial speed of sound and urinary osteocalcin (U-MidOC and unOC) in premature infants (29-32 weeks PMA). *Bone.* 2012; 51:661-666.
3. Rudnicki J, Boberski M, Butrymowicz E, et al. Recording of amplitude-integrated electroencephalography, oxygen saturation, pulse rate, and cerebral blood flow during massage of premature infants. *Am J Perinatol.* 2012;29:561-566.

NIDCAP: A Systematic Review and Meta-analyses of Randomized Controlled Trials

Ohlsson A, Jacobs SE (Univ of Toronto, Ontario, Canada; Royal Women's Hosp, Melbourne, Victoria, Australia)
Pediatrics 131:e881-e893, 2013

Background and Objective.—The "synactive" theory of neurobehavioral development forms the basis of the Newborn Individualized Developmental Care and Assessment Program (NIDCAP). Our objective was to assess the effectiveness of NIDCAP in improving outcomes in preterm infants.

Methods.—Medline, CINAHL, Embase, PsychInfo, The Cochrane Library, Pediatric Academic Societies' Abstracts and Web of Science were searched in July 2010 and February 2012. The studies selected were randomized controlled trials testing the effectiveness of NIDCAP on medical and neurodevelopmental outcomes. The authors abstracted baseline characteristics of infants and outcomes. The risk of bias was assessed by using Cochrane criteria. RevMan 5.1 was used to synthesize data by the use of relative risk and risk difference for dichotomous outcomes and mean or standardized mean difference for continuous outcomes.

Results.—Eleven primary and 7 secondary studies enrolling 627 neonates were included, with 2 of high quality. The composite primary outcomes of death or major sensorineural disability at 18 months corrected age or later in childhood (3 trials, 302 children; relative risk 0.89 [95% confidence interval 0.61 to 1.29]) and survival free of disability at 18 months corrected age or later in childhood (2 trials, 192 infants; relative risk 0.97 [95% confidence interval 0.69 to 1.35]), were not significantly different between the NIDCAP and control groups. With the sensitivity analysis that excluded the 2 statistically heterogeneous outlying studies, there were no significant differences between groups for short-term medical outcomes.

Conclusions.—This systematic review including 627 preterm infants did not find any evidence that NIDCAP improves long-term neurodevelopmental or short-term medical outcomes.

▶ Some 30 years ago, Als conceptualized the synactive theory of child development and established the Newborn Individualized Developmental Care and Assessment Program (NIDCAP).[1,2] This program requires trained caregivers to observe neonatal behaviors before, during, and after caregiving interventions and provide recommendations for care by staff and parents. Over time, these assessments and care protocols include reductions in noise and light levels, clustering of care, aids to promote flexion and self-regulation, and, of course, parental involvement. There have been strong proponents of the concept and vocal opponents who seek the rigid statistical criteria documenting the short- and long-term benefits of NIDCAP.

Symington and Pinelli's[3] Cochrane review regarding NIDCAP in 2006 concluded that the evidence to support NIDCAP as a framework within which to provide developmental care to improve medical and developmental outcomes is inconclusive. In 2009, Ohlsson[4] speculated that the results of the trials of Maguire et al[5] and Peters et al[6] would help clarify the issue. However, Maguire et al concluded that NIDCAP was ineffective for outcomes to term, whereas Peters et al came to the opposite conclusion, reporting that NIDCAP significantly improves short-term and long-term outcomes. Ohlsson went on to note that because both studies were small, differences in results could be a result of chance or baseline characteristics that favored the NIDCAP group in the Peters et al study. Also, because the intervention cannot possibly be masked, this too could be a source of bias. Indeed, trials that are not double blinded yield larger effect estimates. Ohlsson recommended that "before additional research of NIDCAP is initiated, consideration should be given to reports that many NIDCAP behaviors are rarely or never seen among preterm infants, that only a few are associated with stressful/painful interventions, and that clustering of care can result in important behavioral and autonomic reactions. Any innovative, developmentally sensitive intervention should start at birth in the resuscitation room, where neonates are exposed to excessive noise and light levels and painful/stressful stimuli to body parts (mouth, nose, throat, larynx, and hands) represented by large areas in the sensory cortex."

As noted above, Ohlsson and Jacobs have gone through the literature with a fine-tooth comb and also contacted the authors of published studies for clarification to answer the following questions: (1) Does NIDCAP compared with standard care improve neurodevelopmental and medical outcomes in preterm infants? (2) Should NIDCAP become the standard of care in the NICU? What is the evidence? This systematic review and meta-analyses show that the answer to both questions is "no." This does not mean that we should not be sensitive to the needs and aware of the cues from the babies, but the rigidly applied NIDCAP protocols have not shown benefits. It is disappointing given the long history of this intervention that so few subjects had been included in trials. Much can be done to make the environment for the babies in the intensive care units more pleasant and to reduce the pain and stress.

A. A. Fanaroff, MBBCh, FRCPE

References

1. Als H. Towards a synactive theory of development: promise for the assessment of infant individuality. *Infant Ment Health J.* 1982;3:229-243.
2. Als H. A synactive model of neonatal behavioral organization: framework for the assessment of neurobehavioral development in the premature infant and for support of infants and parents in the neonatal intensive care environment. *Phys Occup Ther Pediatr.* 1986;6:3-55.
3. Symington AJ, Pinelli J. Developmental care for promoting development and preventing morbidity in preterm infants. *Cochrane Database Syst Rev.* 2006;2: CD001814.
4. Ohlsson A. NIDCAP: new controversial evidence for its effectiveness. *Pediatrics.* 2009;124:1213-1215.
5. Maguire CM, Walther FJ, Sprij AJ, Le Cessie S, Wit JM, Veen S. Effects of individualized developmental care in a randomized trial of preterm infants <32 weeks. *Pediatrics.* 2009;124:1021-1030.
6. Peters KL, Rosychuk RJ, Hendson L, Coté JJ, McPherson C, Tyebkhan JM. Improvement of short- and long-term outcomes for very low birth weight infants: Edmonton NIDCAP Trial. *Pediatrics.* 2009;124:1009-1020.

NIDCAP: A Systematic Review and Meta-analyses of Randomized Controlled Trials

Ohlsson A, Jacobs SE (Univ of Toronto, Ontario Canada; Royal Women's Hosp, Melbourne, Victoria, Australia)
Pediatrics 131:e881-e893, 2013

Background and Objective.—The "synactive" theory of neurobehavioral development forms the basis of the Newborn Individualized Developmental Care and Assessment Program (NIDCAP). Our objective was to assess the effectiveness of NIDCAP in improving outcomes in preterm infants.

Methods.—Medline, CINAHL, Embase, PsychInfo, The Cochrane Library, Pediatric Academic Societies' Abstracts and Web of Science were searched in July 2010 and February 2012. The studies selected were randomized controlled trials testing the effectiveness of NIDCAP on medical and neurodevelopmental outcomes. The authors abstracted baseline characteristics of infants and outcomes. The risk of bias was assessed by using Cochrane criteria. RevMan 5.1 was used to synthesize data by the use of relative risk and risk difference for dichotomous outcomes and mean or standardized mean difference for continuous outcomes.

Results.—Eleven primary and 7 secondary studies enrolling 627 neonates were included, with 2 of high quality. The composite primary outcomes of death or major sensorineural disability at 18 months corrected age or later in childhood (3 trials, 302 children; relative risk 0.89 [95% confidence interval 0.61 to 1.29]) and survival free of disability at 18 months corrected age or later in childhood (2 trials, 192 infants; relative risk 0.97 [95% confidence interval 0.69 to 1.35]), were not significantly different between the NIDCAP and control groups. With the sensitivity analysis that excluded the 2 statistically heterogeneous outlying studies, there were no significant differences between groups for short-term medical outcomes.

Conclusions.—This systematic review including 627 preterm infants did not find any evidence that NIDCAP improves long-term neurodevelopmental or short-term medical outcomes.

▶ In one of the earliest randomized, controlled trials of the Newborn Individualized Developmental Care and Assessment Program (NIDCAP), which enrolled only 35 infants, my colleagues and I reported that infants managed using individualized developmental care plans in accordance with NIDCAP principles had fewer days of assisted ventilation, fewer days of continuous positive airway pressure, earlier achievement of full enteral feedings, shorter hospital stays, and lower hospital charges.[1] At the end of that article, we commented that "additional studies are needed to elucidate the mechanism of action of these interventions and to determine their applicability to other populations." Several other groups have fulfilled that request, adding nearly 600 infants to the collection of those studied in randomized trials.

This meta-analysis indicates that our enthusiasm for this system of individualized care was unwarranted, however. In a series of similar reviews by these authors and others over the past decade, the apparent benefits of NIDCAP have progressively faded, as is often the case when small initial trials showing large effects are followed by much larger studies. The potential for such shifting results is enhanced when the intervention, such as NIDCAP, cannot be blinded to treating care providers. This most recent analysis now finds no evidence for any consequential improvements in short-term medical or long-term neurodevelopmental outcomes with NIDCAP. Although it seems obvious to adapt the neonatal intensive care unit environment and routines to individualize care for each infant in response to his or her changing physiologic and behavioral states, neither NIDCAP nor other formulations of the broad concept of developmental care have been proven effective in rigorously designed clinical trials. Given the imprecise definition of developmental care, the challenge of implementing those concepts uniformly throughout a hospitalization, and the diversity of other factors that contribute to outcomes for care of preterm infants, it may be too much to ask to insist on a demonstration of benefits in controlled trials. Nonetheless, until there is a better understanding of the specific elements of developmental care (if any) that actually do lead to improved long-term outcomes, efforts to bring these ideas to the bedside need to be tempered by circumspection and humility.

W. E. Benitz, MD

Reference

1. Fleisher BE, VandenBerg K, Constantinou J, et al. Individualized developmental care for very-low-birth-weight premature infants. *Clin Pediatr (Phila)*. 1995;34: 523-529.

The Effects of Music Therapy on Vital Signs, Feeding, and Sleep in Premature Infants

Loewy J, Stewart K, Dassler A-M, et al (Beth Israel Med Ctr, NY)
Pediatrics 131:902-918, 2013

Objectives.—Recorded music risks overstimulation in NICUs. The live elements of music such as rhythm, breath, and parent-preferred lullabies may affect physiologic function (eg, heart and respiratory rates, O_2 saturation levels, and activity levels) and developmental function (eg, sleep, feeding behavior, and weight gain) in premature infants.

Methods.—A randomized clinical multisite trial of 272 premature infants aged ≥32 weeks with respiratory distress syndrome, clinical sepsis, and/or SGA (small for gestational age) served as their own controls in 11 NICUs. Infants received 3 interventions per week within a 2-week period, when data of physiologic and developmental domains were collected before, during, and after the interventions or no interventions and daily during a 2-week period.

Results.—Three live music interventions showed changes in heart rate interactive with time. Lower heart rates occurred during the lullaby ($P < .001$) and rhythm intervention ($P = .04$). Sucking behavior showed differences with rhythm sound interventions ($P = .03$). Entrained breath sounds rendered lower heart rates after the intervention ($P = .04$) and differences in sleep patterns ($P < .001$). Caloric intake ($P = .01$) and sucking behavior ($P = .02$) were higher with parent-preferred lullabies. Music decreased parental stress perception ($P < .001$).

Conclusions.—The informed, intentional therapeutic use of live sound and parent-preferred lullabies applied by a certified music therapist can influence cardiac and respiratory function. Entrained with a premature infant's observed vital signs, sound and lullaby may improve feeding behaviors and sucking patterns and may increase prolonged periods of quiet—alert states. Parent-preferred lullabies, sung live, can enhance bonding, thus decreasing the stress parents associate with premature infant care.

▶ What is the impact of music on the fetus? Although the fetus will respond to music with various movements, their long-term significance in terms of neurodevelopment are uncertain. Anecdotal reports suggest that the fetus may move in a synchronous manner to the music, and it has been suggested that newborns show recognition of music they have heard in utero by showing a significant decrease in heart rate and movements and either perking up (shifting into a more alert state) or going to sleep. In 3- to 4-year-old children, piano lessons enhance children's math and spatial reasoning skills, so it has been surmised that fetuses and newborns may benefit from music too.

The maturation of fetal response to music was characterized over the last trimester of pregnancy by Kisilevsky et al[1] using a 5-minute piano recording of Brahms' Lullaby, played at an average of 95, 100, 105, or 110 dB. Within 30 seconds of the onset of the music, the youngest fetuses (28—32 weeks of gestational age [GA]) showed a heart rate increase limited to the 2 highest decibel levels; over gestation, the threshold level decreased and a response shift from acceleration to deceleration was observed for the lower decibel levels, indicating attention to the stimulus. Over 5 minutes of music, fetuses older than 33 weeks of GA showed a sustained increase in heart rate; body movement changes occurred at 35 weeks of GA. These findings suggest a change in processing of complex sounds at around 33 weeks of GA, with responding limited to the acoustic properties of the signal in younger fetuses but attention playing a role in older fetuses.

Music therapy (MT) has positive effects on basic vital signs, the reduction of pain, and neurologic development. Furthermore, it grants the parents' wishes to participate in the well-being of their child.

In a meta-analysis, Standley[2] noted that evidence-based neonatal intensive care unit (NICU) MT was highly beneficial. Benefits were greatest for live MT and for use early in the infant's NICU stay (birth weight < 1000 g, birth postmenstrual age < 28 weeks). Results justify strong consideration for the inclusion of the following evidence-based NICU—MT protocols in best practice standards for NICU treatment of preterm infants: music listening for pacification, music reinforcement of sucking, and music pacification as the basis for multilayered, multimodal stimulation. Keith et al[3] reported that mothers assigned to music groups produced more milk with a richer fat content.

The study by Loewy et al reported above adds to the body of knowledge on music therapy. They recommend trained music therapists playing parent-preferred melodies. Music can alter cardiorespiratory responses, change states (induce quiet—alert and sleep states), stimulate suck response, and improve oxygen saturation in premature infants and significantly reduce fear and anxiety perception in parents. It should be an integral part of the low-tech aspects of neonatal intensive care.

A. A. Fanaroff, MBBCh, FRCPE

References

1. Kisilevsky S, Hains SM, Jacquet AY, Granier-Deferre C, Lecanuet JP. Maturation of fetal responses to music. *Dev Sci.* 2004;7:550-559.
2. Standley J. Music therapy research in the NICU: an updated meta-analysis. *Neonatal Netw.* 2012;31:311-316.
3. Keith DR, Weaver BS, Vogel RL. The effect of music-based listening interventions on the volume, fat content, and caloric content of breast milk-produced by mothers of premature and critically ill infants. *Adv Neonatal Care.* 2012;12:112-119.

Living with a Crucial Decision: A Qualitative Study of Parental Narratives Three Years after the Loss of Their Newborn in the NICU
Caeymaex L, Speranza M, Vasilescu C, et al (Paris-South Univ, Creteil, France; Centre Hospitalier de Versailles, Le Chesnay, France; Centre Hospitalier Universitaire Antoine Beclère (AP-HP), Clamart, France; et al)
PLoS One 6:e28633, 2011

Background.—The importance of involving parents in the end-of-life decision-making-process (EOL DMP) for their child in the neonatal intensive care unit (NICU) is recognised by ethical guidelines in numerous countries. However, studies exploring parents' opinions on the type of involvement report conflicting results. This study sought to explore parents' experience of the EOL DMP for their child in the NICU.

Methods.—The study used a retrospective longitudinal design with a qualitative analysis of parental experience 3 years after the death of their child in four NICUs in France. 53 face-to-face interviews and 80 telephone interviews were conducted with 164 individuals. Semi-structured interviews were conducted to explore how parents perceived their role in the decision process, what they valued about physicians' attitudes in this situation and whether their long-term emotional well-being varied according to their perceived role in the EOL DMP.

Findings.—Qualitative analysis identified four types of perceived role in the DMP: shared, medical, informed parental decision, and no decision. Shared DM was the most appreciated by parents. Medical DM was experienced as positive only when it was associated with communication. Informed parental DM was associated with feelings of anxiousness and abandonment. The physicians' attitudes that were perceived as helpful in the long term were explicit sharing of responsibility, clear expression of staff preferences, and respectful care and language toward the child.

Interpretation.—Parents find it valuable to express their opinion in the EOL DMP of their child. Nonetheless, they do need continuous emotional support and an explicit share of the responsibility for the decision. As involvement preferences and associated feelings can vary, parents should be able to decide what role they want to play. However, our study suggests that fully autonomous decisions should be misadvised in these types of tragic choices.

▶ There is wide variability in the distribution of roles between physicians and parents as surrogate decision makers in end-of-life (EOL) decisions for dying newborns. This in-depth interview study in France sought to improve our knowledge of this variability by focusing on parents' perceptions of their role and the impact 3 years after the process had taken place. Four neonatal intensive care units (NICUs) in different areas of the country, all of which had no specific protocol for EOL decision making, participated in the study. Interestingly, the researchers disclosed their a priori opinions about the theme of interest before the interview, varying from "parents should decide with staff" to "parents should not be included," as this would generate parental guilt feelings.

Eighty families agreed to be interviewed, of which 53 were face-to-face interviews. The perceived role of the parents was determined only from the face-to-face interviews and not from telephone contact, as this enabled parents the opportunity to extensively describe their involvement. Three types of decision making were described: (1) a shared decision between parents and physicians, (2) a medical decision in which it was perceived that the decision was made by the physician without explicit parental involvement, and (3) an informed parental decision in which the parents considered the situation and made a decision after receiving full information from the doctor. The shared decision was the most common; it was appreciated by the parents, as it allowed them to express themselves without having to decide alone and it showed respect for their personal values. Even so, the weight of the decision persisted for many parents. The medical decision was also largely positive, as parents stated that they had reached the same conclusion as the medical team but expressed relief that they did not have to decide themselves. The informed parent role was least common and was largely a negative experience because of parental feeling of abandonment by the staff. In some it was perceived as positive.

From the details given, it seems that only 6% of the decisions were what we might label quality-of-life decisions, as 46 (33%) infants died without a decision being made. There is one statement that parents expressed that this was acceptable, as it confirmed their view that "we were right to go all the way," but one could be concerned (as voiced by some parents themselves) that in most cases parents, in reality, did not have much of a choice, as the infants had no or only a theoretical chance of survival with intensive care, and no real decision making was required.

It appears from this study that the shared and medical models of decision making are both well accepted by most parents in French NICUs. This is congruent with the fact that in France most neonatologists believe that parents should not be required, or even allowed, to make the EOL decision alone. In this regard, it is worth rereading the study by Orfali and Gordon, "Autonomy Gone Awry,"[1] highlighted in the 2005 YEAR BOOK.

With regard to residual guilt, most parents did report these feelings, but these were mostly independent of their perceived role in the decision-making process. Parents' views of what they desired in regard to physicians' actions and attitudes emphasized what is evident in many studies—that parents want a trusting relationship with staff who should be involved in a nonjudgmental way. They also want continuity and consistency and frank and overt conversations between humans on an equal footing, using respectful language.

J. Hellmann, MBBCh, FCP(SA), FRCPC, MHSc

Reference

1. Orfali K, Gordon EJ. Autonomy gone awry: a cross-cultural study of parents' experiences in neonatal intensive care units. *Theor Med Bioeth*. 2004;25:329-365.

10 Gastrointestinal Health and Nutrition

A pattern-based approach to bowel obstruction in the newborn
Maxfield CM, Bartz BH, Shaffer JL (Duke Univ Med Ctr, Durham, NC)
Pediatr Radiol 43:318-329, 2013

Intestinal obstruction is common in newborns, and the radiologist plays a critical role in the care of these children. Diagnosing and managing the potentially obstructed newborn can be challenging, especially given the myriad underlying pathologies that range from benign to acutely life-threatening. A familiarity with the most common diagnoses is essential, but equally important to the radiologist is a systematic approach to management of the child in this setting. We propose an approach based on the recognition of eight radiographic patterns, five upper gastrointestinal examination (UGI) patterns and four contrast enema patterns. Recognition of these patterns directs further imaging when necessary and allows triage of children who can be managed medically, those requiring elective or urgent surgery and those requiring emergent surgery (Fig 19).

▶ This is a practical review of radiographic signs that will help distinguish various forms of intestinal obstruction in the newborn that often present with vomiting. We are taught that vomiting in the newborn, especially if it is bilious, should be considered an emergency, and radiologic studies need to be done to aid in this diagnosis. Nevertheless, there are numerous other diagnoses that could present in a similar manner, and certain findings on a plain radiograph may be able to obviate further workup. In this review, through identification of 8 patterns on abdominal radiograph, 5 patterns on upper gastrointestinal examination, and 4 patterns on contrast enema, the radiologist and neonatologist can competently and confidently manage common and potentially life-threatening clinical presentations. On supine radiograph, several examples are presented that include single, double, and triple bubbles; single bubble plus distal scattered air; and dilated with separated or nonseparated loops. Diagrams are then provided for upper gastrointestinal studies that help rule in or rule out malrotation with volvulus, and examples of contrast enema studies that provide evidence for a microcolon, distal atresia, and aganglionosis are provided. Finally, a very

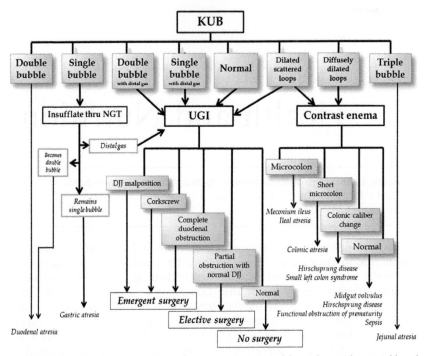

FIGURE 19.—The algorithm for the diagnostic imaging workup of the newborn with potential bowel obstruction. (With kind permission from Springer Science+Business Media. Maxfield CM, Bartz BH, Shaffer JL. A pattern-based approach to bowel obstruction in the newborn. *Pediatr Radiol.* 2013;43:318-329, Copyright 2013.)

useful algorithm with a suggested workup for intestinal obstruction is provided (Fig 19).

J. Neu, MD

Spontaneous intestinal perforation in extremely low birth weight infants: association with indometacin therapy and effects on neurodevelopmental outcomes at 18–22 months corrected age
Wadhawan R, Oh W, Vohr BR, et al (All Children's Hosp, St Petersburg, FL; Women & Infants Hosp, Providence, RI; et al)
Arch Dis Child Fetal Neonatal Ed 98:F127-F132, 2013

Background.—Spontaneous intestinal perforation (SIP) is associated with the use of postnatal glucocorticoids and indometacin in extremely low birth weight (ELBW) infants. The authors hypothesised: 1) an association of SIP with the use of antenatal steroids (ANS) and indometacin either as prophylaxis for intraventricular hemorrhage (IVH) (P Indo) or for treatment of PDA (Indo/PDA) and 2) an increased risk of death or abnormal neurodevelopmental outcomes in infants with SIP at 18–22 months corrected age.

Design/Methods.—The authors retrospectively identified ELBW infants with SIP in the Neonatal Research Network's generic database. Unadjusted analysis identified the differences in maternal, neonatal and clinical variables between infants with and without SIP. Logistic regression analysis identified the adjusted OR for SIP with reference to ANS, P Indo and Indo/PDA. Neurodevelopmental outcomes were assessed among survivors at 18–22 months corrected age.

Results.—Indo/PDA was associated with an increased risk of SIP (adjusted OR 1.61; 95% CI 1.25 to 2.08), while P Indo and ANS were not. SIP was independently associated with an increased risk of death or neurodevelopmental impairment (NDI) (adjusted OR 1.85; 95% CI 1.32 to 2.60) and NDI among survivors (adjusted OR 1.75, 95% CI 1.20 to 2.55).

Conclusion.—Indometacin used for IVH prophylaxis and ANS were not associated with the occurrence of SIP in ELBW infants. Indometacin used for treatment of symptomatic PDA was however associated with an increased risk of SIP. ELBW infants with SIP have an increased risk of poor neurodevelopmental outcomes.

▶ The well-recognized association between spontaneous intestinal perforation (SIP) and the combination of postnatal steroids and indomethacin led to speculation by Wadhawan et al of the Eunice Kennedy Shriver National Institutes of Child Health and Human Development Neonatal Research Network (NRN) that maternal treatment with antenatal steroids combined with neonatal administration of indomethacin for intraventricular hemorrhage (IVH) prophylaxis or treatment of patent ductus arteriosus (PDA) also might predispose to SIP and that SIP would be associated with increased risk of death or neurodevelopmental disability. They were partially correct. In this retrospective cohort study of 11 960 infants born at NRN institutions between 1998 and 2005, 280 of whom had SIP diagnosed, a diagnosis of SIP indeed was associated with increased risk of the composite outcome death or neurodevelopmental impairment at 18 to 22 months of age. Univariate analyses of the relationships among antenatal steroids, indomethacin treatment, and SIP showed antenatal steroids to be associated with reduced risk of SIP and the use of indomethacin, either as IVH prophylaxis or for treatment of PDA, to be linked with increased SIP risk. In logistic regression analyses, indomethacin treatment of PDA was associated with increased risk of SIP (adjusted odds ratio [OR], 1.61; 95% confidence interval [CI], 1.25–2.08); however, the combination of antenatal steroids and indomethacin for IVH prophylaxis was not (OR, 1.21; 95% CI, 0.88–1.66). Biologically plausible explanations for the study findings include the possibility that infants in the PDA treatment group were sicker than those receiving indomethacin prophylaxis, and this was incompletely adjusted in the logistic regression or, alternatively, that indomethacin treatment of PDA might accentuate hypoperfusion associated with the aortic steal of symptomatic PDA. On the other hand, the OR point estimate for the association of prophylactic indomethacin and SIP is in a direction indicating increased risk and, despite the large study population, it is possible that study power remains insufficient to achieve statistical significance for a more modest increase in risk. It's intriguing that early prophylactic indomethacin might have a more favorable safety profile than the use of indomethacin for treatment of PDA, yet the study results must be interpreted with caution.

L. J. Van Marter, MD, MPH

Spontaneous intestinal perforation in extremely low birth weight infants: association with indometacin therapy and effects on neurodevelopmental outcomes at 18–22 months corrected age
Wadhawan R, Oh W, Vohr BR, et al (All Children's Hosp, St Petersburg, FL; Women & Infants Hosp, Providence, RI; et al)
Arch Dis Child Fetal Neonatal Ed 2012 [Epub ahead of print]

Background.—Spontaneous intestinal perforation (SIP) is associated with the use of postnatal glucocorticoids and indometacin in extremely low birth weight (ELBW) infants. The authors hypothesised: 1) an association of SIP with the use of antenatal steroids (ANS) and indometacin either as prophylaxis for intraventricular hemorrhage (IVH) (P Indo) or for treatment of PDA (Indo/PDA) and 2) an increased risk of death or abnormal neurodevelopmental outcomes in infants with SIP at 18–22 months corrected age.

Design/Methods.—The authors retrospectively identified ELBW infants with SIP in the Neonatal Research Network's generic database. Unadjusted analysis identified the differences in maternal, neonatal and clinical variables between infants with and without SIP. Logistic regression analysis identified the adjusted OR for SIP with reference to ANS, P Indo and Indo/PDA. Neurodevelopmental outcomes were assessed among survivors at 18–22 months corrected age.

Results.—Indo/PDA was associated with an increased risk of SIP (adjusted OR 1.61; 95% CI 1.25 to 2.08), while P Indo and ANS were not. SIP was independently associated with an increased risk of death or neurodevelopmental impairment (NDI) (adjusted OR 1.85; 95% CI 1.32 to 2.60) and NDI among survivors (adjusted OR 1.75, 95% CI 1.20 to 2.55).

Conclusion.—Indometacin used for IVH prophylaxis and ANS were not associated with the occurrence of SIP in ELBW infants. Indometacin used for treatment of symptomatic PDA was however associated with an increased risk of SIP. ELBW infants with SIP have an increased risk of poor neurodevelopmental outcomes.

▶ Postnatal steroid use, either alone or when combined with early postnatal indomethacin therapy, has been associated with an increased risk of spontaneous intestinal perforation (SIP).[1] The risk of SIP with postnatal indomethacin treatment alone is less clear. In this article, the authors examined the association of early and late postnatal indomethacin exposure and SIP.

Study data were abstracted from the Eunice Kennedy Shriver National Institute of Child Health and Human Development Neonatal Research Network's generic database for extremely low birth weight (ELBW) infants (1998—2005). Infants were categorized into 2 groups: infants with and without SIP. Intestinal perforation was restricted to perforation that occurred during the first 14 postnatal days without evidence of necrotizing enterocolitis (NEC). ELBW infants with SIP were compared to those without SIP with respect to the use of prophylactic indomethacin within 24 hours of birth, indomethacin for medical treatment of patent ductus arteriosus (PDA) after 24 hours of age, or antenatal steroid (ANS) exposure. In addition, the combined outcome of death or neurodevelopmental impairment (NDI) at 18 to 22 months corrected age was compared among ELBW infants with and without SIP.

Significantly more mothers of infants with SIP had hypertension and received antibiotic therapy before delivery compared to mothers of infants without SIP. In addition, there were significant differences between infants with and without SIP for each of the infant demographic and clinical variables measured. Adjusted odds ratio for SIP vs no SIP revealed that a higher gestational age and being inborn was associated with a lower risk of SIP, whereas male sex, maternal receipt of antibiotics, and indomethacin treatment for PDA were associated with a higher risk. On unadjusted analysis, ANS exposure to greater than 1 dose of steroids and indomethacin, whether used prophylactically or for the treatment of PDA, was associated with a significant risk for SIP. However, on logistic regression analysis, only indomethacin therapy for PDA was significant. Interestingly, infants who received both prophylactic indomethacin and indomethacin for PDA were not at increased risk for SIP. Not surprisingly, the incidence of death or NDI at 18 to 22 months corrected age was higher among infants with SIP.

The authors' conclusion that indomethacin administered for the treatment of PDA is associated with an increased risk of SIP needs to be interpreted cautiously. Because the analysis compared infants with and without SIP with respect to indomethacin exposure and not infants with and without indomethacin exposure with respect to SIP, a more appropriate interpretation would be that infants with SIP are more likely to have received indomethacin for PDA closure than infants without SIP. The latter interpretation is supported by the results of a Cochrane review of indomethacin for asymptomatic PDA closure in preterm infants in which the risk for NEC did not differ among treated and untreated infants.[2] Thus, the increased risk of SIP among infants who received indomethacin treatment for PDA in this study may simply be a reflection of increased severity of illness in this group.

L. A. Papile, MD

References

1. Stark AR, Carlo A, Tyson JE, et al. Adverse effects of early dexamethasone in extremely-low-birth-weight infants. *N Engl J Med.* 2001;344:95-101.
2. Cooke L, Steer P, Woodgate P. Indomethacin for asymptomatic patent ductus arteriosus in preterm infants. *Cochrane Database Syst Rev.* 2003;2:CD003745.

Gut microbiota of healthy Canadian infants: profiles by mode of delivery and infant diet at 4 months

Azad MB, on behalf of the CHILD Study Investigators (Univ of Alberta, Edmonton, Canada; et al)

CMAJ 185:385-394, 2013

Background.—The gut microbiota is essential to human health throughout life, yet the acquisition and development of this microbial community during infancy remains poorly understood. Meanwhile, there is increasing concern over rising rates of cesarean delivery and insufficient exclusive breastfeeding of infants in developed countries. In this article, we characterize the gut microbiota of healthy Canadian infants and describe the influence of cesarean delivery and formula feeding.

Methods.—We included a subset of 24 term infants from the Canadian Healthy Infant Longitudinal Development (CHILD) birth cohort. Mode of delivery was obtained from medical records, and mothers were asked to report on infant diet and medication use. Fecal samples were collected at 4 months of age, and we characterized the microbiota composition using high-throughput DNA sequencing.

Results.—We observed high variability in the profiles of fecal microbiota among the infants. The profiles were generally dominated by Actinobacteria (mainly the genus *Bifidobacterium*) and Firmicutes (with diverse representation from numerous genera). Compared with breastfed infants, formula-fed infants had increased richness of species, with overrepresentation of *Clostridium difficile*. *Escherichia–Shigella* and *Bacteroides* species were underrepresented in infants born by cesarean delivery. Infants born by elective cesarean delivery had particularly low bacterial richness and diversity.

Interpretation.—These findings advance our understanding of the gut microbiota in healthy infants. They also provide new evidence for the effects of delivery mode and infant diet as determinants of this essential microbial community in early life.

▶ The number of cesarean deliveries performed in certain areas of the world appears to be out of control. One needs to question the necessity of many of these and also whether this may end up creating a public health problem with significant increases in allergies, autoimmune diseases, and obesity, all now associated with cesarean vs vaginal delivery.[1,2] The mechanism of this association remains unclear, but recent research has shown that the microbial ecology of the infant intestine differs depending on the route of delivery.[3]

This study used high throughput DNA sequencing of fecal samples from 24 term infants to compare intestinal microbial colonization patterns and to determine the effect of breast milk vs formula feeding in infants who were cesarean delivered vs vaginally delivered. The samples were collected from these infants at 4 months of age. The formula-fed infants had increased richness of species, with *Clostridium difficile* being highly represented. Those infants born by cesarean delivery had an underrepresentation of *Escherichia-Shigella* and *Bacteroides*. This research raises several questions. Is there some significance to the underrepresentation of *Bacteroides* in the cesarean delivered infants? Previous studies have shown that *Bacteroides* may protect against inflammatory conditions in the gut through a single molecule, polysaccharide-A, found in the cell wall of these microbes.[4] Although speculative, this is a highly intriguing relationship that deserves further scrutiny. The richness scores (obtained by the Chao1 method, which estimates the number of different species present) were higher for the formula-fed compared with the breastfed infants, and Shannon diversity (which evaluates both the number of species and their distribution) also trended to be higher in the formula-fed infants. Diversity is usually considered a beneficial trait in an ecosystem. Why it was lower in the exclusively breastfed infants and whether this has any relevance is not known. The possibility that the gut microbiota differences seen after mode of delivery may be related to development of health vs immune, inflammatory, and metabolic diseases in later life is intriguing, and it will be clearly important to merge the developing concepts in mucosal immunology with these findings in the near future.

J. Neu, MD

References

1. Neu J, Rushing J. Cesarean versus vaginal delivery: long-term infant outcomes and the hygiene hypothesis. *Clin Perinatol.* 2011;38:321-331.
2. Blustein J, Attina T, Liu M, et al. Association of caesarean delivery with child adiposity from age 6 weeks to 15 years. *Int J Obes (Lond).* 2013 Apr 8 [Epub ahead of print].
3. Dominguez-Bello MG, Costello EK, Contreras M, et al. Delivery mode shapes the acquisition and structure of the initial microbiota across multiple body habitats in newborns. *Proc Natl Acad Sci U S A.* 2010;107:11971-11975.
4. Mazmanian SK, Round JL, Kasper DL. A microbial symbiosis factor prevents intestinal inflammatory disease. *Nature.* 2008;29:620-625.

Intestinal proteome changes during infant necrotizing enterocolitis
Jiang P, Smith B, Qvist N, et al (Univ of Hong Kong, China; State Serum Inst, Copenhagen, Denmark; Odense Univ Hosp, Denmark; et al)
Pediatr Res 73:268-276, 2013

Background.—Changes in the intestinal and colonic proteome in patients with necrotizing enterocolitis (NEC) may help to characterize the disease pathology and identify new biomarkers and treatment targets for NEC.

Methods.—Using gel-based proteomics, proteins in NEC-affected intestinal and colonic sections were compared with those in adjacent, near-normal tissue sections within the same patients. Western blot and immunohistochemistry were applied to crossvalidate proteomic data and histological location of some selected proteins.

Results.—Thirty proteins were identified with differential expression between necrotic and vital small-intestine sections and 23 proteins were identified for colon sections. Five proteins were similarly affected in the small intestine and colon: histamine receptors (HRs), actins, globins, immunoglobulin, and antitrypsin. Two heat shock proteins (HSPs) were affected in the small intestine. Furthermore, proteins involved in antioxidation, angiogenesis, cytoskeleton formation, and metabolism were affected. Finally, secretory proteins such as antitrypsin, fatty-acid binding protein 5, and haptoglobin differed between NEC-affected and vital tissues.

Conclusion.—NEC progression affects different pathways in the small intestine and colon. HSPs may play an important role, especially in the small intestine. The identified secretory proteins should be investigated as possible circulating markers of NEC progression in different gut regions.

▶ In this study, segments of intestine resected for necrotizing enterocolitis (NEC) in preterm infants were analyzed using 2-dimensional gel separation and subsequent matrix-assisted laser desorption/ionisation-time-of-flight mass spectroscopy for protein identification. A comparison was made between frankly necrotic regions of the intestine and an adjacent region that was thought to still comprise vital tissue. Several proteins were found to be up- or downregulated in the small and large intestine, and 5 were found to be similarly differential in the small and large intestine. The authors conclude that the data of the current study could serve as the basis for developing new circulating biomarkers of region-specific NEC.

There are several aspects of this study that make the results difficult to interpret, thus leading to a fuzzy conclusion. For example, does the necrotic tissue, even though it is found in patients with NEC, represent anything special other than dying tissue? Is there something that might be considered special about the proteins that are found in this dying tissue other than dying tissue from causes other than NEC? There are some proteins that are found to show surprising directions in the dying tissue compared with the vital tissue. For example, intestinal fatty acid binding protein is thought to reflect injured intestinal epithelium, but yet is higher in the vital pieces of intestine.

Another issue that needs to be taken into account with this study is that the techniques used are commonly utilized in the discovery phase of proteomics. Thus, there are several protein candidates that are up- and downregulated. Assuming these represent a specific alteration that would be seen principally in NEC-related necrotic tissue and not just any dying intestine, they would still need to be subjected to more quantitative testing using enzyme-linked adsorbent antibody tests or perhaps even Western blotting for further validation.

J. Neu, MD

A metagenomic study of diet-dependent interaction between gut microbiota and host in infants reveals differences in immune response

Schwartz S, Friedberg I, Ivanov IV, et al (Texas A&M Univ, College Station; Miami Univ, Oxford, OH; et al)
Genome Biol 13:r32, 2012

Background.—Gut microbiota and the host exist in a mutualistic relationship, with the functional composition of the microbiota strongly affecting the health and well-being of the host. Thus, it is important to develop a synthetic approach to study the host transcriptome and the microbiome simultaneously. Early microbial colonization in infants is critically important for directing neonatal intestinal and immune development, and is especially attractive for studying the development of human-commensal interactions. Here we report the results from a simultaneous study of the gut microbiome and host epithelial transcriptome of three-month-old exclusively breast- and formula-fed infants.

Results.—Variation in both host mRNA expression and the microbiome phylogenetic and functional profiles was observed between breast- and formula-fed infants. To examine the interdependent relationship between host epithelial cell gene expression and bacterial metagenomic-based profiles, the host transcriptome and functionally profiled microbiome data were subjected to novel multivariate statistical analyses. Gut microbiota metagenome virulence characteristics concurrently varied with immunity-related gene expression in epithelial cells between the formula-fed and the breast-fed infants.

Conclusions.—Our data provide insight into the integrated responses of the host transcriptome and microbiome to dietary substrates in the early neonatal period. We demonstrate that differences in diet can affect, via gut colonization, host expression of genes associated with the innate immune system. Furthermore, the methodology presented in this study can be adapted to assess other host-commensal and host-pathogen interactions using genomic and transcriptomic data, providing a synthetic genomics-based picture of host-commensal relationships.

▶ The establishment of the intestinal microbiome after birth is critical for immune ontogeny. However, the microbiome can also predispose the host to disease through dysregulated immunity and inflammation in response to antigens, including those in the diet. Although technologies continue to evolve, allowing us to define the specific composition of the microbiome (pyrosequencing) as well as its metabolic and functional role (metabolomics and metagenomics), one can argue that the most important aspect is to understand the link between the microbiome and the host epithelium and how this interaction is altered through our medical and nutritional practices, such as medications and nutrient delivery, through the diet. However, for obvious reasons, directly examining the host epithelium in the human preterm infant is unlikely, as intestinal biopsies or biopsies of other epithelial tissues are not routinely done. Schwartz et al present novel integration of multiple technologies, allowing them to isolate shed intestinal epithelial cells from fecal samples and interrogate epithelial gene expression as a function of the microbiome and diet. In this study, fecal samples were collected at 3 months in 12 infants, half receiving breast milk and the other half formula. From these samples, correlations were made between the epithelium transcriptome and the microbial metagenome as a function of diet. The authors found that in comparison to breastfed infants, infants fed formula had lower phylogenetic heterogeneity (and decreased diversity) of the microbiome; lower overall gene expression by the intestinal epithelium; lower expression of genes regulating intestinal motility, proliferation, and angiogenesis; and higher expression of genes regulating transcription, inflammation, and cytotoxicity. There is controversy regarding whether shed epithelial cells are reflective of healthy native intestinal epithelium; however, in the absence of biopsies of intact intestinal tissue, this methodology currently gives us the best snapshot of these dynamic interactions in an in vivo setting.

C. Martin, MD

Gut microbial colonisation in premature neonates predicts neonatal sepsis
Madan JC, Salari RC, Saxena D, et al (Dartmouth Hitchcock Med Ctr, Lebanon, NH; Dartmouth Med School, Lebanon, NH; et al)
Arch Dis Child Fetal Neonatal Ed 97:F456-F462, 2012

Background.—Neonatal sepsis due to intestinal bacterial translocation is a major cause of morbidity and mortality. Understanding microbial colonisation of the gut in prematurity may predict risk of sepsis to guide future strategies to manipulate the microbiome.

Methods.—Prospective longitudinal study of premature infants. Stool samples were obtained weekly. DNA was extracted and the V6 hypervariable region of *16S rRNA* was amplified followed by high throughput pyrosequencing, comparing subjects with and without sepsis.

Results.—Six neonates were 24—27 weeks gestation at birth and had 18 samples analysed. Two subjects had no sepsis during the study period, two developed late-onset culture-positive sepsis and two had culturenegative systemic inflammation. 324 350 sequences were obtained. The meconium was not sterile and had predominance of *Lactobacillus, Staphylococcus* and Enterobacteriales. Overall, infants who developed sepsis began life with low microbial diversity, and acquired a predominance of *Staphylococcus*, while healthy infants had more diversity and predominance of *Clostridium, Klebsiella* and *Veillonella*.

Conclusions.—In very low birth weight infants, the authors found that meconium is not sterile and is less diverse from birth in infants who will develop lateonset sepsis. Empiric, prolonged antibiotics profoundly decrease microbial diversity and promote a microbiota that is associated not only with neonatal sepsis, but the predominant pathogen previously identified in the microbiome. Our data suggest that there may be a 'healthy microbiome' present in extremely premature neonates that may ameliorate risk of sepsis. More research is needed to determine whether altered antibiotics, probiotics or other novel therapies can re-establish a healthy microbiome in neonates.

▶ Among today's hottest topics in the field of neonatology is the potential for gut microbial colonization to influence neonatal health and disease. The advent of technologies that permit rapid and affordable DNA isolation and sequencing has made possible detailed studies of the neonatal intestinal microbiome. Madan et al conducted a longitudinal study of intestinal colonization and associations with neonatal disorders among 6 infants born at 24 to 27 weeks of gestation, making several important observations, including the following: among this high-risk population, meconium is not sterile; broad-spectrum antibiotic treatment profoundly affects gut colonization; and infants with low microbial diversity are at highest risk of late-onset sepsis. These findings underscore the need to advance our understanding of the neonatal gastrointestinal microbiome and potentially influential modifiable factors, such as feeding practices[1] and the use of broad-spectrum antibiotics.[2] Also of interest is the potential influence of maternal health on neonatal microbiota. In this study, maternal chorioamnionitis was associated with lower gut microbiome diversity, a finding that could be attributable either to maternal antibiotic treatment or to an overabundance of primary pathogens. In another recently published study, Collado et al[3] reported that microbiota and inflammatory markers in breast milk varied by maternal body mass index and pregnancy weight gain, with lower levels of protective *Bifidobacterium* species and predominance of *Staphylococcus* and other potentially pathogenic species in breast milk produced by mothers who were overweight or who experienced excessive weight gain during pregnancy compared with the normal weight group. As in so many aspects of neonatal health, it appears that establishing a healthy intestinal microbiome requires optimal maternal health and perinatal-neonatal care.

L. J. Van Marter, MD, MPH

References

1. Westerbeek EA, van den Berg A, Lafeber HN, Knol J, Fetter WP, van Elburg RM. The intestinal bacterial colonisation in preterm infants: a review of the literature. *Clin Nutr.* 2006;25:361-368.
2. Cotten CM, Taylor S, Stoll B, et al. Prolonged duration of initial empirical antibiotic treatment is associated with increased rates of necrotizing enterocolitis and death for extremely low birth weight infants. *Pediatrics.* 2009;123:58-66.
3. Collado MC, Laitinen K, Salminen S, Isolauri E. Maternal weight and excessive weight gain during pregnancy modify the immunomodulatory potential of breast milk. *Pediatr Res.* 2012;72:77-85.

The human milk microbiome changes over lactation and is shaped by maternal weight and mode of delivery

Cabrera-Rubio R, Collado MC, Laitinen K, et al (Univ of Valencia, Spain; Spanish Natl Res Council (IATA-CSIC), Paterna, Valencia, Spain; Univ of Turku, Finland)
Am J Clin Nutr 96:544-551, 2012

Background.—Breast milk is recognized as the most important post-partum element in metabolic and immunologic programming of health of neonates. The factors influencing the milk microbiome and the potential impact of microbes on infant health have not yet been uncovered.

Objective.—Our objective was to identify pre- and postnatal factors that can potentially influence the bacterial communities inhabiting human milk.

Design.—We characterized the milk microbial community at 3 different time points by pyrosequencing and quantitative polymerase chain reaction in mothers ($n = 18$) who varied in BMI, weight gain, and mode of delivery.

Results.—We found that the human milk microbiome changes over lactation. *Weisella, Leuconostoc, Staphylococcus, Streptococcus,* and *Lactococcus* were predominant in colostrum samples, whereas in 1- and 6-mo milk samples the typical inhabitants of the oral cavity (eg, *Veillonella, Leptotrichia,* and *Prevotella*) increased significantly. Milk from obese mothers tended to contain a different and less diverse bacterial community compared with milk from normal-weight mothers. Milk samples from elective but not from nonelective mothers who underwent cesarean delivery contained a different bacterial community than did milk samples from individuals giving birth by vaginal delivery, suggesting that it is not the operation per se but rather the absence of physiological stress or hormonal signals that could influence the microbial transmission process to milk.

Conclusions.—Our results indicate that milk bacteria are not contaminants and suggest that the milk microbiome is influenced by several factors that significantly skew its composition. Because bacteria present in breast milk are among the very first microbes entering the human body, our data emphasize the necessity to understand the biological role that the milk microbiome could potentially play for human health.

▶ Studies over the past few years are suggesting that human milk is a natural source of microbes and that these microbes are not contaminants from the skin of the mother. Additionally, the types of microbes being found in mother's milk are being analyzed through the use of new high-throughput sequencing technologies that do not rely on culturing the microbes by conventional means. The objective of this study was to identify pre- and postnatal factors that can potentially influence the bacterial communities inhabiting human milk. In this study, the milk microbial community was characterized by pyrosequencing and quantitative polymerase chain reaction in mothers who varied in body mass index, weight gain, and mode of delivery. It was found that the milk microbiome changed over lactation and that it differed depending on whether the mothers were obese and whether the babies were delivered by cesarean-section or vaginal delivery. These are important observations in that they support the concept that environment is an important stimulus to the type of ecosystem that will eventually populate the neonates' gastrointestinal tract. The development of the immune system is thought to be closely linked to these microbes. Furthermore, the metabolic activities of these microbes could play an essential role in the development of leanness or obesity. Identification of these microbes in human milk under various conditions as done in this study is just the beginning of understanding how these microbes may affect the infant not only during the immediate lactation period, but also for the individual's lifetime.

J. Neu, MD

Paneth cell ablation in the presence of *Klebsiella pneumoniae* induces necrotizing enterocolitis (NEC)-like injury in the small intestine of immature mice
Zhang C, Sherman MP, Prince LS, et al (Vanderbilt Univ School of Medicine, Nashville, TN; Univ of Missouri Health System, Columbia)
Dis Model Mech 5:522-532, 2012

Necrotizing enterocolitis (NEC) is a leading cause of morbidity and mortality in premature infants. During NEC pathogenesis, bacteria are able to penetrate innate immune defenses and invade the intestinal epithelial layer, causing subsequent inflammation and tissue necrosis. Normally, Paneth cells appear in the intestinal crypts during the first trimester of human pregnancy. Paneth cells constitute a major component of the innate immune system by producing multiple antimicrobial peptides and proinflammatory mediators. To better understand the possible role of Paneth cell disruption in NEC, we quantified the number of Paneth cells present in infants with NEC and found that they were significantly decreased compared with age-matched controls. We were able to model this loss in the intestine of postnatal day (P)14-P16 (immature) mice by treating them with the zinc chelator dithizone. Intestines from dithizone-treated animals retained approximately half the number of Paneth cells compared with controls. Furthermore, by combining dithizone treatment with exposure to *Klebsiella pneumoniae*, we were able to induce intestinal injury and inflammatory induction that resembles human NEC. Additionally, this novel Paneth cell ablation model produces NEC-like pathology that is consistent with other currently used animal models, but this technique is simpler to use, can be used in older animals that have been dam fed, and represents a novel line of investigation to study NEC pathogenesis and treatment.

▶ Not unlike many animal models of human disease, a model that emulates the developmental susceptibilities of the premature infant to necrotizing enterocolitis (NEC) is hard to capture. NEC is likely a culmination of multiple factors during postnatal intestinal development rather than an acute sentinel event. Factors involved in this convergence include establishment of the intestinal microbiota, development of innate immunity of the gut, and introduction to enteral feedings. Some distinguishing (although not universal) features include a risk that is directly related to the degree of immaturity (thus, innate immunity) and the specificity of gut involvement to the ileum. Zhang et al offer a nice alternative to the traditional rodent models of NEC. The murine model of NEC proposed by Zhang et al captured both of these critical features. In their model, 2-week-old neonatal mice were given intraperitoneal dithizone to selectively ablate Paneth cells. Six hours later, the mice were given enterally administered *Klebsiella pneumoniae* and observed for another 10 hours. This model resulted in the development of NEC at rates and severity similar to those of other traditional models. Additionally, the injury was isolated to the ileum. Another interesting aspect of this model was the ability to maintain the mice on dam milk rather than introducing formula. Although it is clear that formula is a contributing factor to NEC, it is not an essential requirement for the development of NEC. Neonatal intensive care units are increasing their use of breast milk and moving away from diets that are all or mostly formula. Although we expect this to reduce the NEC occurrence, NEC will not be eliminated as we have learned from cases of NEC in infants fed only breast milk. Thus, it will be critical for us to understand the pathophysiologic changes leading to NEC in breastfed models of disease.

C. Martin, MD

Probiotics prevent necrotizing enterocolitis by modulating enterocyte genes that regulate innate immune-mediated inflammation

Ganguli K, Meng D, Rautava S, et al (Massachusetts General Hosp for Children, Boston; Harvard Med School, Boston, MA)
Am J Physiol Gastrointest Liver Physiol 304:G132-G141, 2013

Necrotizing enterocolitis (NEC), an extensive intestinal inflammatory disease of premature infants, is caused, in part, by an excessive inflammatory response to initial bacterial colonization due to the immature expression of innate immune response genes. In a randomized placebo-controlled clinical trial, supplementation of very low birth weight infants with probiotics significantly reduced the incidence of NEC. The primary goal of this study was to determine whether secreted products of these two clinically effective probiotic strains, *Bifidobacterium infantis and Lactobacillus acidophilus*, prevented NEC by accelerating the maturation of intestinal innate immune response genes and whether both strains are required for this effect. After exposure to probiotic conditioned media (PCM), immature human enterocytes, immature human intestinal xenografts, and primary enterocyte cultures of NEC tissue (NEC-IEC) were assayed for an IL-8 and IL-6 response to inflammatory stimuli. The latter two models were also assayed for innate immune response gene expression. In the immature xenograft, PCM exposure significantly attenuated LPS and IL-1β-induced IL-8 and IL-6 expression, decreased TLR2 mRNA and TLR4 mRNA, and increased mRNA levels of specific negative regulators of inflammation, SIGIRR and Tollip. In NEC-IEC, PCM decreased TLR2-dependent IL-8 and IL-6 induction and increased SIGIRR and Tollip expression. The attenuated inflammatory response with PCM was reversed with Tollip siRNA-mediated knockdown. The anti-inflammatory secreted factor is a 5- to 10-kDa molecule resistant to DNase, RNase, protease, heat stress, and acid exposure. *B. infantis*-conditioned media showed superior anti-inflammatory properties to that of *L. acidophilus* in immature human enterocytes, suggesting a strain specificity to this effect. We conclude that PCM promotes maturation of innate immune response gene expression, potentially explaining the protective effects of probiotics in clinical NEC.

▶ Multiple studies have found the potential benefit of probiotic administration to reduce the occurrence of necrotizing enterocolitis in very-low-birth-weight infants. Although these studies have not reported significant adverse events, many were not adequately designed to evaluate secondary complications such as sepsis. There is reason for potential concern in providing the immunoincompetent premature infant with live bacterial organisms. Case studies have reported probiotic-induced bacteremia in premature infants. Furthermore, premature infants have an immature innate immune system leading to an exaggerated inflammatory response when compared with adults with intestinal antigens, including from bacterial organisms thought to be commensal rather than pathogenic.[1] Ganguli et al report encouraging results that would allow the preterm infant to benefit from the positive effects of probiotics but without the need for providing live organisms. Using several different human intestinal models, the authors show that in response to antigenic stimuli, exposure to probiotic-conditioned media (PCM) of 2 commonly used probiotics, *Lactobacillus acidophilus* and *Bifidobacteria infantis*, attenuated the expression of the proinflammatory markers interleukin (IL)-8 and IL-6, decreased mRNA expression of toll-like receptors TLR2 and TLR4, and increased mRNA expression of SIGIRR and Tollip, previously identified negative regulators of inflammation. The specific agent within the PCM responsible for these beneficial effects has not been completely characterized but is thought to be a glycolipid or glycan. The work of Ganguli et al sheds new light on the specific mechanisms by which probiotics exert their beneficial effects and opens new therapeutic avenues in delivering these benefits without the potential concerns of exposing immature infants to live organisms.

C. Martin, MD

Reference

1. Claud EC, Lu L, Anton PM, Savidge T, Walker WA, Cherayil BJ. Developmentally regulated IkappaB expression in intestinal epithelium and susceptibility to flagellin-induced inflammation. *Proc Natl Acad Sci U S A.* 2004;101:7404-7408.

Noninvasive measurement of intestinal epithelial damage at time of refeeding can predict clinical outcome after necrotizing enterocolitis
Reisinger KW, Derikx JPM, Thuijls G, et al (Maastricht Univ Med Ctr, The Netherlands; et al)
Pediatr Res 73:209-213, 2013

Background.—Reintroduction of enteral nutrition in neonates with necrotizing enterocolitis (NEC) should take place when the gut is ready for its normal function. Too early a start of oral feeding might lead to disease relapse, whereas prolonged discontinuation of enteral nutrition is associated with impaired gut function and parenteral nutrition—related complications. This study evaluated whether noninvasive urinary measurement of intestinal fatty acid binding protein (I-FABP) at the time of refeeding can predict clinical outcome in neonates with NEC.

Methods.—Urinary I-FABP concentrations were measured in 21 infants with NEC just before reintroducing enteral nutrition. Poor outcome was defined as unsuccessful reintroduction of enteral feeding (EF), (re)operation for NEC, or death related to NEC after reintroduction of EF.

Results.—Median urinary I-FABP levels in neonates with poor outcome ($n = 5$) were significantly higher as compared with I-FABP levels in neonates with good outcome ($n = 16$) ($P < 0.01$). A clinically significant cutoff value of 963 pg/ml was found to discriminate between infants with poor outcome and those with good outcome (sensitivity 80%, specificity 94%).

Conclusion.—Noninvasive urinary I-FABP measurement at time of refeeding differentiates neonates with poor outcome from neonates with good outcome in NEC. Urinary I-FABP measurement may therefore be helpful in the timing of EF in neonates with NEC.

▶ This study attempts to address whether urinary intestinal fatty acid binding protein (I-FABP) can be used to determine whether a baby can have feedings reintroduced after an episode of necrotizing enterocolitis (NEC). I-FABP is a small (14—15-kDa), water-soluble cytosolic protein found in small and large intestinal epithelial cells. With intestinal cellular damage, it is released into the circulation and passes into the urine where it can be detected. Previous studies have suggested that this might be used as a diagnostic biomarker for NEC.[1,2] In this study, babies who had a good outcome were compared with babies with a bad outcome after NEC in terms of urinary I-FABP concentrations before the re-institution of enteral feedings. Those with a poor outcome had higher concentrations of urinary I-FABP. Unfortunately, this was a very small study, and the groups with poor outcome had a gestational age about 2.5 weeks younger than the good-outcome group. The gestational ages represented babies who were actually somewhat mature (30—32 weeks) with a relatively early onset of NEC (5 and 9 days), hence bringing into question whether the differences between the groups were gestational age related or actually related to gut epithelial damage that would preclude enteral feedings. This report is also difficult to follow. Was the control group matched to the good outcome or the poor outcome group in gestational age? It is difficult to discern how the surgical babies were used to evaluate sensitivity, specificity, and cutoff values with the medical NEC babies. Nevertheless, refeeding after NEC is an important problem. Whether this study actually offers strong data that can be generalized to a larger population is debatable, and I would pick the side that a much more rigorous study needs to be done to support the use of this marker. Nevertheless, it is a good idea and may still hold promise for this indication with larger and better controlled studies.

J. Neu, MD

References

1. Thuijls G, Derikx JP, van Wijck K, et al. Non-invasive markers for early diagnosis and determination of the severity of necrotizing enterocolitis. *Ann Surg.* 2010;251: 1174-1180.
2. Evennett NJ, Hall NJ, Pierro A, Eaton S. Urinary intestinal fatty acid-binding protein concentration predicts extent of disease in necrotizing enterocolits. *J Pediatr Surg.* 2010;45:735-740.

Fecal Phagocyte-Specific S100A12 for Diagnosing Necrotizing Enterocolitis
Däbritz J, Jenke A, Wirth S, et al (Univ Hosp Münster, Germany; Helios Klinikum, Wuppertal, Germany)
J Pediatr 161:1059-1064, 2012

Objective.—To determine whether longitudinal measurements of fecal S100A12, a fecal marker of intestinal inflammation, can identify very low birth weight infants at risk for necrotizing enterocolitis (NEC).

Study Design.—This prospective study included 145 preterm infants with birth weight < 1500 g. Meconium and stool samples (n = 843) were collected prospectively on alternate days for 4 weeks, and fecal S100A12 and calprotectin were measured by enzyme-linked immunosorbent assay.

Results.—Eighteen patients (12.4%) developed NEC. Gestational age and birth weight were significantly lower in the patients with NEC compared with unaffected reference infants. Fecal S100A12 levels were significantly higher in patients with severe NEC at onset of disease and also, in contrast to fecal calprotectin, at 4-10 days before onset of NEC compared with unaffected reference infants (ideal cutoff value, 65 μg/kg; sensitivity, 0.76; specificity, 0.56).

Conclusions.—Fecal S100A12 level may be a helpful marker for predicting disease severity and early risk assessment for subsequent development of NEC. However, the use of fecal S100A12 as a predictive biomarker for NEC in very low birth weight infants may be limited due to a high interindividual and intraindividual variability in S100A12 fecal excretion.

▶ This study evaluates S100A12, a damage-associated protein that is released by activated or damaged cells, primarily neutrophils, or monocyte that has been found in the feces of infants as a potential diagnostic and predictive biomarker for necrotizing enterocolitis (NEC). Of interest is that this biomarker was found in meconium at high levels in babies who subsequently had surgical NEC. However, the use of this as an early predictive biomarker for NEC using meconium was mitigated by the fact that it is actually lower in meconium of those babies who subsequently had medical (stage 2) NEC. Using standard statistical methodologies, such as sensitivity, specificity, and receiver operating characteristic curves, a cutoff point at 65 µg/kg was found. However, this resulted in only an overall sensitivity of 60%, a specificity of 55%, a positive predictive value of 25%, and a negative predictive value of 84%. Overall, this was an improvement when compared with calprotectin, interleukin-6, and C-reactive protein. However, when one compares this with previous studies of intestinal fatty acid binding protein or claudin 3 measured in the urine of preterm infants in a previous study,[1] the S100A12 does not appear to be as good of a marker. The search continues.

J. Neu, MD

Reference

1. Thuijls G, Derikx JP, van Wijck K, et al. Non-invasive markers for early diagnosis and determination of the severity of necrotizing enterocolitis. *Ann Surg.* 2010;251: 1174-1180.

Interleukin 8 correlates with intestinal involvement in surgically treated infants with necrotizing enterocolitis
Benkoe T, Reck C, Gleiss A, et al (Med Univ of Vienna, Austria)
J Pediatr Surg 47:1548-1554, 2012

Purpose.—The aim of this study was to test the predictive value of interleukin (IL) 8 in the assessment of intestinal involvement in necrotizing enterocolitis (NEC).

Methods.—Forty infants with surgically treated NEC were classified into 3 groups based on intestinal involvement during laparotomy: focal (n = 11), multifocal (n = 16), and panintestinal (n = 13). Preoperatively obtained serum levels of IL-8, C-reactive protein, white blood cell count, and platelet count were correlated with intestinal involvement using logistic regression models.

Results.—Interleukin 8 correlated significantly with intestinal involvement in infants with surgically treated NEC (odds ratio, 1.74; confidence interval, 1.27-2.39; $P < .001$). An exploratory IL-8 cutoff value of 449 pg/mL provided a specificity of 81.8% and sensitivity of 82.8% to discriminate focal from multifocal and panintestinal disease. An IL-8 cutoff value of 1388 pg/mL provided a specificity of 77.8% and a sensitivity of 76.9% to discriminate panintestinal disease from focal and multifocal disease.

Conclusions.—To our knowledge, this is the first study to demonstrate a significant correlation of IL-8 with intestinal involvement in advanced NEC in a large patient population. Our results indicate that IL-8 may be a promising biomarker for assessing intestinal involvement in infants with advanced NEC.

▶ This study demonstrates a significant correlation of the chemokine IL-8 with intestinal involvement in advanced necrotizing enterocolitis (NEC). Focal vs multifocal panintestinal NEC were compared in terms of several laboratory parameters, including C-reactive protein, white blood cell, and platelet counts. The latter 3 showed a very poor correlation to these 3 increasing degrees of severity of surgical NEC, whereas interleukin (IL)-8 showed a very significant increase, but still with considerable overlap between the 3 degrees of intestinal involvement. How specific this test will be for differentiating surgical NEC from culture positive sepsis is also questionable because at least one of the studies cited in this article[1] also shows a range of serum IL-8 with considerable overlap. Nevertheless, this test coupled with intestinal fatty acid binding protein, Claudin, and perhaps fecal calprotectin levels may provide the clinician with better tools to help them decide the critical point where these babies have disease that can be treated medically vs surgically.

J. Neu, MD

Reference

1. Harris MC, D'Angio CT, Gallagher PR, Kaufman D, Evans J, Kilpatrick L. Cytokine elaboration in critically ill infants with bacterial sepsis, necrotizing entercolitis, or sepsis syndrome: correlation with clinical parameters of inflammation and mortality. *J Pediatr.* 2005;147:462-468.

Late Onset Necrotizing Enterocolitis in Infants following Use of a Xanthan Gum-Containing Thickening Agent
Beal J, Silverman B, Bellant J, et al (US Food and Drug Administration, Riverdale, MD; Providence St Vincent Med Ctr, Portland, OR; et al)
J Pediatr 161:354-356, 2012

Adverse event reports submitted to the US Food and Drug Administration suggested a possible association between necrotizing enterocolitis and ingestion of a commercial feed thickener by premature infants. Review in 2011 of 22 cases with exposure revealed a distinct illness pattern.

▶ This report of necrotizing enterocolitis (NEC) after the use of this xanthan gum—containing thickening agent should be of major concern to neonatologists, neonatal nurse practitioners, and pediatricians. One obvious concern is that this agent gained such widespread acceptance in neonatal and pediatric care without evidence of safety or efficacy. This is not the first time this has happened and a brief evaluation of many of our current neonatal intensive care unit (NICU) and post-NICU care practices will readily reveal the myriad of common practices that do not have a sound scientific basis and have not been adequately evaluated for safety and efficacy.

The other concern regards the indications provided for use of this agent, which include gastroesophageal (GE) reflux and swallowing disorders. How were these evaluated? Was the diagnosis of GE reflux made on the basis of apnea and/or bradycardia? The cause-and-effect relationship between apnea, bradycardia, and GE reflux is highly questionable. The common use of prokinetics, H2 blockers, and feeding thickeners to prevent and treat apnea and bradycardia are widespread and there is little, if any, information to support safety and efficacy of these agents for this purpose.

Furthermore, how was dysfunctional swallowing evaluated? Nearly half of the infants who received the thickener were diagnosed as having dysfunctional swallowing. Were swallowing radiographs used? What is the evidence that these actually are of benefit in preterm infants? To my knowledge, the evidence for the efficacy of these is sparse and when present can be extremely misleading.

As for the NEC associated with the use of this thickening agent, the mechanism provided by the authors is highly plausible. The high concentration of nonabsorbable carbohydrates in the distal intestine leading to high concentrations of short-chain fatty acids makes sense. For the most part, these are absorbable in the intestine, and butyrate, in particular, can play a very important role in providing energy to colonocytes and improving interepithelial tight junction integrity. However, in high concentrations, these may become toxic and may very well have been at the basis of the development of NEC in these infants.

One other point that needs to be made here is that kudos are deserved to those who first recognized the relationship between the thickener and NEC, networked on the web, and understood that this was indeed not an isolated problem. Kudos also to the US Food and Drug Administration for acting on this issue with warnings that hopefully will prevent additional infants from developing this devastating problem.

J. Neu, MD

Chorioamnionitis as a Risk Factor for Necrotizing Enterocolitis: A Systematic Review and Meta-Analysis
Been JV, Lievense S, Zimmermann LJI, et al (Maastricht Univ Med Ctr, The Netherlands)
J Pediatr 162:236-242.e2, 2013

Objective.—To accumulate available evidence regarding the association between antenatal inflammation and necrotizing enterocolitis (NEC).

Study Design.—A systematic literature search was performed using Medline, Embase, Cochrane Library, ISI Web of Knowledge, and reference hand searches. Human studies published in English that reported associations between chorioamnionitis or other indicators of antenatal inflammation and NEC were eligible. Relevant associations were extracted and reported. Studies reporting associations between histological chorioamnionitis (HC) and NEC, HC with fetal involvement and NEC, and clinical chorioamnionitis and NEC were pooled in separate meta-analyses.

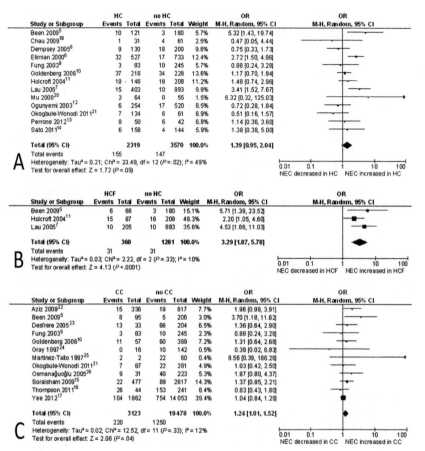

FIGURE 2.—Forest plots for associations between **A**, HC and NEC, **B**, HC with fetal involvement (HCF) and NEC, and **C**, CC and NEC. (Reprinted from Journal Pediatrics. Been JV, Lievense S, Zimmermann LJI, et al. Chorioamnionitis as a risk factor for necrotizing enterocolitis: a systematic review and meta-analysis. *J Pediatr.* 2013;162:236-242.e2, Copyright 2013, with permission from Elsevier.)

Results.—A total of 33 relevant studies were identified. Clinical chorioamnionitis was significantly associated with NEC (12 studies; $n = 22$ 601; OR, 1.24; 95% CI, 1.01-1.52; $P = .04$; $I^2 = 12\%$), but the association between HC and NEC was not statistically significant (13 studies; $n = 5889$; OR, 1.39; 95% CI, 0.95-2.04; $P = .09$; $I^2 = 49\%$). However, HC with fetal involvement was highly associated with NEC (3 studies; $n = 1640$; OR, 3.29; 95% CI, 1.87-5.78; $P \leq .0001$; $I^2 = 10\%$). Selection based on study quality did not affect the results. No indications of publication bias were apparent. Multivariate analyses in single studies generally attenuated the reported associations. Several associations between other markers of antenatal inflammation and NEC are reported.

Conclusion.—Currently available evidence supports a role for antenatal inflammation in NEC pathophysiology. This finding emphasizes the need to further study the underlying mechanisms and evaluate potential interventions to improve postnatal intestinal outcomes (Fig 2).

▶ This is an interesting report from the perspective that meta-analyses can be misleading. The conclusion of this study is that "currently available evidence supports a role for antenatal inflammation in necrotizing enterocolitis (NEC) pathophysiology." This was based on a systematic review and meta-analysis of 33 studies selected from the literature. When all the studies were pooled, no significant overall association with NEC was seen. When the authors then separated studies to include those that included fetal involvement, they found 3 studies. Each of these 3 studies found a significant association among histologic chorioamnionitis, fetal involvement, and NEC, which resulted in a prominent pooled odds ratio of 3.29 with 95% confidence limits of 1.87 and 5.78. When evaluating clinical chorioamnionitis and its association with NEC, the authors found an odds ratio of 1.24 with 95% confidence intervals of 1.01 and 1.52.

Is this an example of "garbage in, garbage out" that is often seen with meta-analyses? Let's look at the 3 studies that related chorioamnionitis that included fetal involvement to NEC (Figure 2). The first of these[1] and the second[2] also had differences in gestational age in the babies who had NEC and had chorioamnionitis. Given the inverse relationship between NEC and gestational age, this finding was not surprising. The third study[3] did not report whether the NEC they saw was definitive (stage 2 or 3, for example). This could be very misleading when signs such as abdominal distention and feeding intolerance may be diagnosed as NEC. When relating NEC to clinical chorioamnionitis alone, a borderline odds ratio was determined. But when one evaluates the studies included, one[4] evaluated mainly term infants and another[5] did not state what criteria were used to diagnose NEC.

Although it remains possible that there is a causal relationship between chorioamnionitis and NEC, using the meta-analysis approach that includes questionable studies makes the results of the meta-analysis questionable.

J. Neu, MD

References

1. Been JV, Rours IG, Kornelisse RF, et al. Histologic chorioamnionitis, fetal involvement, and antenatal steroids: effects on neonatal outcome in preterm infants. *Am J Obstet Gynecol.* 2009;201:587.e1-8.
2. Lau J, Magee F, Qiu Z, Houbé J, Von Dadelszen P, Lee SK. Chorioamnionitis with a fetal inflammatory response is associated with higher neonatal mortality, morbidity, and resource use than chorioamnionitis displaying a maternal inflammatory response only. *Am J Obstet Gynecol.* 2005;193:708-713.
3. Holcroft CJ, Askin FB, Patra A, Allen MC, Blakemore KJ, Graham EM. Are histopathologic chorioamnionitis and funisitis associated with metabolic acidosis in the preterm fetus? *Am J Obstet Gynecol.* 2004;191:2010-2015.
4. Martinez-Tallo E, Claure N, Bancalari E. Necrotizing enterocolitis in full-term or near-term infants: risk factors. *Biol Neonate.* 1997;71:292-298.
5. Aziz N, Cheng YW, Caughey AB. Neonatal outcomes in the setting of preterm premature rupture of membranes complicated by chorioamnionitis. *J Matern Fetal Neonatal Med.* 2009;22:780-784.

A.S.P.E.N. Clinical Guidelines: Nutrition Support of Neonatal Patients at Risk for Necrotizing Enterocolitis

Fallon EM, American Society for Parenteral and Enteral Nutrition (A.S.P.E.N.) Board of Directors (Harvard Med School, Boston, MA; et al)
JPEN J Parenter Enteral Nutr 36:506-523, 2012

Background.—Necrotizing enterocolitis (NEC) is one of the most devastating diseases in the neonatal population, with extremely low birth weight and extremely preterm infants at greatest risk.

Method.—A systematic review of the best available evidence to answer a series of questions regarding nutrition support of neonates at risk of NEC was undertaken and evaluated using concepts adopted from the Grading of Recommendations, Assessment, Development and Evaluation working group. A consensus process was used to develop the clinical guideline recommendations prior to external and internal review and approval by the A.S.P.E.N. Board of Directors.

Results/ Conclusions.—(1) When and how should feeds be started in infants at high risk for NEC? We suggest that minimal enteral nutrition be initiated within the first 2 days of life and advanced by 30 mL/kg/d in infants ≥ 1000 g. (Weak) (2) Does the provision of mother's milk reduce the risk of developing NEC? We suggest the exclusive use of mother's milk rather than bovine-based products or formula in infants at risk for NEC. (Weak) (3) Do probiotics reduce the risk of developing NEC? There are insufficient data to recommend the use of probiotics in infants at risk for NEC. (Further research needed.) (4) Do nutrients either prevent or predispose to the development of NEC? We do not recommend glutamine supplementation for infants at risk for NEC (Strong). There is insufficient evidence to recommend arginine and/or long chain polyunsaturated fatty acid supplementation for infants at risk for NEC. (Further research needed.) (5) When should feeds be reintroduced to infants with NEC? There are insufficient data to make a recommendation regarding time to reintroduce feedings to infants after NEC. (Further research needed.)

▶ This review provides answers from the American Society of Parenteral and Enteral Nutrition to a set of questions that relate to several highly controversial issues surrounding nutritional issues pertaining to infants at risk for the development of necrotizing enterocolitis (NEC). First, I have to applaud the authors for undertaking this challenge, and, second, provide a critique of some of the answers the authors have provided.

There were several questions that were addressed by the authors, to which I would like to offer comments:

1. When and how should feeds be started in infants at high risk for NEC? The authors suggest that minimal enteral nutrition be initiated within the first 2 days of life and advanced by 30 mL/kg/d in infants ≥ 1000 g. They also provide a weak level of evidence for this. There are some issues that need to be raised with this recommendation. Our methods to evaluate feeding readiness in terms of tolerance in these babies remain poor. Babies at the

lower range of > 1000 grams are often very different than babies weighing more than 1500 grams in terms of their intestinal development. To expect the majority of these smaller infants to reach full enteral feeding within the first week after birth as one does in babies closer to 2000 grams is likely to be fraught with hazard if one strictly follows these guidelines without respect for clinical judgment in individual circumstances. Another important point is that these authors do not address feeding issues in preterms less than 1000 grams, who actually represent a significant portion of the babies who develop NEC. Extrapolation of the guidelines to these infants without a caveat that attempting to get these babies to full enteral feedings within the first week would be a major change in most neonatal intensive care units (NICUs) and is also likely to have negative repercussions.

2. Does the provision of mother's milk reduce the risk of developing NEC? The authors suggest the exclusive use of mother's milk rather than bovine-based products or formula in infants at risk for NEC. They provide a weak level of evidence for this. In terms of the use of human milk, especially human milk directly from the babies' own mothers, the evidence for the prevention of NEC in my opinion is quite strong. The use of donor milk in the prevention of NEC relies on meta-analysis of several studies, with no single adequately powered randomized, controlled trials to support the argument that donor milk prevents NEC. Donor milk loses many of its beneficial components in processing and, therefore, would not be expected to be as efficacious as a baby's own mother's milk. The benefits of the use of fortifiers derived from human milk rather than bovine sources is of interest, but the information available is based on a study that did not state NEC as the primary outcome and, therefore, was not adequately powered for this outcome. Nevertheless, the decrease in NEC in this study is of interest. Whether this is adequate to change practice, especially in those NICUs experiencing low NEC rates, remains questionable.

3. Do probiotics reduce the risk of developing NEC? There are insufficient data to recommend the use of probiotics in infants at risk for NEC. The authors state that further research is needed. I agree with this despite the promising outcomes of recent meta-analyses. One must remember that one probiotic is not representative of all. Introduction of a live agent to a highly susceptible population has many theoretical hazards. Caution in routine introduction of probiotics to preterm infants is warranted.

4. Do nutrients either prevent or predispose to the development of NEC? The authors do not recommend glutamine supplementation for infants at risk for NEC based on a strong level of evidence. There is insufficient evidence to recommend arginine and/or long-chain polyunsaturated fatty acid supplementation for infants at risk for NEC, where they state that "further research is needed." I agree with most of this, with the exception that the evidence against the use of glutamine is strong. In reality, none of the studies in humans were done to evaluate the effects of glutamine in the prevention of NEC. In fact, the largest study of enteral glutamine supplementation did suggest benefits in terms of feeding tolerance, but this study was not powered or intended to evaluate NEC prevention. Furthermore, a very strong

body of evidence shows that glutamine can prevent intestinal injury in animal models. To state that the evidence against the use of glutamine is strong may thwart further research in this area and this, in my opinion, is unwarranted, especially because dosage and mode of delivery (in a milk matrix or in water), for example, has not received adequate scrutiny.

J. Neu, MD

Cholestasis, Bronchopulmonary Dysplasia, and Lipid Profile in Preterm Infants Receiving MCT/ω-3—PUFA—Containing or Soybean-Based Lipid Emulsions
Skouroliakou M, Konstantinou D, Agakidis C, et al (Harokopio Univ, Athens, Greece; "IASO" Maternity Hosp, Athens, Greece; Alexander Technological Education Inst, Thessaloniki, Greece)
Nutr Clin Pract 27:817-824, 2012

Background.—This study aimed to compare the effect of 2 lipid emulsions (LEs), a medium-chain triglyceride (MCT)/ω-3—polyunsaturated fatty acid (PUFA)—containing LE and a soybean-based LE, on the incidence of neonatal cholestasis, bronchopulmonary dysplasia (BPD), and lipid profile of preterm infants.

Patients and Methods.—In this prospective, observational study, 2 groups of preterm neonates, the very low birth weight (VLBW) (n = 129) and the low birth weight (LBW) groups (n = 153), which received parenteral LEs for at least 7 days, were included. Infants received either MCT/ω-3—PUFA—containing LE (SMOFlipid, subgroup I) or soybean-based LE (Intralipid, subgroup II) according to the attending neonatologist's preference and availability. Full biochemical assessment was performed on days of life 15, 30, and 45 and on discharge.

Results.—Of the VLBW infants, 7.4% and 13.3% of infants in subgroups I and II, respectively, developed cholestasis (*P* =.39; odds ratio [OR], 0.52; 95% confidence interval [CI], 0.15—1.76). The duration of LE administration was independently associated with cholestasis (*P* < .001; OR, 0.925; 95% CI, 0.888—0.963). The maximum amounts of lipids administered ranged between 1.6 and 3.6 g/kg/d in both VLBW subgroups. The VLBW subgroup I had lower incidence of BPD, lower alkaline phosphatase and phosphate, higher high-density lipoprotein (HDL), and lower cholesterol-to-HDL ratio on discharge than the VLBW subgroup II. The type of LE was independently associated with BPD and alkaline phosphatase. In the LBW group, the type of LE was not associated with clinical and biochemical parameters.

Conclusion.—In VLBW infants, the MCT/ω-3—PUFA—containing LE administration is associated with decreased BPD and more favorable lipoprotein profile. Although a trend toward a lower incidence of cholestasis was observed, a preventive effect of MCT/ω-3—PUFA—containing LE on parenteral nutrition-associated cholestasis is not supported.

▶ Accruing data clearly demonstrate that the current soy-based lipid emulsion used commonly in North America is insufficient in meeting the specific fatty acid requirements for the preterm infant and is potentially harmful. Although trials in the United States comparing different lipid emulsions await appropriate Food and Drug Administration approval, such trials have been conducted over the past few years outside North America. Their results provide insight as to which lipid emulsion blends may be more appropriate but raise further questions that need to be evaluated in greater detail before readily adopting new emulsions. An example of these principles is illustrated in this recent clinical trial. Low-birth-weight and very-low-birth-weight (VLBW) infants were given Intralipid (soy-based) or SMOFlipid (medium-chain triglyceride fish oil—enriched). Among VLBW infants, SMOFlipid resulted in lower rates of bronchopulmonary dysplasia, higher serum levels of high-density lipoprotein (HDL) cholesterol, and a lower total cholesterol-to-HDL ratio. This study and other comparative lipid emulsion studies show a significant trend toward improved clinical outcomes, hinting that we can do better; however, a comprehensive evaluation of the biologic effects of different lipid emulsions is often lacking. Do the alternative lipid emulsions reduce the inevitable postnatal deficit in critical fatty acids such as docosahexaenoic acid? How do systemic levels of other essential and critical fatty acid levels change compared with birth levels (levels at which the infant would have been exposed to throughout gestation if he/she had not been born early)? Although fish oil reduces cholesterol synthesis and has hematologic effects that benefit the adult with cardiovascular disease, are these effects desirable or safe in the developing preterm infant? What are the specific nutrigenetic changes with different lipid emulsion blends? The comprehensive answers to these questions will be worth the effort and get us closer to the optimal lipid emulsion for the preterm infant.

C. Martin, MD

Early Enteral Fat Supplement and Fish Oil Increases Fat Absorption in the Premature Infant with an Enterostomy
Yang Q, Ayers K, Chen Y, et al (Wake Forest Univ Health Science, Winston-Salem, NC)
J Pediatr 2013 [Epub ahead of print]

Objective.—To test the hypothesis that in the premature infant with an enterostomy, early enteral supplementation with Microlipid (fat supplement) and fish oil increases enteral fat absorption and decreases the requirement for Intralipid (intravenous fat emulsion).

Study Design.—Premature infants (<2 months old) with an enterostomy after surgical treatment for necrotizing enterocolitis or spontaneous intestinal perforation and tolerating enteral feeding at 20 mL/kg/day were randomized to usual care (control 18 infants) or early supplementing enteral fat and fish oil (treatment 18 infants). Intravenous fat emulsion was decreased as enteral fat intake was increased. Daily weight, ostomy output, and nutrition data were recorded. Weekly 24-hour ostomy effluent was collected until bowel reanastomosis, and fecal fat, fecal liquid, and dry feces were measured. Fat absorption (g/kg/d) was calculated by subtracting fecal fat from dietary fat. The fecal liquid and dry feces were reported as mg/g wet stool. Date were analyzed by using ANOVA and mixed-effects model.

Results.—The interval from initial postoperative feeding to bowel reanastomosis varied from 2 to 10 weeks. The treatment group received more dietary fat and less intravenous fat emulsion and had higher enteral fat absorption, less fecal liquid, and drier feces than the control group. These effects were greater among infants with a high ostomy compared with those with a low ostomy. Enteral fat intake was significantly correlated with fat absorption.

Conclusion.—Early enteral fat supplement and fish oil increases fat absorption and decreases the requirement for intravenous fat emulsion. This approach could be used to promote bowel adaptation and reduce the use of intravenous fat emulsion in the premature infant with an enterostomy.

▶ Transition to enteral feedings after an ostomy is often a difficult process, with infants exhibiting feeding intolerance and increased watery stool output. This results in a vicious cycle of prolonged absence of enteral substrate, leading to intestinal maladaptation and extended exposure to parenteral nutrition (PN) and increasing the risk of other undesirable outcomes, such as cholestasis and PN-associated liver disease.

These authors studied a cohort of premature infants with enterostomies to determine whether early enteral fat and fish oil supplements would increase fat absorption and decrease the requirements for intravenous fat infusion. The infants were given usual care or a dietary supplement of a Microlipid and fish oil. Compared with the group with usual care, the treatment group tolerated a greater volume of enteral feedings and had less watery ostomy effluents. The other reported differences were expected, as defined by the intervention, and it is unclear whether these findings reflect a true physiologic benefit. For example, the treatment group had greater dietary fat intake (thus, less intravenous lipid infusion), greater fat excretion, and greater enteral calories, but there was no difference in weight gain. Despite this, the clinical findings of better feeding tolerance and improved ostomy output warrant further evaluation of the efficacy of enterally administered lipids in promoting intestinal adaptation and reducing the reliance on intravenous lipid infusions for all premature infants, not just those with ostomies. Of particular note is the finding that the total percentage of fat absorption was similarly low in both groups, with values consistent with disorders of exocrine pancreatic insufficiency. This is a critical variable that needs to be considered as therapeutic options are evaluated. Further studies of lipid polyunsaturated fatty acids (PUFA) enteral supplements for all preterm infants should include the effect of high-fat PUFA diets on the microbiome, total fat and specific fatty acid absorption rates, and systemic fatty acid levels to ensure adequate delivery and absorption of essential and critical fatty acids.

C. Martin, MD

Noninvasive measurement of fecal calprotectin and serum amyloid A combined with intestinal fatty acid–binding protein in necrotizing enterocolitis
Reisinger KW, Van Der Zee DC, Brouwers HAA, et al (Maastricht Univ Med Ctr, the Netherlands; Univ Med Ctr, Utrecht, the Netherlands)
J Pediatr Surg 47:1640-1645, 2012

Background.—Diagnosis of necrotizing enterocolitis (NEC), prevalent in premature infants, remains challenging. Enterocyte damage in NEC can be assessed by intestinal fatty acid–binding protein (I-FABP), with a sensitivity of 93% and a specificity of 90%. Numerous markers of inflammation are known, such as serum amyloid A (SAA) and fecal calprotectin.

Purpose.—The aim of the present study was to evaluate which combination of noninvasive measurement of inflammatory markers and I-FABP improves the diagnostic accuracy in neonates suspected for NEC.

Methods.—In 62 neonates with clinical suspicion of NEC (29 with final diagnosis of NEC), urinary I-FABP, urinary SAA, and fecal calprotectin levels were determined quantitatively. Diagnostic accuracy was calculated for the combinations I-FABP–SAA and I-FABP–fecal calprotectin, using a multivariable logistic regression model.

Results.—The combination of SAA and I-FABP did not increase the diagnostic accuracy of I-FABP. However, the combination of fecal calprotectin and I-FABP improved accuracy significantly. The combination of urinary I-FABP and fecal calprotectin measurement produced a sensitivity of 94%, a specificity of 79%, a positive likelihood ratio of 4.48, and a negative likelihood ratio of 0.08.

Conclusion.—The combination of noninvasive measurement of I-FABP and fecal calprotectin seems promising for diagnosing NEC at an early time point. Prospective analysis is required to confirm this finding and to evaluate better treatment strategies based on noninvasive measurement of I-FABP and calprotectin.

▶ The appropriate early diagnosis of necrotizing enterocolitis (NEC) is one of the major challenges faced in caring for newborns. The commonly used Bell's staging criteria along with its variants are somewhat problematic, especially because Stage 1 usually represents signs and symptoms that should raise concern but does not represent a distinct pathologic entity. Even stages 2 and 3 represent dilemmas. The clinician is commonly faced with a baby with a distended abdomen and a suspicious-appearing radiograph with air-filled loops of bowel but no pneumatosis intestinalis or portal venous gas. This could represent a baby who will subsequently require surgery (and the need for this may progress rapidly) or a baby with sepsis or simply feeding intolerance who will respond nicely to antibiotics and/or alterations in feeding. The need for better diagnostic biomarkers to help distinguish babies who are at highest risk for developing NEC is clear.

This study evaluated 62 neonates with a clinical suspicion of NEC, wherein 29 emerged with a final diagnosis of NEC. Urine and feces were sampled at the onset of suspicion. Serum amyloid A (SAA), intestinal fatty acid binding protein (IFABP), and fecal calprotectin were analyzed in these samples as diagnostic biomarkers. All of these biomarkers have been suggested to be efficacious in previous studies. One rationale for this study was to evaluate a combination of these to determine whether this would improve their diagnostic value.

Of interest, the sensitivity, specificity, likelihood ratios, areas under the curve, and cutoff values for urinary IFABP were quite similar to a study previously published by a group from the same center.[1] The addition of SAA to IFABP did not improve the diagnostic accuracy. This is not surprising because SAA alone does not appear to distinguish sepsis from NEC.[2] In this study, when fecal calprotectin was added to the IFABP measurement, the sensitivity, specificity, LR + and LR− of 94%, 79%, 4.48, and 0.08, respectively, were obtained. This appeared to show improved diagnostic accuracy compared with IFABP alone. However, it is also of interest that in the previous study from Thuijls et al,[1] the sensitivity, specificity, LR + and LR− were 93, 90, 9.3, and 0.08, respectively. The latter numbers were quite good in the previous study and, thus, they mitigate against the need for fecal calprotectin. Furthermore, as seen in this study, fecal calprotectin could be analyzed in only a limited number of babies because these samples are not available when we would like them (babies will not poop when asked to do so), a fact that also minimizes the value of adding the fecal calprotectin.

A caveat that needs to be raised about the design of this study as well as similarly designed studies is that these samples were not collected prospectively, but at the time of suspected onset of the disease. This can introduce bias into the study in which those babies with the most obvious signs and symptoms have their samples collected more readily than those whose signs and symptoms are less obvious. One other issue that needs to be questioned is why the authors chose not to also evaluate urinary claudin 3 levels in addition to the IFABP. This was a marker previously shown to also be promising by Thuijls et al.[1]

As suggested by the authors, this is certainly an important area that requires additional investigation.

J. Neu, MD

References

1. Thuijls G, Derikx JP, van Wijck K, et al. Non-invasive markers for early diagnosis and determination of the severity of necrotizing enterocolitis. *Ann Surg*. 2010;251:1174-1180.
2. Ng PC, Ang IL, Chiu RW, et al. Host-response biomarkers for diagnosis of late-onset septicemia and necrotizing enterocolitis in preterm infants. *J Clin Invest*. 2010;120:2989-3000.

Parenteral lipid administration to very-low-birth-weight infants—early introduction of lipids and use of new lipid emulsions: a systematic review and meta-analysis
Vlaardingerbroek H, Veldhorst MAB, Spronk S, et al (Erasmus MC—Sophia Children's Hosp, Rotterdam, Netherlands; Erasmus MC, Rotterdam, Netherlands; et al)
Am J Clin Nutr 96:255-268, 2012

Background.—The use of intravenous lipid emulsions in preterm infants has been limited by concerns regarding impaired lipid tolerance. As a result, the time of initiation of parenteral lipid infusion to very-low-birth-weight (VLBW) infants varies widely among different neonatal intensive care units. However, lipids provide energy for protein synthesis and supply essential fatty acids that are necessary for central nervous system development.

Objective.—The objective was to summarize the effects of initiation of lipids within the first 2 d of life and the effects of different lipid compositions on growth and morbidities in VLBW infants.

Design.—A systematic review and meta-analysis of publications identified in a search of PubMed, EMBASE, and Cochrane databases was undertaken. Randomized controlled studies were eligible if information on growth was available.

Results.—The search yielded 14 studies. No differences were observed in growth or morbidity with early lipid initiation. We found a weak favorable association of non—purely soybean-based emulsions with the incidence of sepsis (RR: 0.75; 95% CI: 0.56, 1.00).

Conclusions.—The initiation of lipids within the first 2 d of life in VLBW infants appears to be safe and well tolerated; however, beneficial effects on growth could not be shown for this treatment nor for the type of lipid emulsion. Emulsions that are not purely soybean oil-based might be associated with a lower incidence of sepsis. Large-scale randomized controlled trials in preterm infants are warranted to determine whether early initiation of lipids and lipid emulsions that are not purely soybean oil—based results in improved long-term outcomes.

▶ One of the most common nutritional practices in the neonatal intensive care unit that is not based on good evidence is the withholding of intravenous lipids in very-low-birth-weight (VLBW) babies who are not able to feed by the enteral route. Common practice is to not provide lipids for several days, then to begin slowly with increments of 0.5 g/kg/day. This is similar to the practice of withholding intravenous amino acids. However, with recent studies and recommendations,[1] this practice is becoming obsolete, but the practice of limiting lipids remains. This review and meta-analysis of 14 studies concludes that the initiation of lipids within the first 2 days of life in VLBW infants appears to be safe and well tolerated; however, beneficial effects on growth could not be shown for this treatment nor for the type of lipid provided. Nevertheless, lipids provide a major source of energy for these infants who have minimal energy stores and are known to prevent catabolism and improve amino acid utilization. Essential fatty acid deficiency also occurs in the majority of these infants within a week if they are not supplied either enterally or parenterally.[2] We also are finding that energy decrements in the first week after birth in these infants is associated with decrements in mental development indices at 18 months of age.[3] Most of the contraindications to providing lipids early to these babies are dogmas that have been propagated through the years with little-to-no evidence to support them, and evidence suggests that providing up to 3 g/kg/d right after birth is not associated with detrimental effects.[4] Until further studies are done, as suggested in this article, I see no reason to withhold lipids from these infants and to provide them with 3 g/kg/d as soon as possible after birth.

J. Neu, MD

References

1. Hay WW Jr. Strategies for feeding the preterm infant. *Neonatology.* 2008;94: 245-254.
2. Gutcher GR, Farrell PM. Intravenous infusion of lipid for the prevention of essential fatty acid deficiency in premature infants. *Am J Clin Nutr.* 1991;54:1024-1028.
3. Stephens BE, Walden RV, Gargus RA, et al. First-week protein and energy intakes are associated with 18-month developmental outcomes in extremely low birth weight infants. *Pediatrics.* 2009;123:1337-1343.
4. Ibrahim HM, Jeroudi MA, Baier RJ, Dhanireddy R, Krouskop RW. Aggressive early total parental nutrition in low-birth-weight infants. *J Perinatol.* 2004;24:482-486.

Creamatocrit Analysis of Human Milk Overestimates Fat and Energy Content When Compared to a Human Milk Analyzer Using Mid-infrared Spectroscopy

O'Neill EF, Radmacher PG, Sparks B, et al (Univ of Louisville, KY)
J Pediatr Gastroenterol Nutr 56:569-572, 2013

Background and Objective.—Human milk (HM) is the preferred feeding for human infants but may be inadequate to support the rapid growth of the very-low-birth-weight infant. The creamatocrit (CMCT) has been widely used to guide health care professionals as they analyze HM fortification; however, the CMCT method is based on an equation using assumptions for protein and carbohydrate with fat as the only measured variable. The aim of the present study was to test the hypothesis that a human milk analyzer (HMA) would provide more accurate data for fat and energy content than analysis by CMCT.

Methods.—Fifty-one well-mixed samples of previously frozen expressed HM were obtained after thawing. Previously assayed "control" milk samples were thawed and also run with unknowns. All milk samples were prewarmed at 40°C and then analyzed by both CMCT and HMA. CMCT fat results were substituted in the CMCT equation to reach a value for energy (kcal/oz). Fat results from HMA were entered into a computer model to reach a value for energy (kcal/oz). Fat and energy results were compared by paired t test with statistical significance set at $P < 0.05$. An additional 10 samples were

TABLE 2.—Comparison of Human Milk Fat and Energy by 3 Methods

	Fat content, g/dL			Energy, kcal/oz		
Sample	Human milk Analyzer*	Creamatocrit	Lab[†]	Human milk Analyzer*	Creamatocrit	Lab[‡]
1	4.0	6.1	4.0	19.6	22.5	19.8
2	2.6	5.0	2.5	15.4	20.5	15.7
3	3.8	6.9	3.7	19.5	23.9	19.5
4	5.8	10.5	5.7	24.4	30.2	24.2
5	2.8	5.1	2.6	15.9	20.8	16.1
6	3.7	7.6	3.9	18.7	25.1	19.0
7	2.9	4.9	2.9	16.2	20.2	16.8
8	3.1	5.0	3.0	17.0	20.5	17.0
9	3.2	5.4	3.3	17.2	21.2	17.8
10	3.2	4.7	3.1	17.3	20.0	17.5
Mean	3.5 ± 0.9	6.1 ± 1.8[§]	3.5 ± 0.9	18.1 ± 2.6	22.5 ± 3.2[‖]	18.3 ± 2.5

*Calais Human Milk Analyzer, Metron Instruments, Solon, OH.
[†]DQCI, Mounds View, MN.
[‡]Energy calculation: kcal/oz = ([9 × fat] + [4 × lactose] + [4 × protein])/3.34.
[§]$P < 0.001$ creamatocrit vs laboratory and HMA.
[‖]$P = 0.002$ creamatocrit vs laboratory and HMA.

analyzed locally by both methods and then sent to a certified laboratory for quantitative analysis. Results for fat and energy were analyzed by 1-way analysis of variance with statistical significance set at $P < 0.05$.

Results.—Mean fat content by CMCT (5.8 ± 1.9 g/dL) was significantly higher than by HMA (3.2 ± 1.1 g/dL, $P < 0.001$). Mean energy by CMCT (21.8 ± 3.4 kcal/oz) was also significantly higher than by HMA (17.1 ± 2.9, $P < 0.001$). Comparison of biochemical analysis with HMA of the subset of milk samples showed no statistical difference for fat and energy, whereas CMCT was significantly higher than for both fat ($P < 0.001$) and energy ($P = 0.002$).

Conclusions.—The CMCT method appears to overestimate fat and energy content of HM samples when compared with HMA and biochemical methods (Table 2).

▶ The creamatocrit technique for measuring fat and energy in milk has been used for more than 30 years. Similar in technique to measuring a hematocrit level, this method uses the percentage of cream to total volume, which is then substituted into an equation to yield energy (kcal/oz). The equation assumes constant protein and carbohydrate content, with fat being the only variable nutrient, which is not a correct assumption. Nevertheless, with fat providing a large percentage of the energy from human milk, the energy composition may vary somewhat but remains most dependent on fat concentration. This study compares fat and energy concentrations that are derived from a laboratory to a bedside commercially available human milk analyzer and the creamatocrit. The creamatocrit overestimated the human milk analyzer as well as the laboratory-derived fat concentration and energy content in most cases (Table 2).

Despite the overestimation, it was so consistent that it actually validated utility of the creamatocrit. One could readily adjust for the few extra points that were so consistently elevated. However, it shows that there are more accurate techniques available, especially when protein values are also desired as mentioned by the author. Adjusting the protein levels probably is just as valuable, if not more so, than the fat concentrations to obtain better growth. It is to be remembered that each infant is different and may still respond differently to intake, so measures of a baby's growth and responses to nutrients remain the most important criteria for adjusting feedings.

J. Neu, MD

Breast-feeding vs Formula-feeding for Infants Born Small-for-Gestational-Age: Divergent Effects on Fat Mass and on Circulating IGF-I and High-Molecular-Weight Adiponectin in Late Infancy

de Zegher F, Sebastiani G, Diaz M, et al (Univ of Leuven, Belgium; Univ of Barcelona, Esplugues, Spain; et al)
J Clin Endocrinol Metab 98:1242-1247, 2013

Context.—Fetal growth restraint, if followed by rapid weight gain, confers risk for adult disease including diabetes. How breast-feeding may lower such risk is poorly understood.

Objective, Study Participants, Intervention, Outcomes.—In infants born small-for-gestational-age (SGA), we studied the effects of nutrition in early infancy (breast-feeding vs formula-feeding; BRF vs FOF) on weight partitioning and endocrine markers in late infancy. Body composition (by absorptiometry), fasting glycemia, insulin, IGF-I, and high-molecular-weight (HMW) adiponectin were assessed at 4 and 12 months in BRF controls born appropriate-for-GA (N = 31) and in SGA infants receiving BRF (N = 48) or FOF (N = 51), the latter being randomized to receive a standard formula (FOF1) or a protein-rich formula (FOF2).

Setting.—The study was conducted in a University Hospital.

Results.—SGA-BRF infants maintained a low fat mass and normal levels of IGF-I and HMW adiponectin. In contrast, SGA-FOF infants normalized their body composition by gaining more fat; this normalization was accompanied by a marked fall in HMW adiponectinemia and, in FOF2 infants, by elevated IGF-I levels. In late infancy, SGA-BRF infants were most sensitive to insulin, even more sensitive than appropriate-for-GA—BRF controls.

Conclusions.—Because the health perspectives are better for SGA-BRF than for SGA-FOF infants, the present results suggest that FOF for SGA infants should aim at maintaining normal IGF-I and HMW-adiponectin levels rather than at normalizing body composition. Nutriceutical research for SGA infants may thus have to be redirected.

▶ Television commercials constantly bombard us with the concept that bigger is better. This is not necessarily so. Particularly for an intrauterine growth—restricted infant catching up with or surpassing his or her peers in weight, which looks good in the short term but may have dire consequences, such as the metabolic syndrome and diabetes, in the long term. These Spanish investigators, in comparing breast feeding with formula feeding for term infants born small for gestational age, show the underlying differences in fat mass and on circulating IGF-I and high-molecular-weight adiponectin in late infancy. Literally, you cannot have your cake and it eat too. The formula-fed infants gain weight and adipose tissue more readily, whereas the breast-fed infants catch up at a slower pace but retain a better metabolic profile.

I knew very little about adiponectin, so I looked it up and learned that it is a protein hormone secreted from adipose tissue that modulates a number of metabolic processes, including glucose regulation and fatty acid oxidation. The adiponectin gene is localized to chromosome 3q27, a region highlighted as affecting genetic susceptibility to type 2 diabetes and obesity. A low level of adiponectin is an independent risk factor for developing metabolic syndrome and diabetes mellitus. Surprisingly, low levels are found in obese individuals. Adiponectin has many functions, such as increasing glucose uptake, decreasing gluconeogenesis, enhancing lipid catabolism including triglyceride clearance and protection from endothelial dysfunction, and control of energy metabolism. It has direct effects on the brain in regulating appetite.

After reading this article, the logical and inevitable conclusion is that the use of human milk is highly desirable for growth-restricted babies. They will not catch up as quickly as formula-fed babies, but the risks of diabetes and the metabolic syndrome should be substantially reduced.

A. A. Fanaroff, MBBCh, FRCPE

A New Liquid Human Milk Fortifier and Linear Growth in Preterm Infants
Moya F, Sisk PM, Walsh KR, et al (Coastal Carolina Neonatology, Wilmington, NC; Wake Forest Univ School of Medicine, Winston-Salem, NC; Mead Johnson Nutrition, Evansville, IN)
Pediatrics 130:e928-e935, 2012

Objectives.—To evaluate the growth, tolerance, and safety of a new ultraconcentrated liquid human milk fortifier (LHMF) designed to provide optimal nutrients for preterm infants receiving human breast milk in a safe, nonpowder formulation.

Methods.—Preterm infants with a body weight ≤1250 g fed expressed and/or donor breast milk were randomized to receive a control powder human milk fortifier (HMF) or a new LHMF for 28 days. When added to breast milk, the LHMF provided ∼20% more protein than the control HMF. Weight, length, head circumference, and serum prealbumin, albumin, blood urea nitrogen, electrolytes, and blood gases were measured. The occurrence of sepsis, necrotizing enterocolitis, and serious adverse events were monitored.

Results.—This multicenter, third party–blinded, randomized controlled, prospective study enrolled 150 infants. Achieved weight and linear growth rate were significantly higher in the LHMF versus control groups ($P = .04$ and 0.03, respectively). Among infants who adhered closely to the protocol, the LHMF had a significantly higher achieved weight, length, head circumference, and linear growth rate than the control HMF ($P = .004$, $P = .003$, $P = .04$, and $P = .01$, respectively). There were no differences in measures of feeding tolerance or days to achieve full feeding volumes. Prealbumin, albumin, and blood urea nitrogen were higher in the LHMF group versus the control group (all $P < .05$). There was no difference in the incidence of confirmed sepsis or necrotizing enterocolitis.

Conclusions.—Use of a new LHMF in preterm infants instead of powder HMF is safe. Benefits of LHMF include improvements in growth and avoidance of the use of powder products in the NICU.

▶ Optimization of human milk fortification for very-low-birth-weight infants (VLBW, <1500 g birth weight) remains challenging. A Cochrane review reported that fortification of human milk improved short-term growth and increased nitrogen retention.[1] However, there were no long-term advantages in growth or neurodevelopmental outcomes. In fact, there wasn't even a clear effect on bone mineral content.[1]

Furthermore, comparisons between fortified human milk vs preterm formula fed to preterm infants showed slower growth despite the fortification.[2-5] Fifty-eight percent of VLBW infants fed predominantly fortified human milk had extra-uterine growth restriction at discharge.[6] Because postnatal growth failure is a surrogate for inadequate nutrition, which may lead to neurocognitive impairment, further refinements with human milk fortification are needed.

Short-term benefits of feeding human milk to preterm infants include protection against sepsis and necrotizing enterocolitis.[5,7-10] Longer-term benefits include less respiratory disease the first year of life and, of course, improved neurocognitive development.[11-14] Therefore, human milk is the preferred feeding for preterm infants as recently endorsed by the American Academy of Pediatrics.[15]

The conundrum for the VLBW infant is that human milk provides inadequate amounts of several nutrients, especially protein, vitamin D, calcium, phosphorus, and sodium. Donor milk has even less protein than a mother's own milk for her preterm infants. Human milk must, therefore, be fortified for many VLBW infants. Postnatal growth failure of VLBW infants is associated with poor neurocognitive outcome.[16,17] Inadequate protein is most likely responsible for the slow growth and poor outcomes.[18] Fortification with protein poses substantial challenges. It is limiting for growth and neurocognitive development. Therefore, shortfalls of protein, even modest ones, are not acceptable. However, protein intakes in excess of needs have been considered dangerous. To prevent poor neurocognitive outcomes as well as other specific nutrient deficiencies, such as osteopenia (inadequate calcium and phosphorus intake), nutrient fortification of human milk is necessary.[18]

Human milk fortifiers have been either liquid or powder. The Centers for Disease Control have recommended that all formulas used with high-risk infants be sterile because powder formulas may be contaminated and convey infections.[19] Liquid formulations are processed to be sterile, but powder formulations are not.[19]

A new liquid human milk fortifier providing approximately 20% more protein than the powdered fortifier was fed to 72 VLBW infants less than 1250 g birth weight for 28 days while controls were fed the powder human milk fortifier in a randomized, controlled, prospective study.[20] Both donor and mothers' own milk were used. Achieved weight gain and linear growth were significantly higher with the liquid fortifier. Head circumference was also greater among infants who adhered closely to the protocol. However, there were no significant differences in rates of mean weight growth between the liquid and powder, 15.8 + 0.5 g/kg/d vs 15.7 + 0.5 g/kg/d, respectively.[20] Mean length growth rate was higher for the liquid 0.16 + 0.006 cm/d vs 0.14 + 0.006 cm/d for powder.[20] The study concludes that feeding a traditional powdered fortifier or the new liquid was safe and well tolerated.

A traditional method used to sterilize a liquid formulation is to acidify the product. This new fortifier has been acidified to a pH of approximately 4.3 and also acidifies the human milk to approximately 4.7. The pH on blood gases was slightly higher in the controls in the liquid human milk fortifier trial, and means for HCO_3 were higher in the controls on day 6 (25.9 + 0.62 mEq/L vs 22.3 + 0.62 mEq/L; $P < .001$).[20]

Erickson et al tested the effects of acidification on human milk's cellular and nutritional content.[21] They divided 100 frozen samples of milk, collected from 8 mothers with infants in the neonatal intensive care unit, into 2 equal aliquots, control and acidified. They used citric acid to acidify.[21] Acidification caused significant reduction in white cells, lipase activity, and total protein but an increase in creamatocrit.[21] They speculate that acidification caused an increase in triglycerides and fewer free fatty acids and, therefore, decreased lipase activity in the milk, which may cause fat malabsorption.[21] Furthermore, they suggested that casein protein denaturation and precipitation explained the reduction in protein.[21]

Fortification of human milk has become more complex and controversial. Inadequate protein, slower growth, nonsterile powders, and acidification of liquids remain issues.[18]

Another controversy around fortification with bovine milk–based products is whether these increase the risk of necrotizing enterocolitis (NEC).[22] An exclusively human milk–based diet was associated with lower rates of medical and surgical NEC in a randomized trial.[22]

Finally, human milk analyzers using infrared spectroscopy that provide real-time rapid measures of fat, protein, lipase, and energy are being used to measure individual milk samples to customize and individualize human milk fortification.[23]

Growth, protein, acidification, bovine-based vs human milk–based, analyze and individualize—it is more complex than we thought. We are making progress realizing it really is all about the protein to grow lean and promote neurodevelopment. We just have to figure out how!

D. Adamkin, MD

References

1. Kuschel CA, Harding JE. Multicomponent fortified human milk for promoting growth in preterm infants. *Cochrane Database Syst Rev.* 2004;(1):CD000343.
2. Carlson SJ, Ziegler EE. Nutrient intakes and growth of very low birth weight infants. *J Perinatol.* 1998;18:252-258.

3. Olsen IE, Richardson DK, Schmid CH, Ausman LM, Dwyer JT. Intersite differences in weight growth velocity of extremely premature infants. *Pediatrics.* 2002;110:1125-1132.
4. Pieltain C, De Curtis M, Gérard P, Rigo J. Weight gain composition in preterm infants with dual energy X-ray absorptiometry. *Pediatr Res.* 2001;49:120-124.
5. Schanler RJ, Shulman RJ, Lau C. Feeding strategies for premature infants: beneficial outcomes of feeding fortified human milk versus preterm formula. *Pediatrics.* 1999;103:1150-1157.
6. Henriksen C, Westerberg AC, Rønnestad A, et al. Growth and nutrient intake among very-low-birth-weight infants fed fortified human milk during hospitalisation. *Br J Nutr.* 2009;102:1179-1186.
7. Furman L, Taylor G, Minich N, Hack M. The effect of maternal milk on neonatal morbidity of very low-birth-weight infants. *Arch Pediatr Adolesc Med.* 2003; 157:66-71.
8. Henderson G, Anthony MY, McGuire W. Formula milk versus maternal breast milk for feeding preterm or low birth weight infants. *Cochrane Database Syst Rev.* 2007;(4):CD002972.
9. Henderson G, Craig S, Brocklehurst P, McGuire W. Enteral feeding regimens and necrotising enterocolitis in preterm infants: a multicentre case-control study. *Arch Dis Child Fetal Neonatal Ed.* 2009;94:F120-F123.
10. Sisk PM, Lovelady CA, Dillard RG, Gruber KJ, O'Shea TM. Early human milk feeding is associated with a lower risk of necrotizing enterocolitis in very low birth weight infants. *J Perinatol.* 2007;27:428-433.
11. Blaymore Bier JA, Oliver T, Ferguson A, Vohr BR. Human milk reduces outpatient upper respiratory symptoms in premature infants during their first year of life. *J Perinatol.* 2002;22:354-359.
12. Bier JA, Oliver T, Ferguson AE, Vohr BR. Human milk improves cognitive and motor development of premature infants during infancy. *J Hum Lact.* 2002;18: 361-367.
13. O'Connor DL, Jacobs J, Hall R, et al. Growth and development of premature infants fed predominantly human milk, predominantly premature infant formula, or a combination of human milk and premature formula. *J Pediatr Gastroenterol Nutr.* 2003;37:437-446.
14. Vohr BR, Poindexter BB, Dusick AM, et al. Beneficial effects of breast milk in the neonatal intensive care unit on the developmental outcome of extremely low birth weight infants at 18 months of age. *Pediatrics.* 2006;118:e115-e123.
15. Section on Breastfeeding. Breastfeeding and the use of human milk. *Pediatrics.* 2012;129:e827-e841.
16. Ehrenkranz RA, Dusick AM, Vohr BR, Wright LL, Wrage LA, Poole WK. Growth in the neonatal intensive care unit influences neurodevelopmental and growth outcomes of extremely low birth weight infants. *Pediatrics.* 2006;117:1253-1261.
17. Weisglas-Kuperus N, Hille ET, Duivenvoorden HJ, et al; Dutch POPS-19 Collaborative Study Group. Intelligence of very preterm or very low birthweight infants in young adulthood. *Arch Dis Child Fetal Neonatal Ed.* 2009;94:F196-F200.
18. Arslanoglu S, Moro GE, Ziegler EE. Preterm infants fed fortified human milk receive less protein than they need. *J Perinatol.* 2009;29:489-492.
19. Baker RD. Infant formula safety. *Pediatrics.* 2002;110:833-835.
20. Moya F, Sisk PM, Walsh KR, Berseth CL. A new liquid human milk fortifier and linear growth in preterm infants. *Pediatrics.* 2012;130:e928-e935.
21. Erickson T, Gill G, Chan GM. The effects of acidification on human milk's cellular and nutritional content. *J Perinatol.* 2012;33:371-373.
22. Sullivan S, Schanler RJ, Kim JH, et al. An exclusively human milk-based diet is associated with a lower rate of necrotizing enterocolitis than a diet of human milk and bovine milk-based products. *J Pediatr.* 2010;156:562-567.e1.
23. Sauer CW, Kim JH. Human milk macronutrient analysis using point-of-care near-infrared spectrophotometry. *J Perinatol.* 2011;31:339-343.

Bacteriological, Biochemical, and Immunological Modifications in Human Colostrum After Holder Pasteurisation

Espinosa-Martos I, Montilla A, Gómez de Segura A, et al (Universidad Complutense de Madrid, Spain; CEI (CSIC+UAM), Madrid, Spain; et al)

J Pediatr Gastroenterol Nutr 56:560-568, 2013

Objective.—The objective of this work was to evaluate the effect of Holder pasteurisation of human colostrum on a variety of microbiological, biochemical, and immunological parameters.

Methods.—Colostrum samples from 10 donors, and 8 samples of mature milk used as controls, were heated at 62.5 °C for 30 minutes. Bacterial counts and the concentration of furosine, lactose, myoinositol, glucose, lactulose, cytokines, and immunoglobulins were determined before and after the heat treatment.

Results.—Mean bacterial counts in nonpasteurised colostrum samples oscillated between 2.72 and 4.13 $\log_{10}$ colony-forming units per millilitre in the agar media tested. Holder pasteurisation led to the destruction of the bacteria originally present in the samples. Furosine was detected in all samples before pasteurisation and increased significantly after the heat treatment (from 6.60 to 20.59 mg/100 g protein). Lactulose content was below the detection limit in nonpasteurised colostrum, but it was detected in all samples and quantified in 7 of them (from 10.68 to 38.02 mg/L) after Holder pasteurisation. Lactose, glucose, and myoinositol concentrations did not change after Holder pasteurisation. The concentrations of most cytokines and immunoglobulins were significantly higher in colostrum than in mature milk samples. Immunoglobulin content, both in colostrum and in milk samples, was reduced during pasteurisation, whereas, among cytokines, only macrophage inflammatory protein-1β, interleukin-7, and granulocyte-macrophage-colony-stimulating factor concentrations were affected by this heat treatment.

Conclusions.—Lactulose and furosine content could be used as heat treatment indicators in colostrum samples. Holder pasteurisation modified the immunological profile of both colostrum and mature milk.

▶ Holder pasteurization involves heating of donor human milk to 62.5°C for 30 minutes and is the technique required by the Human Milk Banking Association of North America and several other human milk banking associations.[1] Although considerable research already exists on the effects of pasteurization on mature human milk, the focus of this article is on its effect on colostrum with a comparison to mature human milk. Several take-home messages can be derived from this article:

1. Protein concentration is significantly higher in colostrum than in mature milk; thus the results of previous studies on mature milk cannot be directly extrapolated to colostrum.

2. Pasteurization eliminated growth of all bacteria studied in colostrum. The fact that many of the bacteria recently found in colostrum may actually be

commensal with beneficial effects on the host may actually be a negative effect of pasteurization.

3. Most of the nutritional value of lactose, myoinositol, and glucose appear to be unaffected.

4. Most cytokine and chemokine concentrations are considerably higher in colostrum compared with mature milk, but are minimally, if at all, affected by pasteurization.

5. Immunoglobulin M and A are present in higher concentrations in colostrum than in mature milk, and both are significantly decreased with pasteurization.

Overall, it remains obvious that colostrum contains numerous bioactive components that could be beneficial for the infant. Whatever is available should be provided to the infant from the baby's own mother when feasible. Pasteurized colostrum is still higher in certain factors, such as immunoglobulin A and M, transforming growth factor-β, and macrophage inflammatory protein, when compared with mature human milk, so if it is available (often it is a very precious and rare commodity), it should be used in the most vulnerable infants.

J. Neu, MD

Reference

1. Tully DB, Jones F, Tully MR. Donor milk: what's in it and what's not. *J Hum Lact.* 2001;17:152-155.

Prevention of Invasive *Cronobacter* Infections in Young Infants fed Powdered Infant Formulas

Jason J (Jason and Jarvis Associates, Hilton Head Island, SC)
Pediatrics 130:e1076-e1084, 2012

Background.—Invasive *Cronobacter* infection is rare, devastating, and epidemiologically/microbiologically linked to powdered infant formulas (PIFs). In 2002—2004, the US Food and Drug Administration advised health care professionals to minimize PIF and powdered human milk fortifier (HMF)'s preparation, feeding, and storage times and avoid feeding them to hospitalized premature or immunocompromised neonates. Labels for PIF used at home imply PIF is safe for healthy, term infants if label instructions are followed.

Methods.—1) Medical, public health, Centers for Disease Control and Prevention, US Food and Drug Administration, and World Health Organization records, publications, and personal communications were used to compare 68 (1958—2003) and 30 (2004—2010) cases of invasive *Cronobacter* disease in children without underlying disorders. 2) The costs of PIFs and ready-to-feed formulas (RTFs) were compared.

Results.—Ninety-nine percent (95/96) of all infected infants were <2 months old. In 2004—2010, 59% (17/29) were term, versus 24% (15/63) in 1958—2003; 52% (15/29) became symptomatic at home, versus

21% (13/61). Of all infected infants, 26% (22/83) had received breast milk (BM), 23% (19/82) RTF, and 90% (76/84) PIF or HMF. Eight percent received BM and not PIF/HMF; 5%, RTF without PIF/HMF. For at least 10 PIF-fed infants, label instructions were reportedly followed. Twenty-four ounces of milk-based RTF cost $0.84 more than milk-based PIF; 24 ounces of soy-based RTF cost $0.24 less than soy-based PIF.

Conclusions.—*Cronobacter* can infect healthy, term (not just hospitalized preterm) young infants. Invasive *Cronobacter* infection is extremely unusual in infants not fed PIF/HMF. RTFs are commercially sterile, require minimal preparation, and are competitively priced. The exclusive use of BM and/or RTF for infants <2 months old should be encouraged.

▶ *Cronobacter* is a multispecies genus of gram-negative microbes that, before 2007, was classified as *Enterobacter sakazakii*. Numerous outbreaks of *Cronobacter* have been reported in neonatal intensive care units (NICUs) and in those evaluated, all of the affected infants received some form of powdered infant formula. The disease manifested by infants infected with this pathogen resembles meningitis, necrotizing enterocolitis, and/or sepsis. This retrospective study evaluated records from several sources, including the Centers for Disease Control and Prevention, the US Food and Drug Administration, and the World Health Organization, to better determine the scope of this problem beyond that seen in NICUs and to determine the effects of safety labeling on prevention of the disease.

The results showed that the vast majority of these infants were younger than 2 months of age and more than 50% were term in the years 2004—2010. Only 8% of the infants who had the disease received breast milk without powdered infant formula/human milk fortifier. In many of the infected infants, US Food and Drug Administration guidelines and labeling instructions reportedly were followed.

The author of this article states several caveats that may have biased her studies, including reporting bias between formula-fed and breast-fed babies and problems with parental recall that may implicate the feeding rather than an exogenous source (eg, contaminated water, nipples). However, it is highly important that *Cronobacter* has never been isolated from breast milk, unopened bottled water, treated US municipal drinking water, unopened ready-to-feed formula, or unopened concentrates.

As suggested in the article, babies should be exclusively breast fed, but if commercial supplements are given, they should be in the form of ready-to-feed bottles. The cost of this is higher than powdered preparations, but at a cost of approximately $0.84 per day for ready-to-feed preparations.

J. Neu, MD

Association Between Maternal Use of Folic Acid Supplements and Risk of Autism Spectrum Disorders in Children
Surén P, Roth C, Bresnahan M, et al (Norwegian Inst of Public Health, Nydalen, Oslo, Norway; Columbia Univ, NY; et al)
JAMA 309:570-577, 2013

Importance.—Prenatal folic acid supplements reduce the risk of neural tube defects in children, but it has not been determined whether they protect against other neurodevelopmental disorders.

Objective.—To examine the association between maternal use of prenatal folic acid supplements and subsequent risk of autism spectrum disorders (ASDs) (autistic disorder, Asperger syndrome, pervasive developmental disorder—not otherwise specified [PDD-NOS]) in children.

Design, Setting, and Patients.—The study sample of 85 176 children was derived from the population-based, prospective Norwegian Mother and Child Cohort Study (MoBa). The children were born in 2002-2008; by the end of follow-up on March 31, 2012, the age range was 3.3 through 10.2 years (mean, 6.4 years). The exposure of primary interest was use of folic acid from 4 weeks before to 8 weeks after the start of pregnancy, defined as the first day of the last menstrual period before conception. Relative risks of ASDs were estimated by odds ratios (ORs) with 95% CIs in a logistic regression analysis. Analyses were adjusted for maternal education level, year of birth, and parity.

Main Outcome Measure.—Specialist-confirmed diagnosis of ASDs.

Results.—At the end of follow-up, 270 children in the study sample had been diagnosed with ASDs: 114 with autistic disorder, 56 with Asperger syndrome, and 100 with PDD-NOS. In children whose mothers took folic acid, 0.10% (64/61 042) had autistic disorder, compared with 0.21% (50/24 134) in those unexposed to folic acid. The adjusted OR for autistic disorder in children of folic acid users was 0.61 (95% CI, 0.41-0.90). No association was found with Asperger syndrome or PDD-NOS, but power was limited. Similar analyses for prenatal fish oil supplements showed no such association with autistic disorder, even though fish oil use was associated with the same maternal characteristics as folic acid use.

Conclusions and Relevance.—Use of prenatal folic acid supplements around the time of conception was associated with a lower risk of autistic disorder in the MoBa cohort. Although these findings cannot establish causality, they do support prenatal folic acid supplementation.

▶ More than 20 years ago, an inverse association between maternal folate status and incidence of infants born with neural tube defects (NTDs) was recognized. This led US health agencies to recommend that women of childbearing age consume 400 μg of folic acid each day. Of interest is that the increased use of folic acid supplementation directly coincided with the time that many feel is the apparent beginning and continuous increase in the prevalence of autism and related autism spectrum disorders in the United States. Are these similar time frames of changes in maternal folate status and possible autism prevalence a random event, or has improved maternal (and fetal) folate status during pregnancy played a role? This has caused concern that folic acid supplementation may be a double-edged sword.

This study used a large Norwegian cohort to evaluate the effects of periconceptional folic acid supplementation on the subsequent development of autism and related disorders. The controls included a cohort that was studied for fish oil consumption, which did not show an effect on autism, whereas folic acid supplementation resulted in a significant odds ratio of 0.6. Overall, this is a well-done study, albeit with limitations of such large epidemiologic studies that do not prove causality but, rather, associations. Adding to the credibility of the association of folic acid on decreased autism, other studies suggest that folic acid antagonists such as valproate may increase embryopathy and also has been suggested to increase autism.

Folic acid—related molecular nutrition is complex with too numerous biochemical spheres of influence to predict effects in a generalizable way. Several gene variants and other nutrients are interactive factors. Despite all the good news on folic acid supplementation, it should still be a focus of active investigation, and we need to keep an open mind when it comes to public policy for routine supplementation.

J. Neu, MD

Oral L-arginine supplementation and faecal calprotectin levels in very low birth weight neonates

Polycarpou E, Zachaki S, Papaevangelou V, et al ('Alexandra' Hosp, Athens, Greece; NCSR 'Demokritos', Athens, Greece; Athens Univ, Greece; et al)
J Perinatol 33:141-146, 2013

Objective.—The objective of this study is to determine the potential effect of oral L-arginine supplementation on intestinal inflammation in very low birth weight (VLBW) neonates, as estimated by faecal calprotectin levels.

Study Design.—The study enrolled 83 VLBW neonates with birth weight ≤ 1500 g and gestational age ≤ 34 weeks. In this double-blind study, 40 neonates received daily oral L-arginine supplementation of 1.5 mmol kg^{-1} per day between the 3rd and 28th day of life, and 43 neonates placebo. Stool samples were collected on days 3, 14 and 28, and calprotectin was measured by enzyme-linked immunosorbent assay.

Result.—Calprotectin values significantly decreased over time in both groups ($P = 0.032$). No difference in faecal calprotectin values was recorded between neonates receiving arginine supplementation and neonates receiving placebo at days 3, 14 and 28.

Conclusion.—Faecal calprotectin values decrease with increasing postnatal age in VLBW infants, but this is not related to arginine supplementation.

▶ It has been known for more than a decade that plasma arginine concentrations in babies who subsequently have necrotizing enterocolitis (NEC) are low when compared with those who do not.[1] A study by Amin et al[2] suggested that supplementation with a combination of parenteral and enteral arginine could prevent NEC. It was suggested that more studies were needed to support this notion. This study by Polycarpou et al was not adequately powered to determine whether NEC could be prevented by enteral arginine supplementation but aimed at a reduction of fecal calprotectin, an inflammatory marker previously found to be elevated before the development of NEC. Calprotectin levels were measured on days 3, 14, and 28, and NEC incidence was monitored. Fecal calprotectin levels did not differ at any of the time points between arginine-supplemented or control infants. Of interest was that the concentration of fecal calprotectin did decrease during this time, suggesting a fecal inflammation in the meconium of these infants that was not found in the later specimens. Two other findings were of interest. The NEC incidence was 23% and 10% in the controls and arginine-treated infants, respectively, suggesting a benefit of arginine, but this did not reach statistical significance. Four of the control infants, but none in the arginine-supplemented group, died of NEC-related causes ($P = .045$). There was also a trend for lower calprotectin levels in the breast milk—fed group compared with the control group at 28 days, but this did not reach statistical significance.

Although the results of this study are largely negative from a statistical perspective, the reduction in NEC remains intriguing in light of the previous results of Amin et al.[2] Such a percentage reduction, if supported in a larger trial, could result in a number needed to treat of about 8 to prevent 1 case of NEC.

J. Neu, MD

References

1. Becker RM, Wu G, Galanko JA, et al. Reduced serum amino acid concentrations in infants with necrotizing enterocolitis. *J Pediatr.* 2000;137:785-793.
2. Amin HJ, Zamora SA, McMillan DD, et al. Arginine supplementation prevents necrotizing enterocolitis in the premature infant. *J Pediatr.* 2002;140:425-431.

Selected Macro/Micronutrient Needs of the Routine Preterm Infant
Bhatia J, Griffin I, Anderson D, et al (Georgia Health Sciences Univ, Augusta; Univ of California Davis Med Ctr, Sacramento; Baylor College of Medicine, Houston TX; et al)
J Pediatr 162:S48-S55, 2013

Requirements for optimal nutrition, especially for micronutrients, are not well defined for premature infants. The "reference fetus," developed by Ziegler et al,[1] has served as a model to define nutritional needs and studies designed to determine nutrient requirements. Revision of nutrient requirements and provision of optimal nutrition may lead to improved outcomes in preterm infants. Appropriate provision of nutrients also may help prevent nutritional disorders, such as metabolic bone disease and anemia. In this review, we discuss calcium, phosphorus, magnesium, vitamin D, iron, and copper, and define optimal intakes based on the available published data.

▶ One of the most confusing areas of nutrition for preterm infants involves the requirement of various micronutrients, such as calcium, phosphorus, magnesium, zinc, vitamin D, copper, and iron. This article reviews the physiology and function of these micronutrients, their estimated requirements, their enteral absorption, and difficulties with parenteral administration. Some of the most recent studies that have researched the requirements for these micronutrients are reviewed, and gaps in our knowledge that still remain about these critical nutrients are discussed. Previous guidelines are provided as well as a rationale for areas wherein these guidelines needed to be revised, and new guidelines are provided where appropriate. Comparisons are made wherein the guidelines may differ depending on the source of these differences (eg, American Academy of Pediatrics, European Society of Pediatric Gastroenterology, Hepatology, and Nutrition and World Health Organization). Finally, recommendations are made depending on gestational age, geographical considerations, and concomitant conditions (eg, previous blood loss, erythropoietin use). Overall, this is a very useful article that provides an excellent update in the area of micronutrient needs and recommended provision in the preterm infant.

J. Neu, MD

Copper Levels in Cholestatic Infants on Parenteral Nutrition
Corkins MR, Martin VA, Szeszycki EE (Indiana Univ School of Medicine, Indianapolis)
JPEN J Parenter Enteral Nutr 37:92-96, 2013

Background.—Copper levels are primarily regulated by biliary excretion. In cholestatic patients, there is a concern that the standard dose of copper in parenteral nutrition (PN) will result in excessive copper levels. This study looked retrospectively at cholestatic infants receiving PN with measured copper levels to ascertain if this is an actual clinical concern.

Methods.—All infants from the previous 10 years receiving PN who had a copper level checked and were cholestatic were reviewed. Children with metabolic or liver structural anomalies were excluded from the review. Of the 28 patients found, 26 had gastrointestinal disorders, and 82% of these infants were on the standard PN copper dose (20 µg/kg/d).

Results.—Only one elevated copper level was found in a child with congenital heart disease, but 13 low levels were found. A smaller number of follow-up copper levels demonstrated that despite cholestasis, some patients require copper supplementation above standard recommendations.

Conclusion.—Cholestasis does not appear to impair copper excretion enough to result in elevated levels. In fact, infants with gastrointestinal disorders may require higher than standard dosing. Monitoring copper levels appears to be necessary to appropriately regulate copper dosing for cholestatic infants receiving PN.

▶ It is common practice to reduce or eliminate copper (Cu) supplementation in the parenteral nutrition of infants with cholestasis because of the increased risk of hepatotoxicity. This practice of providing "cholestatic total parenteral nutrition" (TPN) that is devoid of Cu partially stems from the realization that trace minerals such as Cu and manganese are normally excreted in the bile. This prompted a cautionary note from the American Society for Clinical Nutrition Subcommittee on Pediatric Parenteral Nutrient Requirements: "Considerable caution is required in administering intravenous Cu to patients with impaired biliary excretion including those with TPN cholestasis."[1]

This article and another recent study[2] both suggest that supplementation of parenteral Cu at 20 μg/kg/day does not lead to a significant increase in Cu toxicity or worsening of liver disease in cholestatic infants. In fact, the current study, which evaluated infants who were receiving standard Cu dosing and had Cu levels drawn once, twice, and occasionally 3 times, shows no significant correlation between Cu levels and cholestasis as determined by concentrations of direct bilirubin. In fact, several patients actually required increased Cu dosing because of low serum levels, even if they were cholestatic. These authors provide sage advice that may change the practice in many neonatal intensive care units caring for cholestatic children. They state that cholestatic infants do not appear to require an automatic reduction of the Cu in their parenteral nutrition. In fact, some infants appear to require increased Cu supplementation despite being cholestatic. They recommend using standard dosing in cholestatic children but monitoring Cu levels.

J. Neu, MD

References

1. Greene HL, Hambidge KM, Schanler R, Tsang RC. Guidelines for the use of vitamins, trace elements, calcium, magnesium, and phosphorus in infants and children receiving total parenteral nutrition: report of the Subcommittee on Pediatric Parenteral Nutrient Requirements from the Committee on Clinical Practice Issues of the American Society for Clinical Nutrition. *Am J Clin Nutr.* 1988;48: 1324-1342.
2. Frem J, Sarson Y, Sternberg T, Cole CR. Copper supplementation in parenteral nutrition of cholestatic infants. *J Pediatr Gastroenterol Nutr.* 2010;50: 650-654.

A randomized trial of vitamin D supplementation in 2 community health center networks in South Carolina

Wagner CL, McNeil R, Hamilton SA, et al (Med Univ of South Carolina, Charleston; Durham Veterans Affairs Med Ctr, NC; Eau Claire Cooperative Health Ctrs, Columbia, SC)

Am J Obstet Gynecol 208:137.e1-137.e13, 2013

Objective.—We sought to determine whether 4000 IU/d (vs 2000 IU/d) of vitamin D during pregnancy is safe and improves maternal/neonatal 25-hydroxyvitamin D [25(OH)D] in a dose-dependent manner.

Study Design.—A total of 257 pregnant women 12-16 weeks' gestation were enrolled. Randomization to 2000 vs 4000 IU/d followed 1-month run-in at 2000 IU/d. Participants were monitored for hypercalciuria, hypercalcemia, and 25(OH)D status.

Results.—Maternal 25(OH)D (n = 161) increased from 22.7 ng/mL (SD 9.7) at baseline to 36.2 ng/mL (SD 15) and 37.9 ng/mL (SD 13.5) in the 2000 and 4000 IU groups, respectively. While maternal 25(OH)D change from baseline did not differ between groups, 25(OH)D monthly increase differed between groups ($P < .01$). No supplementation-related adverse events occurred. Mean cord blood 25(OH)D was 22.1 ± 10.3 ng/mL in 2000 IU and 27.0 ± 13.3 ng/mL in 4000 IU groups ($P = .024$). After controlling for race and study site, preterm birth and labor were inversely associated with predelivery and mean 25(OH)D, but not baseline 25(OH)D.

Conclusion.—Maternal supplementation with vitamin D 2000 and 4000 IU/d during pregnancy improved maternal/neonatal vitamin D status. Evidence of risk reduction in infection, preterm labor, and preterm birth was suggestive, requiring additional studies powered for these endpoints.

▶ Vitamin D deficiency shares several risk factors with poor birth outcomes, including young maternal age, obesity, and African-American race. Because of its potential modifiability, manipulation of vitamin D status during pregnancy has become an area of active research. Wagner et al performed a randomized, double-blind trial of 2000 IU/d vs 4000 IU/d during pregnancy to show safety and dose response of high doses of vitamin D. Randomization resulted in no significant differences in baseline characteristics or in complications of pregnancy. However, among trial completers, 28.9% (24 of 83) of women in the lower-dose group experienced preterm labor compared with 16.7% (13 of 78) in the higher-dose group ($P = .09$). Preterm delivery did not differ in the 2 groups ($P = 1.0$). Increase in maternal serum 25-hydroxyvitamin D level was similar in the 2 groups (from 22.7 ng/mL to 36.2 ng/mL and 37.9 ng/mL in the low- and high-risk groups, respectively); however, umbilical cord 25-hydroxyvitamin D was significantly higher in the 4000-IU group (vs 2000-IU group) (27.0 vs 22.1, $P = .024$.) Maternal calcium levels were similar (8.9 mg/dL in the 2000-IU group and 9.0 mg/dL in the 4000-IU group), but parathyroid hormone differed (17.5 pg/mL in the low-dose group vs 15.2 in the high-dose group). The authors conclude that these doses are safe because there were no cases of hypervitaminosis D. Secondary analyses showed that for every 10-ng/mL increment of 25-hydroxyvitamin D, there were decreased odds of preterm delivery (odds ratio [OR], 0.46; $P = .001$) and infection (OR, 0.74; $P = .026$). This study is of clinical relevance because some pregnant women are already taking high doses of vitamin D during pregnancy before safety and efficiency have been established. Findings of the study of Wagner et al should be interpreted cautiously, especially because the investigators did not adjust for body mass index, which can significantly confound such findings.

H. Burris, MD

Development of Pyloric Stenosis After a 4-Day Course of Oral Erythromycin
Lozada LE, Royall MJ, Nylund CM, et al (Univ of the Health Sciences, Bethesda, MD)
Pediatr Emerg Care 29:498-499, 2013

Early exposure to oral erythromycin in young infants, particularly in the first 2 weeks of life, has previously been associated with the development of hypertrophic pyloric stenosis. We report a case of an infant who received an abbreviated 4-day course of oral erythromycin for suspected *Chlamydia* conjunctivitis at 5 days of life then underwent pyloromyotomy for pyloric stenosis less than 2 weeks later. Health care providers should use erythromycin judiciously in neonates because only a few days of exposure to this medication may lead to the development of a surgical condition of gastric outlet obstruction.

▶ This report of a case of pyloric stenosis in an infant who received oral erythromycin for only 4 days should serve as a reminder of the potential complications of using this drug. In this particular instance, it was used for conjunctivitis. In neonatal intensive care, oral erythromycin is being used more commonly in preterm infants, in whom its use in moderate-to-high doses may promote feeding tolerance and decrease cholestasis.[1] However, it is to be noted that this complication seems to be rare and has not been reported in preterm infants receiving it for improvement of gastric emptying and feeding tolerance. Nevertheless, these occasional reports of pyloric stenosis, in addition to the unknown effects on the intestinal microbiota, should raise enough concern to refrain from routine use of this drug, reserving it for those babies for whom other nonpharmacologic techniques (eg, positioning, longer feeding intervals) have been tried. Furthermore, if a trial of this drug is used for the purpose of improving feeding tolerance for a few days and a benefit is not clear, it should be discontinued. If it shows benefit, a trial of discontinuance after a couple of weeks of maturation in the baby is warranted.

J. Neu, MD

Reference

1. Ng PC. Use of oral erythromycin for the treatment of gastrointestinal dysmotility in preterm infants. *Neonatology.* 2009;95:97-104.

Maternal exposure to bisphenol A and genistein has minimal effect on A^{vy}/a offspring coat color but favors birth of agouti over nonagouti mice

Rosenfeld CS, Sieli PT, Warzak DA, et al (Univ of Missouri, Columbia)
Proc Natl Acad Sci U S A 110:537-542, 2013

Reports that maternal diet influences coat color in mouse offspring carrying the agouti A^{vy} allele have received considerable attention because the range, from pseudoagouti (brown) to yellow, predicts adult health outcomes, especially disposition toward obesity and diabetes, in yellower mice. Bisphenol A (BPA), an endocrine-disrupting compound with estrogenic properties, fed to a/a dams harboring A^{vy}/a conceptuses has been reported to induce a significant shift toward yellower mice, whereas consumption of either genistein (G) alone or in combination with BPA led to greater numbers of healthy, brown offspring. Groups of C57/B6 a/a females, which are nonagouti, were fed either a phytoestrogen-free control diet or one of six experimental diets: diets 1−3 contained BPA (50 mg, 5 mg, and 50 µg BPA/kg food, respectively); diet 4 contained G (250 mg/kg food); diet 5 contained G plus BPA (250 and 50 mg/kg food, respectively); and diet 6 contained 0.1 µg of ethinyl estradiol (EE)/kg food. Mice were bred to A^{vy}/a males over multiple parities. In all, 2,824 pups from 426 litters were born. None of the diets provided any significant differences in relative numbers of brown, yellow, or intermediate coat color A^{vy}/a offspring. However, BPA plus G ($P < 0.0001$) and EE diets ($P = 0.005$), but not the four others, decreased the percentage of black (a/a) to A^{vy}/a offspring from the expected Mendelian ratio of 1:1. Data suggest that A^{vy}/a conceptuses, which may possess a so-called "thrifty genotype," are at a competitive advantage over a/a conceptuses in certain uterine environments.

▶ Whether the effects of toxic exposures in pregnancy could be mitigated by dietary interventions remains an unknown but active area of animal research. The agouti mouse model is ideal for studying environmental effects on phenotype. Agouti mice have different phenotypes despite identical genotypes thought to be a result of DNA methylation differences of the agouti A^{vy} locus. They can range from having yellow to brown coat colors, with yellow A^{vy}/a mice having a predisposition to obesity and tumors compared with the brown healthier mice (more similar to a/a mice). Prior studies have found that supplementing dams with phytoestrogens (genistein) during pregnancy alters offspring coat color to brown and improves health outcomes.[1] Bisphenol A (BPA) has been shown to shift the coat color to yellow with the less-healthy phenotype. Most exciting was the discovery that exposure to BPA could be mitigated by supplementing dams with genistein or a diet high in methyl-group donors (folic acid and others).[2] However, Rosenfeld et al were unable to replicate these findings in a recent study of 426 litters and 2824 pups. These authors were unable to detect differences in coat color by maternal diet in A^{vy}/a offspring. They compared 6 diets with a phytoestrogen-free control diet, including 3 tiers of BPA exposure, high-dose BPA plus genistein, genistein alone, and ethinyl estradiol. Notably, they found that the genotypes of offspring were not evenly distributed as Mendelian genetics would predict. Instead, in the BPA plus genistein and in the ethyl estradiol—supplemented pregnancies, a significantly higher proportion of the offspring were A^{vy}/a (68.3% and 59.2%, respectively). This finding raises the possibility of in utero, competitive advantage (as opposed to epigenetic alteration) of fetuses with the potentially thrifty A^{vy} genotype, despite the potential for later-in-life adverse health consequences.

L. J. Van Marter, MD, MPH

References

1. Dolinoy DC, Weidman JR, Waterland RA, Jirtle RL. Maternal genistein alters coat color and protects Avy mouse offspring from obesity by modifying the fetal epigenome. *Environ Health Perspect.* 2006;114:567-572.
2. Dolinoy DC, Huang D, Jirtle RL. Maternal nutrient supplementation counteracts bisphenol A-induced DNA hypomethylation in early development. *Proc Natl Acad Sci U S A.* 2007;104:13056-13061.

The next generation of disease risk: Are the effects of prenatal nutrition transmitted across generations? Evidence from animal and human studies
Roseboom TJ, Watson ED (Academic Med Centre, Amsterdam, The Netherlands; Univ of Cambridge, UK)
Placenta 33:e40-e44, 2012

Suboptimal intrauterine conditions, including poor nutrition, during critical periods of growth may lead to lifelong changes in the body's organs and tissues, thus providing a physiological basis for adult-onset disease. Remarkably, recent evidence suggests that the long-term consequences of adverse conditions during early development may not be limited to one generation, but may lead to poor health in the generations to follow, even if these individuals develop in normal conditions themselves. For example, the diet of a pregnant mother may affect the development and disease risk of her children and even her grandchildren. There is limited evidence for this in humans since studies of multiple generations are difficult to maintain. However, recent animal models have been generated to investigate this phenomenon and will be instrumental in the future for assessing the underlying mechanisms of intergenerational and transgenerational transmission of disease. These mechanisms remain unclear, though environmental, metabolic and epigenetic factors are likely involved. Researchers have begun to address how changes in metabolism and epigenetic regulation of gene expression caused by poor nutrition can be passed from one generation to the next. Ultimately, these findings will shed light on the transmission of diabetes, obesity and cardiovascular disease that are rapidly expanding in Western countries. Public health strategies that focus on improved maternal nutrition may provide a means of promoting cardiovascular and metabolic health. However, the full impact of these strategies may not be apparent for decades.

▶ The cliché "you are what you eat" is rapidly evolving into "you are what your mother ate" or "you are what your great-great grandfather ate." This review provides a nice overview of the current state of understanding of what for decades has been termed "nutritional programming." Since the time of Lamarck, it has been thought that one's environment may play a role in the phenotype and health of subsequent generations. Numerous examples in plants and non-human animals support this notion. However, the classical theories of Darwin and the 25 000 or so genes that are expressed from our DNA do not appear to provide a reasonable explanation for these environmentally altered traits. In this article, the authors discuss several of the studies, including those from the Dutch famine, where phenotypic alterations are occurring in subsequent generations in those exposed as fetuses to undernutrition during various phases of pregnancy. Also discussed are studies of Saudi women who fast during Ramadan and show alterations in their offspring that differ depending on the sex of the offspring and also the timing of the fasting during gestation.

The authors differentiate between intergenerational and transgenerational alterations, where the intergenerational affect only the F1 and F2 progeny, whereas transgenerational affect F3 and F4 progeny and beyond. The difference between these effects is that the intergenerational progeny are directly affected during gestation by the environmental agent, either as a fetus or as the gamete harbored by the fetus. The transgenerational effect needs to evoke epigenetic mechanisms such as DNA or histone alterations (methylation, acetylation) or gene silencing. Although an in-depth description of these mechanisms is not described in this article, the reference[1] describes some of these mechanisms in much greater depth.

Of note, although a bit discouraging, is that this article very correctly mentions how shallow our understanding of the mechanism of these nutrition-induced alterations in phenotype really is and emphasizes the importance of obtaining a better understanding. The authors discuss the huge epidemic about to emerge in India, where generations have been exposed to undernutrition and now with adequate nutrition, obesity and type 2 diabetes are beginning to emerge. Another example given by the authors is the US African-American population where undernutrition likely extends back to the days of slavery or even before, but now, metabolic syndrome is rampant.

J. Neu, MD

Reference

1. Daxinger L, Whitelaw E. Understanding transgenerational epigenetic inheritance via the gametes in mammals. *Nat Rev Genet*. 2012;13:152-162.

Extremely low birthweight infants: how neonatal intensive care unit teams can reduce postnatal malnutrition and prevent growth retardation
Loÿs C-M, Maucort-Boulch D, Guy B, et al (Hôpital de la Croix-Rousse, Hospices Civils de Lyon, France; Université Claude-Bernard Lyon 1, France)
Acta Paediatr 102:242-248, 2013

Aim.—To evaluate the impact of an improved nutritional policy for extremely low birthweight (ELBW) infants on nutritional deficits and postnatal growth.

Method.—We compared two groups of 37 ELBW infants, born before and after the introduction of an improved nutritional policy in April 2006. Group A (born 2005 to early 2006) and group B (born 2009) stayed in a French neonatal intensive care unit (NICU) for at least 7 weeks. Optimal energy and protein intakes were 120 and 3.5 g/kg/day, respectively, and used to calculate cumulative deficits. Delta z-scores for weight, length and head circumference were calculated between birth and 36 weeks of postmenstrual age (PMA). The improved nutritional policy focused on earlier and higher parenteral intake of lipids and proteins, earlier and higher human milk fortification and earlier transition to preterm formula.

Results.—The two groups did not differ in gestational age and birthweight. However, protein and energy deficits were significantly reduced in group B. Between birth and 36 weeks of PMA, delta z-scores were significantly reduced for length ($p = 0.012$) but not for weight ($p = 0.09$) or head circumference ($p = 0.83$).

Conclusion.—Higher parenteral intake and close attention to enteral feeding reduced nutritional deficits and linear growth restriction in infants admitted to a French NICU.

▶ How, when, and what to feed preterm infants have been matters of debate since the inception of neonatal intensive care. Over the past 2 decades, there has been a significant shift in our concern for not only poor growth but also suboptimal subsequent neurodevelopment in these infants. Numerous beliefs have existed about providing the same levels of lipids and amino acids to those babies born prematurely and the metabolic imbalances these may incur. We now know that some of the practices based on these beliefs can place these babies in a state of starvation, with nutritional deficits that cannot be retrieved.

This study evaluated a more aggressive team approach to both parenteral and enteral feedings that was instituted in the authors' neonatal intensive care unit and compared this with a previous epoch. Although this is not an optimal design because of the likelihood of many covariates over the 2 epochs, it does provide interesting data. This study showed very significant differences in length of time on total parenteral nutrition (TPN), improved growth (including length), and a significant minimization of nutritional deficits. The more aggressive approach appears to be reasonable, but why limit the babies to less than 3 g/kg/day and increase to 3 g incrementally? Why not just start at 3 g/kg/day? Although I think their guidelines could use some tweaking and certainly the composition of lipids and amino acids in TPN solutions that we have available to us could be improved, these authors make a very important point: We can do better with nutritional support of these babies. It takes effort and a team approach.

J. Neu, MD

The human milk microbiome changes over lactation and is shaped by maternal weight and mode of delivery

Cabrera-Rubio R, Collado MC, Laitinen K, et al (Univ of Valencia, Spain; the Inst of Agrochemistry and Food Science, Paterna, Valencia, Spain; Univ of Turku, Finland; et al)

Am J Clin Nutr 96:544-551, 2012

Background.—Breast milk is recognized as the most important post-partum element in metabolic and immunologic programming of health of neonates. The factors influencing the milk microbiome and the potential impact of microbes on infant health have not yet been uncovered.

Objective.—Our objective was to identify pre- and postnatal factors that can potentially influence the bacterial communities inhabiting human milk.

Design.—We characterized the milk microbial community at 3 different time points by pyrosequencing and quantitative polymerase chain reaction in mothers ($n = 18$) who varied in BMI, weight gain, and mode of delivery.

Results.—We found that the human milk microbiome changes over lactation. *Weisella, Leuconostoc, Staphylococcus, Streptococcus*, and *Lactococcus* were predominant in colostrum samples, whereas in 1- and 6-mo milk samples the typical inhabitants of the oral cavity (eg, *Veillonella, Leptotrichia*, and *Prevotella*) increased significantly. Milk from obese mothers tended to contain a different and less diverse bacterial community compared with milk from normal-weight mothers. Milk samples from elective but not from nonelective mothers who underwent cesarean delivery contained a different bacterial community than did milk samples from individuals giving birth by vaginal delivery, suggesting that it is not the operation per se but rather the absence of physiological stress or hormonal signals that could influence the microbial transmission process to milk.

Conclusions.—Our results indicate that milk bacteria are not contaminants and suggest that the milk microbiome is influenced by several factors that significantly skew its composition. Because bacteria present in breast milk are among the very first microbes entering the human body, our data emphasize the necessity to understand the biological role that the milk microbiome could potentially play for human health (Fig 4).

▶ The complexity of human milk seems to have no limits. This groundbreaking article describes a new look at the bacteriology of human milk using the powerful technique of quantitative polymerase chain reaction analysis of the bacterial 16S rRNA genes. This methodology allows quantitative description of the entire microbiome of any biological specimen. These authors have demonstrated that

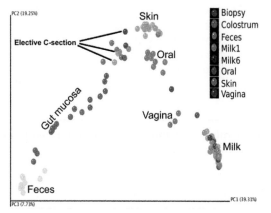

FIGURE 4.—Relatedness between milk bacteria and the rest of the human microbiome. The graph shows a principal components analysis of the bacterial composition of milk from colostrum and at 1 and 6 mo compared with available adult female sequences from the same 16S gene region (hypervariable regions V1 and V2) from skin, vagina, feces, gut mucosa, and oral epithelium. Milk samples from the 3 time points clustered together and separately from the rest, except for samples collected from mothers who gave birth by elective and nonelective cesarean section, which overlap with oral samples. Data from the human microbiome are from fecal samples (26); from skin, vagina, and oral samples (15); and from Durban et al (27). C-section, cesarean section; Milk1, milk at 1 mo; Milk6, milk at 6 mo; PC, principal components; PC1, first component of the principal components analysis; PC2, second component of the principal components analysis; PC3, third component of the principal components analysis. *Editor's Note*: Please refer to original journal article for full references. (Reprinted from the American Journal of Clinical Nutrition. Cabrera-Rubio R, Collado MC, Laitinen K, et al. The human milk microbiome changes over lactation and is shaped by maternal weight and mode of delivery. *Am J Clin Nutr.* 2012;96:544-551, with permission from American Society for Nutrition.)

the microbial constituents of human milk are specific and distinct from those of other body sites (Fig 4). These data should make it apparent that human milk is not normally sterile. Profiles change as milk production progresses from colostrum to mature milk and are substantially influenced by the experience of labor. These observations indicate that the bacterial constituents of human milk are not merely incidental contaminants from the mother's skin or the infant's mouth, but are highly regulated, both with respect to their bacterial constituents and over time. Therefore, it is very likely that there are specific mechanisms by which milk is seeded with healthy commensal organisms. Recent evidence that dendritic cells penetrate the intestinal epithelium, take up commensal bacteria from the gut lumen, then reach the systemic circulation and retain even live bacteria for several days has led to the proposition that intestinal bacteria may be actively transferred to the mammary glands within dendritic cells. This may be an important component of acquisition of normal bowel microflora by newborn infants. This hypothesis may help explain why there has been so little success in demonstrating beneficial effects of pasteurized human milk comparable to those of unpasteurized expressed maternal milk, for preterm infants, in particular, because pasteurization eliminates these commensal bacteria. This characterization of the human milk microbiome might also provide a useful guide to selection of candidate organisms for use as probiotics, in the long tradition of trying to match the composition of proprietary infant formulas to that of natural human milk. The diversity of the normal flora of human milk, as demonstrated in this article, suggests that use of a single or even 2 organisms as supplemental probiotics may not be sufficient and raises the concern that such approaches may disrupt normal acquisition of flora from maternal milk. Perhaps human milk is the best probiotic.

W. E. Benitz, MD

Effect of Early Limited Formula on Duration and Exclusivity of Breastfeeding in At-Risk Infants: An RCT

Flaherman VJ, Aby J, Burgos AE, et al (Univ of California, San Francisco; Stanford Univ, CA; Kaiser Permanente Med Ctr, Downey, CA)
Pediatrics 131:1059-1065, 2013

Background and Objectives.—Recent public health efforts focus on reducing formula use for breastfed infants during the birth hospitalization. No previous randomized trials report the effects of brief early formula use. The objective of the study was to determine if small formula volumes before the onset of mature milk production might reduce formula use at 1 week and improve breastfeeding at 3 months for newborns at risk for breastfeeding problems.

Methods.—We randomly assigned 40 exclusively breastfeeding term infants, 24 to 48 hours old, who had lost ≥5% birth weight to early limited formula (ELF) intervention (10 mL formula by syringe after each breastfeeding and discontinued when mature milk production began) or control (continued exclusive breastfeeding). Our outcomes were breastfeeding and formula use at 1 week and 1, 2, and 3 months.

Results.—Among infants randomly assigned to ELF during the birth hospitalization, 2 (10%) of 20 used formula at 1 week of age, compared with 9 (47%) of 19 control infants assigned during the birth hospitalization to continue exclusive breastfeeding ($P = .01$). At 3 months, 15 (79%) of 19 infants assigned to ELF during the birth hospitalization were breastfeeding exclusively, compared with 8 (42%) of 19 controls ($P = .02$).

Conclusions.—Early limited formula may reduce longer-term formula use at 1 week and increase breastfeeding at 3 months for some infants. ELF may be a successful temporary coping strategy for mothers to support breastfeeding newborns with early weight loss. ELF has the potential for increasing rates of longer-term breastfeeding without supplementation based on findings from this RCT.

▶ This study found that small controlled volumes of formula, before the onset of mature milk production, may benefit exclusive breastfeeding at 1 week and 3 months in full-term infants who have ≥5% weight loss in the first 36 hours (Table 2 of the original article).

These findings appear to contradict much current thinking about the detrimental effects of formula use and breastfeeding success, where breast milk feeding should be exclusive. However, the essence of this research finding is that the methodology used to supplement breastfeeding is what has led to increased breastfeeding success and not the use of formula. Specifically, the intervention consisted of offering a limited volume of formula (10 mL) after each breast feeding, using a syringe rather than nipple bottle, and for a limited duration (until the mother has established full milk production). The implementation of a specific protocol for supplementing breastfeeding in specific babies who were in apparent trouble (loss of ≥5% birth weight) is the important finding in this study because essentially the supplement could be formula, donor milk, or other suitable fluid.

Moreover, the study provided an intervention that empowers the mother. Mothers who are breastfeeding, particularly first-time mothers, are anxious that they do not produce enough milk, as mentioned by the author. It is possible that provision of an intervention that can alleviate a mother's anxiety, such as the one in this study (ie, formula feeding), can lead to improved breastfeeding success. To ensure the results are not driven by such an effect, replication of the study wherein the control receives a sham intervention, such as a whole body massage after each breastfeeding session, could shed light on the mechanism underlying the benefits of providing limited amounts of supplement on breastfeeding.

It is our opinion that breastfeeding is best and should be encouraged. There are times when an alternative such as formula is needed and may actually be of benefit for breastfeeding, as this study supports. Public policy that bans formula feeding altogether is extreme and can be detrimental. Some mothers find reassurance that there is formula in case they can't breastfeed. Some can't breastfeed (such as previous breast cancer or cosmetic surgery patients). There are also mothers who do not want to breastfeed (for personal reasons), and they should not be made to feel guilty.

This article serves as a first step on how to use formula as a supplement to enhance breastfeeding and not as a replacement.

S. Fucile, OTR, PhD

Oral Microbial Profile Discriminates Breast-fed From Formula-fed Infants
Holgerson PL, Vestman NR, Claesson R, et al (Umeå Univ, Sweden; et al)
J Pediatr Gastroenterol Nutr 56:127-136, 2013

Objectives.—Little is known about the effect of diet on the oral microbiota of infants, although diet is known to affect the gut microbiota. The aims of the present study were to compare the oral microbiota in breast-fed and formula-fed infants, and investigate growth inhibition of streptococci by infant-isolated lactobacilli.

Methods.—A total of 207 mothers consented to participation of their 3-month-old infants. A total of 146 (70.5%) infants were exclusively and 38 (18.4%) partially breast-fed, and 23 (11.1%) were exclusively formula-fed. Saliva from all of their infants was cultured for *Lactobacillus* species, with isolate identifications from 21 infants. *Lactobacillus* isolates were tested for their ability to suppress *Streptococcus mutans* and *S sanguinis*.

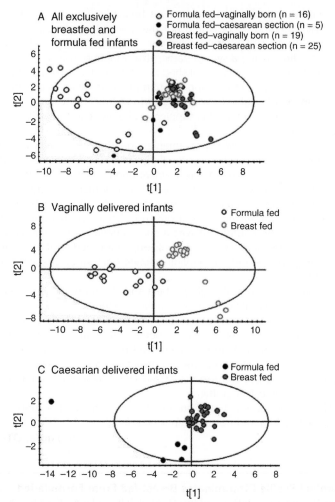

FIGURE 1.—Partial least-squares discriminant analysis score scatterplots illustrating clustering of exclusively breast-fed (red symbols) compared with exclusively formula-fed (black symbols) 3-month-old infants by oral microbiota. Clustering was derived by multivariate partial least squares modelling using dichotomous Human Oral Microbe Identification Microarray (HOMIM) signals, lactobacilli cultured from saliva, and selected individual characteristics as the X-block and mode of feeding as the Y-block. A, Model 2 (all 65 exclusively breast- and formula-fed infant samples used for HOMIM microarray); B, model 3 (samples from vaginally delivered infants used for HOMIM microarray); and C, model 4 (samples from caesarean section—delivered infants used for HOMIM microarray). Red symbols with unfilled circles indicate vaginally and filled dots caesarean-delivered infants. Black symbols with unfilled circles indicate vaginally and filled dots caesarean-delivered infants. For interpretation of the references to color in this figure legend, the reader is referred to web version of this article. (Reprinted from Holgerson PL, Vestman NR, Claesson R, et al. Oral microbial profile discriminates breast-fed from formula-fed infants. *J Pediatr Gastroenterol Nutr.* 2013;56:127-136, © 2013, with permission by the AAP.)

Oral swabs from 73 infants were analysed by the Human Oral Microbe Identification Microarray (HOMIM) and by quantitative polymerase chain reaction for *Lactobacillus gasseri*.

Results.—Lactobacilli were cultured from 27.8% of exclusively and partially breast-fed infants, but not from formula-fed infants. The prevalence of 14 HOMIM-detected taxa, and total salivary lactobacilli counts differed by feeding method. Multivariate modelling of HOMIM-detected bacteria and possible confounders clustered samples from breast-fed infants separately from formula-fed infants. The microbiota of breast-fed infants differed based on vaginal or C-section delivery. Isolates of *L planta-rum*, *L gasseri*, and *L vaginalis* inhibited growth of the cariogenic *S mutans* and the commensal *S sanguinis*: *L plantarum* >*L gasseri* >*L vaginalis*.

Conclusions.—The microbiota of the mouth differs between 3-month-old breast-fed and formula-fed infants. Possible mechanisms for microbial differences observed include species suppression by lactobacilli indigenous to breast milk (Fig 1).

▶ This is an important study in that it not only addresses the differences in oral microbiota in babies who are breastfed vs formula fed, it also shows interesting data on babies who were delivered by cesarean section vs vaginal delivery under breast-feeding or formula-feeding conditions at 3 months after birth. Using culture of oral microbiota, the authors found that approximately 30% breastfed and partially breast-fed infants, but none of the exclusively formula-fed babies, had *Lactobacillus* in their saliva. This finding suggested that the *Lactobacilli* might have an inhibitory effect on oral *streptococci*. These investigators used a targeted microarray technique that evaluates approximately 300 microbial taxa clustered differentially depending on mode of delivery (vaginal vs cesarean section) and whether the babies were formula or breastfed (Fig 1). This is highly reminiscent of another recent study[1] in which fecal microbiota were analyzed depending on mode of delivery and formula vs breastmilk feeding at 4 months after birth. Although it is difficult to make any firm conclusions based on these data, it is clear that feeding type and mode of delivery interact to form a different mouth as well as gastrointestinal microbiota several months after birth. The implications of this in terms of development of the gastrointestinal tract and immunity remain to be discovered.

J. Neu, MD

Reference

1. Azad MB, Konya T, Maughan H, et al. Gut microbiota of healthy Canadian infants: profiles by mode of delivery and infant diet at 4 months. *CMAJ*. 2013; 185:385-394.

11 Hematology and Bilirubin

Anemia, Apnea of Prematurity, and Blood Transfusions

Zagol K, Lake DE, Vergales B, et al (Univ of Virginia, Charlottesville; et al)

J Pediatr 161:417-421.e1, 2012

Objective.—To compare the frequency and severity of apneic events in very low birth weight (VLBW) infants before and after blood transfusions using continuous electronic waveform analysis.

Study Design.—We continuously collected waveform, heart rate, and oxygen saturation data from patients in all 45 neonatal intensive care unit beds at the University of Virginia for 120 weeks. Central apneas were detected using continuous computer processing of chest impedance, electrocardiographic, and oximetry signals. Apnea was defined as respiratory pauses of >10, >20, and >30 seconds when accompanied by bradycardia (<100 beats per minute) and hypoxemia (<80% oxyhemoglobin saturation as detected by pulse oximetry). Times of packed red blood cell transfusions were determined from bedside charts. Two cohorts were analyzed. In the transfusion cohort, waveforms were analyzed for 3 days before and after the transfusion for all VLBW infants who received a blood transfusion while also breathing spontaneously. Mean apnea rates for the previous 12 hours were quantified and differences for 12 hours before and after transfusion were compared. In the hematocrit cohort, 1453 hematocrit values from all VLBW infants admitted and breathing spontaneously during the time period were retrieved, and the association of hematocrit and apnea in the next 12 hours was tested using logistic regression.

Results.—Sixty-seven infants had 110 blood transfusions during times when complete monitoring data were available. Transfusion was associated with fewer computer-detected apneic events ($P < .01$). Probability of future apnea occurring within 12 hours increased with decreasing hematocrit values ($P < .001$).

Conclusions.—Blood transfusions are associated with decreased apnea in VLBW infants, and apneas are less frequent at higher hematocrits.

▶ Cardiorespiratory events in preterm infants, namely various combinations of apnea, bradycardia, and desaturation, remain nagging problems that defy simple solution. This is probably one reason why several studies over the past 25 years have examined the role of packed red blood cell transfusion on the incidence of such episodes. These studies have shown only variable benefit on apnea incidence and duration,[1-4] and one study suggested that just volume expansion can provide the same benefit.[5] Over the past decade, the threshold for transfusion of preterm infants has fallen considerably; however, packed cell transfusion is still a frequent option in infants with apnea and hematocrit levels in the mid-20s.

Zagol et al at the University of Virginia have developed expertise in algorithms designed for longer-term neonatal cardiorespiratory monitoring. In this study, they confirm earlier impressions that transfusion does benefit apnea when accompanied by bradycardia and hypoxemia. There are 2 likely explanations: The first is that hypoxic depression of breathing and resultant apnea may benefit from improved oxygen-carrying capacity. The second is that apnea incidence is unchanged but that each apnea is less likely to result in desaturation (and bradycardia) with improved oxygen-carrying capacity. Perhaps the most striking observation in this article is that nursing records of apneic episodes greatly underestimate their true incidence; not surprising, given the busy neonatal intensive care unit environment and the limitations of bedside respiratory monitoring by impedance techniques.

R. J. Martin, MD

References

1. Joshi A, Gerhardt T, Shandloff P, Bancalari E. Blood transfusion effect on the respiratory pattern of preterm infants. *Pediatrics.* 1987;80:79-84.
2. DeMaio JG, Harris MC, Deuber C, Spitzer AR. Effect of blood transfusion on apnea frequency in growing premature infants. *J Pediatr.* 1989;114:1039-1041.
3. Westkamp E, Soditt V, Adrian S, Bohnhorst B, Groneck P, Poets CF. Blood transfusion in anemic infants with apnea of prematurity. *Biol Neonate.* 2002;82:228-232.
4. Stute H, Greiner B, Linderkamp O. Effect of blood transfusion on cardiorespiratory abnormalities in preterm infants. *Arch Dis Child Fetal Neonatal Ed.* 1995; 72:F194-F196.
5. Bifano EM, Smith F, Borer J. Relationship between determinants of oxygen delivery and respiratory abnormalities in preterm infants with anemia. *J Pediatr.* 1992;120:292-296.

Effect of Fresh Red Blood Cell Transfusions on Clinical Outcomes In Premature, Very Low-Birth-Weight Infants: The ARIPI Randomized Trial
Fergusson DA, Hébert P, Hogan DL, et al (Univ of Ottawa, Ontario, Canada; et al)
JAMA 308:1443-1451, 2012

Context.—Even though red blood cells (RBCs) are lifesaving in neonatal intensive care, transfusing older RBCs may result in higher rates of organ dysfunction, nosocomial infection, and length of hospital stay.

Objective.—To determine if RBCs stored for 7 days or less compared with usual standards decreased rates of major nosocomial infection and organ dysfunction in neonatal intensive care unit patients requiring at least 1 RBC transfusion.

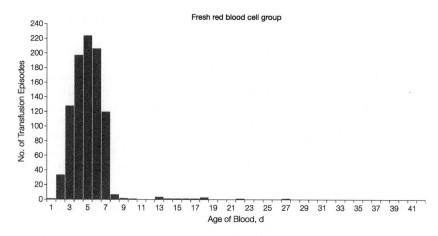

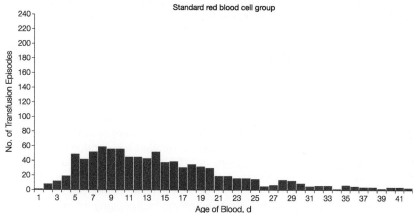

FIGURE 2.—Distribution of Age of Red Blood Cell Transfusion Episodes in Fresh and Standard Groups. For interpretation of the references to color in this figure legend, the reader is referred to web version of this article. (Reprinted from Fergusson DA, Hébert P, Hogan DL, et al. Effect of fresh red blood cell transfusions on clinical outcomes in premature, very low-birth-weight infants: the ARIPI randomized trial. *JAMA*. 2012;308:1443-1451, Copyright 2012, American Medical Association. All rights reserved.)

Design, Setting, and Participants.—Double-blind, randomized controlled trial in 377 premature infants with birth weights less than 1250 g admitted to 6 Canadian tertiary neonatal intensive care units between May 2006 and June 2011.

Intervention.—Patients were randomly assigned to receive transfusion of RBCs stored 7 days or less (n = 188) vs standard-issue RBCs in accordance with standard blood bank practice (n = 189).

Main Outcome Measures.—The primary outcome was a composite measure of major neonatal morbidities, including necrotizing enterocolitis, retinopathy of prematurity, bronchopulmonary dysplasia, and intraventricular hemorrhage, as well as death. The primary outcome was measured within the entire period of neonatal intensive care unit stay up to 90 days after randomization. The rate of nosocomial infection was a secondary outcome.

Results.—The mean age of transfused blood was 5.1 (SD, 2.0) days in the fresh RBC group and 14.6 (SD, 8.3) days in the standard group. Among neonates in the fresh RBC group, 99 (52.7%) had the primary outcome compared with 100 (52.9%) in the standard RBC group (relative risk, 1.00; 95% CI, 0.82-1.21). The rate of clinically suspected infection in the fresh RBC group was 77.7% (n = 146) compared with 77.2% (n = 146) in the standard RBC group (relative risk, 1.01; 95% CI, 0.90-1.12), and the rate of positive cultures was 67.5% (n = 127) in the fresh RBC group compared with 64.0% (n = 121) in the standard RBC group (relative risk, 1.06; 95% CI, 0.91-1.22).

Conclusion.—In this trial, the use of fresh RBCs compared with standard blood bank practice did not improve outcomes in premature, very low-birth-weight infants requiring a transfusion.

Trial Registration.—clinicaltrials.gov Identifier: NCT00326924; Current Controlled Trials Identifier: ISRCTN65939658 (Fig 2).

▶ Red blood cells (RBCs) undergo physiologic and biochemical changes during ex vivo storage. Some of these changes include reduction in 2,3-diphospho-glycerate; increase in nitric oxide levels; release of cytokines; and increases in fragility, adhesiveness, and aggregation. These effects of storage may result in pro-inflammatory effects and impaired oxygen delivery. Studies in children and adults have found that selective use of blood stored for shorter intervals was associated with decreased rates of infection, organ failure, and death and in-creased length of stay. This double-blind, controlled trial randomly assigned 377 premature patients (birth weight < 1250 g) to transfusion using fresh RBCs (stored for ≤7 days) or standard RBCs (stored for 2—42 days). Use of fresher blood did not decrease or increase rates of major complications (necro-tizing enterocolitis, intraventricular hemorrhage, retinopathy of prematurity, bronchopulmonary dysplasia) or death, either individually or collectively; the composite outcome was observed in 52.7% of patients with fresh RBCs vs 52.9% in the standard RBC group. Rates of suspected or confirmed infection did not differ between groups, but the prevalence of confirmed infection in both groups was high (> 60%). Length of hospitalization also was not different. Strengths of the trial include an adequate sample size, careful randomization, and near universal protocol completion and outcome ascertainment. The ability of the trial to detect differences between groups may have been limited by extensive overlap between the ages of transfused blood (Fig 2) with mean storage times of 5.1 ± 2.0 days and 14.6 ± 8.3 days in fresh RBC and standard RBC groups, respectively. As noted by the authors, this choice of experimental design, which was driven by considerations of feasibility, limited the potential for detec-tion of benefits from use of even fresher blood (eg, stored for ≤2 days). Another concern is that the enrolled subjects represent only 33% of the 1138 potentially eligible subjects who required transfusion and whose parents did not decline to participate; among the excluded subjects were 236 who received directed donor blood, 218 who underwent transfusion before randomization, and 39 who died.

This selection process and the apparently anomalously high infection rate among enrolled infants suggest that this sample may not be representative of the underlying population of all infants with birth weights less than 1250 g. Consequently, the broader implications for practice remain somewhat uncertain. It is also important that this trial was not intended to address the potential role of fresh blood in massive transfusion circumstances, such as acute exsanguination, exchange transfusion, or initiation of cardiopulmonary bypass. The investigators should be congratulated on completion of this very well-designed clinical trial to address this important clinical practice question.

V. P. Akula, MD

Effect of Fresh Red Blood Cell Transfusions on Clinical Outcomes in Premature, Very Low-Birth-Weight Infants: The ARIPI Randomized Trial
Fergusson DA, Hébert P, Hogan DL, et al (Univ of Ottawa, Ontario, Canada; et al)
JAMA 308:1443-1451, 2012

Context.—Even though red blood cells (RBCs) are lifesaving in neonatal intensive care, transfusing older RBCs may result in higher rates of organ dysfunction, nosocomial infection, and length of hospital stay.

Objective.—To determine if RBCs stored for 7 days or less compared with usual standards decreased rates of major nosocomial infection and organ dysfunction in neonatal intensive care unit patients requiring at least 1 RBC transfusion.

Design, Setting, and Participants.—Double-blind, randomized controlled trial in 377 premature infants with birth weights less than 1250 g admitted to 6 Canadian tertiary neonatal intensive care units between May 2006 and June 2011.

Intervention.—Patients were randomly assigned to receive transfusion of RBCs stored 7 days or less (n = 188) vs standard-issue RBCs in accordance with standard blood bank practice (n = 189).

Main Outcome Measures.—The primary outcome was a composite measure of major neonatal morbidities, including necrotizing enterocolitis, retinopathy of prematurity, bronchopulmonary dysplasia, and intraventricular hemorrhage, as well as death. The primary outcome was measured within the entire period of neonatal intensive care unit stay up to 90 days after randomization. The rate of nosocomial infection was a secondary outcome.

Results.—The mean age of transfused blood was 5.1 (SD, 2.0) days in the fresh RBC group and 14.6 (SD, 8.3) days in the standard group. Among neonates in the fresh RBC group, 99 (52.7%) had the primary outcome compared with 100 (52.9%) in the standard RBC group (relative risk, 1.00; 95% CI, 0.82-1.21). The rate of clinically suspected infection in the fresh RBC group was 77.7% (n = 146) compared with 77.2% (n = 146) in the standard RBC group (relative risk, 1.01; 95% CI, 0.90-1.12), and the rate of positive cultures was 67.5% (n = 127) in the fresh RBC group compared with 64.0% (n = 121) in the standard RBC group (relative risk, 1.06; 95% CI, 0.91-1.22).

Conclusion.—In this trial, the use of fresh RBCs compared with standard blood bank practice did not improve outcomes in premature, very low-birth-weight infants requiring a transfusion.

Trial Registration.—clinicaltrials.gov Identifier: NCT00326924; Current Controlled Trials Identifier: ISRCTN65939658.

▶ Very-low-birth-weight (VLBW) infants frequently require multiple red blood cell (RBC) transfusions. To reduce blood donor exposures, a dedicated donor policy has been adopted in many US and Canadian neonatal intensive care units (NICUs). This practice allows a single RBC unit to be used for all transfusions given to an infant until the unit's expiration date (up to 42 days).

In recent years, a growing number of observational studies in critically ill adults documented a strong association between prolonged RBC storage time and poor clinical outcomes, including mortality, organ dysfunction, and infections. These adverse consequences have been attributed to the decrease in RBC deformability and 2,3-diphosphoglycerate content as well as the release of free hemoglobin and bioactive substances during storage.

In the Age of Red Cells in Preterm Infants (ARIPI) study, 377 infants born at < 1250 g and admitted to 6 Canadian NICUs were randomized to receive either fresh RBCs (stored ≤7 days) or standard RBCs. In all participating NICUs, standard RBCs were derived from dedicated donor units, with storage times ranging from 2 to 42 days at the time of transfusion. As a consequence, nearly all infants in the standard group received both fresh and older blood transfusions. The mean age of the blood transfused was 5.1 ± 2.0 days in the fresh group and 14.6 ± 8.3 days in the standard group.

Against all predictions, the study showed no significant differences (or even trends) between the 2 groups in any outcome measured. Thus, the authors appropriately concluded that the use of fresh RBCs did not improve outcomes in VLBW infants when compared with the standard blood bank practices of the participating units. Importantly, however, the ARIPI study did not truly compare fresh with old RBCs (only 12 infants exclusively received blood stored for >14 days). Thus, the conclusions of this study cannot be extrapolated to NICUs that might have very different blood banking and transfusion policies.

M. Sola-Visner, MD

Thrombocytopaenia and intraventricular haemorrhage in very premature infants: a tale of two cities
von Lindern JS, Hulzebos CV, Bos AF, et al (Leiden Univ Med Ctr, The Netherlands; Univ Med Ctr Groningen, The Netherlands; et al)
Arch Dis Child Fetal Neonatal Ed 97:F348-F352, 2012

Objective.—To study whether the incidence of intraventricular haemorrhage (IVH) in very premature infants (<32 weeks gestation) with thrombocytopaenia is lower when using a liberal platelet-transfusion guideline compared with a restrictive guideline.

Study Design.—A retrospective cohort study comparing the incidence of IVH in very premature infants with thrombocytopaenia (platelet count < 150×10^9/l) admitted between 2007 and 2008 to two neonatal intensive care unit in The Netherlands. The restrictive platelet-transfusion unit (N = 353 infants < 32 weeks gestation) transfused only in case of active haemorrhage and a platelet count < 50×10^9/l. The liberal-transfusion unit (N = 326 infants < 32 weeks gestation) transfused according to predefined platelet count thresholds. Primary outcome was the incidence and severity of IVH in infants with thrombocytopaenia in both units.

Results.—The number of infants with thrombocytopaenia that received a platelet transfusion was significantly lower in the restrictive-transfusion unit compared with the liberal-transfusion unit, 15% (21/145) versus 31% (41/141), ($p < 0.001$). The incidence of IVH in infants with thrombocytopaenia in the restrictive-transfusion and liberal-transfusion units was 30% (44/145) and 29% (41/141), respectively ($p = 0.81$). The incidence of severe IVH (grade 3 or 4) in the restrictive-transfusion and liberal-transfusion units was 8% (12/145) and 11% (16/141), respectively ($p = 0.38$).

Conclusion.—In the restrictive-transfusion unit, the rate of platelet transfusions was significantly lower, but the incidence and severity of IVH was similar to the liberal-transfusion unit.

▶ Thrombocytopenia, a platelet count <150 000/μL, is a very common finding in very-low-birth-weight (VLBW) newborn infants, but the consequences of and optimal management for this observation remain uncertain. Practice is guided by only a single randomized, controlled trial[1] that demonstrated no benefit from transfusion to achieve platelet counts >150 000/μL, as compared with tolerating counts as low as 50 000/μL. This observational comparison of 2 units in the Netherlands that used different criteria for platelet transfusion for infants born at < 32 weeks' gestation updates and confirms those results. These authors found that thrombocytopenia was associated with an increased risk of intraventricular hemorrhage (IVH), but that IVH risk was not modified by either the severity of thrombocytopenia or by a more liberal policy of treatment with platelet transfusion. Although the more restrictive policy of transfusion only if the platelet count fell below 50 000/μL halved the number of patients who received a transfusion, it was not associated with higher rates of IVH or other bleeding events. Together, these analyses indicate that, at least in the absence of overt signs of bleeding, the threshold for platelet transfusion in VLBW infants should be no greater than 50 000/μL. In both of these studies, all infants with platelet counts < 50 000/μL were transfused, so the role of transfusion in those infants is still untested. Absence of a relationship between severity of thrombocytopenia and risk of IVH, observed by these authors and others, and lack of an effect of transfusion suggest that this association may be mediated by factors other than a simple hemorrhagic diathesis attributable to platelet deficiency. Recent retrospective studies have suggested that platelet transfusions may confer some morbidity, potentially offsetting the postulated benefit of IVH prevention. Additional trials to clarify this picture, perhaps beginning with examination of outcomes and consequences of treatment in VLBW infants with platelet counts between 30 000 and 50 000/μL, are urgently needed.

W. E. Benitz, MD

Reference

1. Andrew M, Vegh P, Caco C, et al. A randomized, controlled trial of platelet transfusions in thrombocytopenic premature infants. *J Pediatr.* 1993;123:285-291.

Venous thromboembolism in neonates and children—Update 2013
Nowak-Göttl U, Janssen V, Manner D, et al (Univ Hosp of Kiel & Lubbock, Germany; et al)
Thromb Res 131:S39-S41, 2013

Thromboses (VTE) in children were associated with medical diseases with and without acquired or inherited thrombophilic risk factors (IT). Disease recurrence rates vary between 3% in children with a first event during the neonatal period and 21% in children with idiopathic VTE. Recently reported systematic reviews showed significant associations between VTE and factor V G1691A or factor II G20210A mutations, protein C, protein S and antithrombin deficiency, more pronounced when combined IT were involved. The factor II G20210A mutation, protein C, protein S, and antithrombin deficiency did also play an important role at VTE recurrence. Primarily asymptomatic family members of pediatric VTE index cases showed annual VTE incidence rates of 2.82% in carriers of antithrombin, protein C, or protein S deficiency, 0.42% and 0.25% in carriers of the factor II G202010A or V G1691A mutation, and 0.10% in relatives with no IT.

▶ The late Maureen Andrew[1] drew attention to the importance of clotting disorders in pediatric patients and was responsible for establishing a registry as well as a hotline to call for consultation. The registry has proved to be of enormous value, and the consultation service is excellent. This article draws our attention to a common but probably unrecognized set of problems in the neonatal period, venous thromboembolism (VTE). Thrombophilic disorders include inherited conditions, such as factor V Leiden, protein C deficiency, protein S deficiency, antithrombin deficiency, and prothrombin 20210A mutations. Factor V Leiden is the most common inherited abnormality in this class. It affects approximately 5% to 7% of the white population of European descent in the United States. An example of acquired thrombophilia is the development of a lupus anticoagulant or antiphospholipid antibody syndrome; these factors, together with antithrombin, protein C, or protein S deficiency; the mutations of coagulation factor V (G1691A); and factor II (G20210A) are risk factors in adults. Neonates with protein S and protein C deficiency may present with purpura fulminans.

The coagulation system of children changes with age, with marked physiologic differences in the concentration of most blood clotting proteins, a concept known as *developmental hemostasis.* Thus, for comparable clinical risk factors, the thrombosis risk is substantially reduced in children compared with adults, which suggests the presence of protective mechanisms.[1] Among children, neonates are at the greatest risk for VTE with the next peak incidence during puberty and adolescence.[1] The yearly incidence of venous events was estimated to be 24 per 10000. In neonates, the most commonly reported VTEs are renal vein thrombosis, vena caval occlusion, and thromboembolic stroke mainly of venous origin. In addition, central line—associated VTEs have been reported.

Duplex sonography, venography, computed tomography, and magnetic resonance imaging can be used to diagnose VTE in neonates.

In the absence of evidence from randomized trials, the treatment of VTE is largely empiric and based on limited data from children and guidelines adapted from adult patients. Unfractionated heparin, low-molecular-weight heparins, and vitamin K antagonists are the commonly used antithrombotic drugs,[2-5] whereas newly developed antithrombotic agents, such as argatroban, bivalirudin, or fondaparinux, are under discussion and are increasingly administered in small pediatric clinical trials. Because of the low frequency of these disorders, there is an urgent need for multicenter, multinational registries and trials.

A. A. Fanaroff, MBBCh, FRCPE

References

1. Andrew M. Developmental hemostasis: relevance to thromboembolic complications in pediatric patients. *Thromb Haemost.* 1995;74:415-425.
2. Monagle P, Chan AK, Goldenberg NA, et al. American College of Chest Physicians. Antithrombotic therapy in neonates and children: Antithrombotic Therapy and Prevention of Thrombosis, 9th ed: American College of Chest Physicians Evidence-Based Clinical Practice Guidelines. *Chest.* 2012;141:e737S-e801S.
3. Bidlingmaier C, Kenet G, Kurnik K, et al. Safety and efficacy of low molecular weight heparin in children: a systematic review of the literature and meta-analysis of single arm studies. *Semin Thromb Hemost.* 2011;37:814-825.
4. Nowak-Göttl U, Dietrich K, Schaffranek D, et al. In pediatric patients, age has more impact on dosing of vitamin K antagonists than VKORC1 or CYP2C9 genotypes. *Blood.* 2010;116:5789-5790.
5. Goldenberg NA, Pounder E, Knapp-Clevenger R, Manco-Johnson MJ. Validation of upper extremity post-thrombotic syndrome outcome measurement in children. *J Pediatr.* 2010;157:852-855.

Incidence of Chronic Bilirubin Encephalopathy in Canada, 2007—2008

Sgro M, Campbell DM, Kandasamy S, et al (Li Ka Shing Knowledge Inst, Toronto, Ontario, Canada; St Michael's Hosp, Toronto, Ontario, Canada; et al)
Pediatrics 130:e886-e890, 2012

Background and Objectives.—Despite the implementation of screening guidelines to identify infants at risk for hyperbilirubinemia, chronic bilirubin encephalopathy (CBE) continues to be reported worldwide in otherwise healthy infants. The incidence of CBE in Canada is unknown. The objectives of this study were to establish the incidence of CBE in Canada and identify epidemiological and medical risk factors associated with its occurrence.

Methods.—Data on infants were collected prospectively through the Canadian Pediatric Surveillance Program. Infants born between January 1, 2007 and December 31, 2008 were included if they either had symptoms of CBE and a history of hyperbilirubinemia, or if they presented in the newborn period with severe hyperbilirubinemia and an abnormal MRI finding as per the reporting physician.

Results.—During the study period, 20 cases were identified; follow-up data were available for 14 of these. The causes for the hyperbilirubinemia included glucose-6-phosphate dehydrogenase deficiency ($n = 5$), sepsis ($n = 2$), ABO incompatibility and other red blood cell antibodies ($n = 7$). Fifteen infants had abnormal brain MRI findings during the neonatal period. At follow-up, 5 infants developed classic choreoathetoid cerebral palsy, 6 had spectrum of neurologic dysfunction and developmental delay (as described by the reporting physician), and 3 were healthy.

Conclusions.—CBE continues to occur in Canada at an incidence that appears to be higher than previously reported.

▶ The Canadian Pediatric Society Surveillance Program (CPSP) is a program that surveys Canadian pediatricians and pediatric subspecialists to obtain data on uncommon pediatric diseases. Similar programs exist elsewhere[1] and are the next best thing to prospectively obtained, population-based data. Using the CPSP database, Sgro et al have reported previously on the number of Canadian newborns whose bilirubin levels exceeded 425 μmol/L (24.8 mg/dL)[2] and how many of these infants presented with acute bilirubin encephalopathy.[3] In this study, the authors provide us with the CPSP data on infants born between January 2007 and December 2008 who met their criteria for chronic bilirubin encephalopathy or kernicterus. To be included, infants had to have had a maximum bilirubin level of greater than 425 μmol/L (24.8 mg/dL) or an exchange transfusion. In addition, they were required to have at least 2 of the classical signs of chronic bilirubin encephalopathy or findings on magnetic resonance imaging that are typical for kernicterus. Of the 20 infants so identified, 3 were later found to have normal development, which left 17 cases. Based on the Canadian birth rates, this represents an incidence of 1 in 44000 or 2.3 in 100000 live births, a rate that is significantly higher than that of about 0.5 of 100000 live births in population-based studies in the United Kingdom, Denmark, and California.[1,4,5] As the authors note, some of these differences might be explained by different methods of case identification.

In this study, in addition to the 3 infants who appeared to have normal development at age 12 to 19 months, 6 cases were lost to follow-up, so there is no way of knowing whether they developed chronic bilirubin encephalopathy. If we exclude these 9 cases, we are left with 11 confirmed cases, which would give a lower incidence of 1 in 67000 or 1.5 in 100000 live births. Based on an incidence of 2.3 in 100000 live births, Canada would have about 8 cases of kernicterus per year (370000 annual births). If we had a similar rate in the United

States (4 million annual births), we would see some 40 cases per year. It is also noteworthy that in 5 of their 20 cases (25%), G6PD deficiency was the cause of the hyperbilirubinemia, an incidence almost identical to that found in the US kernicterus registry.[6] Notwithstanding both the professional and lay publicity devoted to this problem and the publication of several national guidelines,[7-11] kernicterus continues to occur in the industrialized world. All recent guidelines now recommend that we measure a serum or transcutaneous bilirubin level in all newborns before discharge and, in 3 studies,[12-14] the introduction of universal bilirubin screening significantly decreased the frequency of bilirubin levels greater than 25 mg/dL (425 μmol/L). There is anecdotal evidence that more nurseries are adopting this practice, and we know that combining the hour-specific bilirubin level with the infant's gestation provides an excellent prediction of the risk or lack of risk of the infant subsequently having severe hyperbilirubinemia.[15-18] If all of our nurseries did this, and physicians followed the postdischarge management outlined,[8] it is possible that we might see a reduction in the incidence of kernicterus.

M. J. Maisels, MBBCh, DSc

References

1. Manning D, Todd P, Maxwell M, Jane Platt M. Prospective surveillance study of severe hyperbilirubinaemia in the newborn in the UK and Ireland. *Arch Dis Child Fetal Neonatol Ed.* 2007;92:F342-346.
2. Sgro M, Campbell D, Shah V. Incidence and causes of severe neonatal hyperbilirubinemia in Canada. *CMAJ.* 2006;175:587-590.
3. Sgro M, Campbell D, Barozzino T, Shah V. Acute neurological findings in a national cohort of neonates with severe neonatal hyperbilirubinemia. *J Perinatol.* 2011;31: 392-396.
4. Bjerre JV, Petersen JR, Ebbesen F. Surveillance of extreme hyperbilirubinaemia in Denmark. A method to identify the newborn infants. *Acta Paediatr.* 2008;97: 1030-1034.
5. Bjerre JV, Ebbesen F. [Incidence of kernicterus in newborn infants in Denmark] [in Danish]. *Ugeskr Laeger.* 2006;168:686-691.
6. Bhutani VK, Johnson LH, Maisels MJ, et al. Kernicterus: epidemiological strategies for its prevention through systems-based approaches. *J Perinatol.* 2004;24: 650-662.
7. American Academy of Pediatrics, Subcommittee on Hyperbilirubinemia. Management of hyperbilirubinemia in the newborn infant 35 or more weeks of gestation. *Pediatrics.* 2004;114:297-316.
8. Maisels MJ, Bhutani VK, Bogen D, Newman TB, Stark AR, Watchko JF. Hyperbilirubinemia in the newborn infant ≥35 weeks' gestation: an update with clarifications. *Pediatrics.* 2009;124:1193-1198.
9. Guidelines for detection, management and prevention of hyperbilirubinemia in term and late preterm newborn infants (35 or more weeks' gestation) - Summary [Article in English, French]. *Paediatr Child Health.* 2007;12:401-418.
10. Rennie J, Burman-Roy S, Murphy MS. Neonatal jaundice: summary of NICE guidance. *BMJ.* 2010;340:c2409.
11. Bratlid D, Nakstad B, Hansen TWR. National guidelines for treatment of jaundice in the newborn. *Acta Paediatr.* 2011;100:499-505.
12. Eggert L, Wiedmeier SE, Wilson J, Christensen R. The effect of instituting a prehospital-discharge newborn bilirubin screening program in an 18-hospital health system. *Pediatrics.* 2006;117:e855-e862.
13. Mah MP, Clark SL, Akhigbe E, et al. Reduction of severe hyperbilirubinemia after institution of predischarge bilirubin screening. *Pediatrics.* 2010;125:e1143-e1148.

14. Kuzniewicz MW, Escobar GJ, Newman TB. Impact of universal bilirubin screening on severe hyperbilirubinemia and phototherapy use. *Pediatrics.* 2009; 124:1031-1039.

15. Keren R, Luan X, Friedman S, Saddlemire S, Cnaan A, Bhutani VK. A comparison of alternative risk-assessment strategies for predicting significant neonatal hyperbilirubinemia in term and near-term infants. *Pediatrics.* 2008;121:e170-e179.

16. Bhutani VK, Stark AR, Lazzeroni LC, et al. Predischarge screening for severe neonatal hyperbilirubinemia identifies infants who need phototherapy. *J Pediatr.* 2012. Available at: http://dx.doi.org/10.1016/j.jpeds.2012.08.022, Accessed June 10, 2013.

17. Maisels MJ, DeRidder JM, Kring EA, Balasubramaniam M. Routine transcutaneous bilirubin measurements combined with clinical risk factors improve the prediction of subsequent hyperbilirubinemia. *J Perinatol.* 2009;29:612-617.

18. Newman T, Liljestrand P, Escobar G. Combining clinical risk factors with serum bilirubin levels to predict hyperbilirubinemia in newborns. *Arch Pediatr Adolesc Med.* 2005;159:113-119.

An approach to the management of hyperbilirubinemia in the preterm infant less than 35 weeks of gestation

Maisels MJ, Watchko JF, Bhutani VK, et al (Beaumont Children's Hosp, Royal Oak, MI)
J Perinatol 32:660-664, 2012

We provide an approach to the use of phototherapy and exchange transfusion in the management of hyperbilirubinemia in preterm infants of <35 weeks of gestation. Because there are limited data for evidence-based recommendations, these recommendations are, of necessity, consensus-based. The recommended treatment levels are based on operational thresholds for bilirubin levels and represent those levels beyond which it is assumed that treatment will likely do more good than harm. Long-term follow-up of a large population will be needed to evaluate whether or not these recommendations should be modified.

▶ Phototherapy for neonatal jaundice is arguably the most commonly applied treatment in neonatal medicine. Data from the Norwegian Quality Registry for Newborn Medicine for the 4-year period from 2008 to 2011 show that 26.5% of the 23654 infants admitted to neonatal intensive care units in Norway received phototherapy, while 72% of all infants born at less than 28 weeks' gestation were put under the lights (Stensvold HJ, personal communication). We all recognize that the evidence base for our therapeutic guidelines is weak, and for the most immature infants we rely almost entirely on expert opinion. Therefore, many guidelines in current use provide no advice on the management of the smallest preemies.[1] However, most of us believe that the more immature an infant, the more likely he or she is to be vulnerable to the neurotoxic effects of bilirubin. Such infants, therefore, are commonly subjected to phototherapy, albeit the intervention levels are so varied that an international survey some years ago showed that some of us would perform an exchange transfusion at a total serum bilirubin (TSB) level where others would not even switch on the phototherapy lamps.[2]

The American Academy of Pediatrics' guidelines for management of neonatal jaundice are widely used but provide no advice on how to manage jaundiced infants less than 35 weeks' gestation.[3] This current study aimed to remedy this deficiency. The authors recognized up front that there are precious few data on which to base these suggested guidelines. Therefore, the choices are to a large extent pragmatic. These include the levels suggested for intervention and the tabular (and, thus, to some extent stepwise) format, with a lack of adjustment for postnatal age (at least until the infant moves into the next bracket for gestational age). Also, the suggestions to start with lower irradiance in the smallest infants (less than 750 g birth weight) and only increase this if TSB is not controlled at the lower level and the option to use prophylactic phototherapy in infants less than 26 weeks' gestation are similarly pragmatic.

Let me suggest that the extant evidence might also be logically argued to point in a different direction. An important starting point for this argument is the recent reanalysis of the data from Neonatal Research Network,[4] which showed increased mortality for extremely-low-birth-weight (ELBW) infants with a birth weight less than 750 g treated with aggressive phototherapy vs conservative phototherapy. It is important here to note that the term "aggressive" did not apply to irradiance but to the TSB level at which phototherapy was initiated. Thus, the infants treated conservatively were, as might be expected, treated for a significantly shorter period of time (35 ± 31 vs 88 ± 48 h, $P < .001$), but the irradiance did not, by design, differ between the groups.

It is of interest here to consider Maisels'[5] reanalysis of the data from the older Collaborative Phototherapy Trial,[6] in which he calculated the relative risk for mortality among treated ELBW infants to be 1.49 (confidence interval, 0.93 to 2.40). In that trial, all of the infants randomized to phototherapy were treated for 96 hours, while the control infants were not treated. Given the phototherapy equipment available at that time, irradiance was most likely considerably lower than the target irradiance in the Neonatal Research Network study.[4]

Thus, the difference in mortality, if indeed attributable to phototherapy, may perhaps be ascribed to the duration of phototherapy rather than irradiance. If we accept this interpretation of the data, an argument might be made in favor of higher irradiance to reduce the duration of treatment. Similarly, as prophylactic phototherapy will certainly increase the duration of exposure to the lights, it may not be the optimal approach.

However, the question as to the levels of TSB at which we should intervene with treatment should probably consider the findings of significantly reduced impairment in all surviving infants between 500 and 1000 g treated aggressively in the Neonatal Research Network trial.[4] Thus, tolerating higher levels of TSB may be detrimental to the neurodevelopmental outcome of these most immature infants.

The authors of this article conclude: "A long-term follow-up of a large population of such infants might identify which of these suggested approaches is preferred." I believe we can all concur.

T. W. R. Hansen, Md, PhD, MHA, FAAP

References

1. Bratlid D, Nakstad B, Hansen TWR. National guidelines for treatment of jaundice in the newborn. *Acta Paediatr.* 2011;100:499-505.
2. Hansen TWR. Therapeutic approaches to neonatal jaundice: an international survey. *Clin Pediatr (Phila).* 1996;35:309-316.
3. American Academy of Pediatrics Subcommittee on Hyperbilirubinemia. Management of hyperbilirubinemia in the newborn infant 35 or more weeks of gestation. *Pediatrics.* 2004;114:297-316.
4. Tyson JE, Pedroza C, Langer J, et al. Does aggressive phototherapy increase mortality while decreasing profound impairment among the smallest and sickest newborns? *J Perinatol.* 2012;32:677-684.
5. Maisels MJ. Neonatal jaundice. In: Sinclair JC, Bracken MB, eds. *Effective Care of the Newborn Infant.* Oxford, England: Oxford University Press; 1992:507-561.
6. Brown AK, Kim MH, Wu PYK, Bryla DA. Efficacy of phototherapy in prevention and management of neonatal hyperbilirubinemia. *Pediatrics.* 1985;75:393-400. 439-441.

Impact of a Transcutaneous Bilirubinometry Program on Resource Utilization and Severe Hyperbilirubinemia

Wainer S, Parmar SM, Allegro D, et al (Alberta Children's Hosp and Peter Lougheed Centre, Calgary, Alberta, Canada; Calgary Laboratory Services, Alberta, Canada; Post-Partum Community Services, Calgary, Alberta, Canada)
Pediatrics 129:77-86, 2012

Objectives.—Our goal was to assess the impact of programmatic and coordinated use of transcutaneous bilirubinometry (TcB) on the incidence of severe neonatal hyperbilirubinemia and measures of laboratory, hospital, and nursing resource utilization.

Methods.—We compared the neonatal hyperbilirubinemia-related outcomes of 14 796 prospectively enrolled healthy infants ≥35 weeks gestation offered routine TcB measurements in both hospital and community settings by using locally validated nomograms relative to a historical cohort of 14 112 infants assessed by visual inspection alone.

Results.—There was a 54.9% reduction (odds ratio [OR]: 2.219 [95% confidence interval (CI): 1.543–3.193]; $P < .0001$) in the incidence of severe total serum bilirubin values (≥342 μmol/L; ≥20 mg/dL) after implementation of routine TcB measurements. TcB implementation was associated with reductions in the overall incidence of total serum bilirubin draws (134.4 vs 103.6 draws per 1000 live births, OR: 1.332 [95% CI: 1.226–1.446]; $P < .0001$) and overall phototherapy rate (5.27% vs 4.30%, OR: 1.241 [95% CI: 1.122–1.374]; $P < .0001$), a reduced age at readmission for phototherapy (104.3 ± 52.1 vs 88.9 ± 70.5 hours, $P < .005$), and duration of phototherapy readmission (24.8 ± 13.6 vs 23.2 ± 9.8 hours, $P < .05$). There were earlier ($P < .01$) and more frequent contacts with public health nurses (1.33 vs 1.66, $P < .01$) after introduction of the TcB program.

Conclusions.—Integration of routine hospital and community TcB screening within a comprehensive public health nurse newborn follow-up program is associated with significant improvements in resource utilization and patient safety.

▶ Wainer and colleagues have made an important contribution to our understanding of how transcutaneous bilirubin (TcB) measurements can improve the care of newborn infants. They used a public health nurse program that ensures that every infant born at one of the Calgary Health Region nurseries is seen within 1 to 2 days of discharge. The nurses are trained in newborn assessment and, armed with a TcB device, they obtain measurements at the follow-up visit for all infants. Using a nomogram developed in their nurseries, the visiting public health nurse is able to decide whether a TcB measurement is necessary, whether the TcB measurement should be repeated within 24 hours, or whether subsequent routine care is appropriate. Those of us in less supportive environments can only gaze with envy at this ideal example of caring for newborns and their mothers, and the results should not surprise us.

The program significantly enhanced patient safety while it reduced demands on both laboratory and hospital resources. TcB measurements provided noninvasive, instantaneous information about the infant's bilirubin concentration. As with any point-of-care test, however, quality control is essential and Wainer et al point out that "25% of devices did not perform within allowable limits of our quality control procedures... in spite of passing the manufacturer's standard wavelength calibration." Thus, there is clearly a need for more rigorous calibration methods and quality control for these instruments. Currently, clinical laboratories in the United States are not involved in the evaluation of these devices, although they do provide quality control for other point-of-care measurements. Because there is little doubt that the use of TcB measurements both in and out of the hospital will continue to increase, perhaps it is time for our laboratory pathologists to become more involved in this important endeavor.

M. J. Maisels, MB, BCh, DSc

Limitations and Opportunities of Transcutaneous Bilirubin Measurements
Bosschaart N, Kok JH, Newsum AM, et al (Univ of Amsterdam, Netherlands; et al)
Pediatrics 129:689-694, 2012

Objective.—Although transcutaneous bilirubinometers have existed for over 30 years, the clinical utility of the technique is limited to a screening method for hyperbilirubinemia, rather than a replacement for invasive blood sampling. In this study, we investigate the reason for this limited clinical value and address possibilities for improvement.

Methods.—To obtain better insight into the physiology of bilirubin measurements, we evaluated a transcutaneous bilirubinometer that determines not only the cutaneous bilirubin concentration (TcB) but also the blood volume fraction (BVF) in the investigated skin volume. For 49 neonates (gestational age 30 ± 3.1 weeks, postnatal age 6 [4—10] days) at our NICU, we performed 124 TcB and 55 BVF measurements.

Results.—The TcB correlated well with the total serum bilirubin concentration (TSB) ($r = 0.88$) with an uncertainty of 55 μmol/L. The BVF in the measured skin volume ranged between 0.1% and 0.75%.

Conclusions.—The performance of our bilirubinometer is comparable to existing transcutaneous devices. The limited clinical value of current bilirubinometers can be explained by the low BVF in the skin volume that is probed by these devices. Because the TcB depends for over 99% on the contribution of extravascular bilirubin, it is a physiologically different parameter from the TSB. Hence, the standard method of evaluation that compares the TcB to the TSB is insufficient to fully investigate the clinical value of transcutaneous bilirubinometers, ie, their predictive value for kernicterus. We suggest that the clinical value may be improved considerably by changing either the method of evaluation or the technological design of transcutaneous bilirubinometers.

▶ The first commercially available, portable, hand-held instrument to measure transcutaneous bilirubin (TcB) electronically was described by Yamanouchi et al[1] in 1980, and TcB measurements have helped us to manage jaundiced infants for the past 30 years.[2] These instruments measure the yellowness of reflected light after it passes through the skin and subcutaneous tissues. Taking into account the contributions of hemoglobin, melanin, and dermal thickness, an algorithm converts this information into an estimate of the total serum bilirubin (TSB) level, and multiple studies have confirmed that TcB measurements correlate quite nicely with TSB.[2] But it has never been entirely clear what these instruments are measuring.

In this elegant study, these authors describe the use of a new transcutaneous instrument that measures the skin absorption coefficient, a measurement that allows them to calculate what fraction of the skin volume is made up of blood and extravascular tissue. With this information they show that more than 99% of what we are measuring with our TcB measurements is the bilirubin present in the extravascular tissue and not in the blood. Thus, it is not difficult to understand why the TcB is not a direct measurement of TSB but is a measurement primarily of tissue bilirubin. Nevertheless, when used as a screening tool, TcB measurements are of enormous value both in the nursery[3] and the outpatient setting.[4,5]

These investigators note that spectroscopic techniques exist that might allow measurement of bilirubin in the dermal microcirculation, raising the future possibility of a bilirubinometer that can measure the bilirubin directly in the intravascular space, in which case TcB measurements could replace the measurement of TSB in the serum just as pulse oximetry has largely replaced the measurement of partial pressure of arterial oxygen.

A. A. Fanaroff, MBBCh, FRCPE

References

1. Yamanouchi I, Yamauchi Y, Igarashi I. Transcutaneous bilirubinometry: preliminary studies of noninvasive transcutaneous bilirubin meter in the Okayama National Hospital. *Pediatrics*. 1980;65:195-202.
2. Maisels MJ. Transcutaneous bilirubinometry. *Neo Reviews*. 2006;7:217-225.
3. Keren R, Luan X, Friedman S, Saddlemire S, Cnaan A, Bhutani V. A comparison of alternative risk-assessment strategies for predicting significant neonatal hyperbilirubinemia in term and near-term infants. *Pediatrics*. 2008;121:e170-e179.
4. Wainer S, Parmar SM, Allegro D, Rabi Y, Lyon ME. Impact of a transcutaneous bilirubinometry program on resource utilization and severe hyperbilirubinemia. *Pediatrics*. 2012;129:77-86.
5. Maisels MJ, Engle W, Wainer S, Jackson GL, McManus S, Artinian F. Transcutaneous bilirubin levels in an outpatient and office population. *J Perinatol*. 2011; 31:621-624.

Outcome and cost analysis of implementing selective Coombs testing in the newborn nursery

Shahid R, Graba S (Loyola Univ Med Ctr, Maywood, IL)

J Perinatol 32:966-969, 2012

Objective.—(1) To determine whether infants born to O+ mothers who had selective cord-blood testing would have higher rates of clinically significant hyperbilirubinemia compared with those newborns who had routine cord-blood testing. (2) To determine the amount of cost savings by implementing a policy of selective cord-blood testing in newborns born to O+ mothers.

Study Design.—We conducted a retrospective pre/post intervention chart review on all infants in the normal newborn nursery at Loyola, born to blood type O+ women between 1 April 2008 and 1 April 2009. The pre-intervention group (routine testing) included infants born within 6 months before implementation of a new policy. The postintervention group (selective testing) included infants born within 6 months following the implementation of a new policy. Data were collected for each of these groups regarding clinically significant hyperbilirubinemia.

Result.—All 250 of the infants in the routine testing group had a cord-blood type and Coombs done, whereas 42 of 164 (25%) infants in the selective group had testing done. By the end of the 6 months following the policy change, only 8% of infants were undergoing cord testing. When comparing routine vs selective testing, there was no statistically significant difference in the 24-h serum bilirubin, rate of phototherapy during the birth hospitalization, rate of readmission for hyperbilirubinemia or peak serum bilirubin level at readmission. The 92% reduction of cord-blood typing and Coombs testing would lead to a cost saving of $4100 per year to our hospital and $18 900 per year to our patients, and 95 h per year of technician time to perform these tests. When extrapolated to Illinois births in 2008, this would lead to an annual cost saving of almost $800 000 to Illinois hospitals and about $3.6 million to patients.

Conclusion.—Selective newborn cord testing of infants born to O+ mothers can decrease the use of resources and costs without increasing the risk of clinically significant hyperbilirubinemia.

▶ About 20 years ago, the director of our blood bank asked me why we measure the blood type and administer the direct antiglobulin test (DAT) on all infants of group O mothers. Of course, I responded that such measurements were important to identify infants who are at risk for developing hyperbilirubinemia. But the blood bank director, anxious to cut costs, persisted and asked me to provide some data documenting the benefit of this procedure. So I reviewed a number of charts of infants of type O mothers, and I was somewhat surprised to find that nowhere in the chart was there any documentation to indicate that the infants' pediatrician had recorded the result of the blood type and DAT, nor was there any indication that, if known, the results of these tests played a role in the timing of the discharge or the plan for follow-up. Perhaps this information was noted by the pediatrician and just not recorded, but I could find no evidence of this thought process.

By this time, we had already introduced transcutaneous bilirubin (TcB) measurements in our nursery, so I was hard-pressed to make the case that we should continue to perform a blood type and DAT on all of these infants. As a result, we discontinued this practice. Our pediatricians were agreeable and, in the ensuing years, we could not detect any increase in the incidence of severe hyperbilirubinemia in our ABO-incompatible infants. Other publications of that era supported this decision.[1,2]

This article again documents the low yield from the routine performance of these tests, although it should be noted that these authors did perform a predischarge total serum bilirubin (TSB) measurement on all of their infants at age 24 hours. We now know that the predischarge, hour-specific, bilirubin measurement, together with the infant's gestational age, provide the information we need to allow an accurate and clinically relevant prediction of the risk, or lack of risk, of subsequent hyperbilirubinemia.[3-6] Infants with ABO hemolytic disease typically develop early jaundice. Of ABO-incompatible, DAT-positive infants who developed a TSB above the 95th percentile,[3] 67% did so within the first 24 hours.[7] Thus, appropriate clinical monitoring and universal TSB/TcB screening should identify early jaundice and the need for blood typing and DAT testing.

The 2004 American Academy of Pediatrics' guidelines recommend that "it is an option to test the cord blood for the infant's blood type and DAT, but it is not required provided that there is appropriate surveillance, risk assessment before discharge, and follow-up."[8] This is sensible advice, and as long as we comply with this recommendation, we should be able to safely abandon the routine testing of the blood type and DAT in infants of group O mothers.

M. J. Maisels, MB, BCh, DSc

References

1. Leistikow EA, Collin MF, Savastano GD, de Sierra TM, Leistikow BN. Wasted health care dollars. Routine cord blood type and Coombs' testing. *Arch Pediatr Adolesc Med.* 1995;149:1147-1151.

2. Madlon-Kay DJ. Identifying ABO incompatibility in newborns: selective vs automatic testing. *J Fam Pract*. 1992;35:278-280.
3. Bhutani VK, Johnson L, Sivieri EM. Predictive ability of a predischarge hour-specific serum bilirubin for subsequent significant hyperbilirubinemia in healthy term and near-term newborns. *Pediatrics*. 1999;103:6-14.
4. Keren R, Luan X, Friedman S, Saddlemire S, Cnaan A, Bhutani V. A comparison of alternative risk-assessment strategies for predicting significant neonatal hyperbilirubinemia in term and near-term infants. *Pediatrics*. 2008;121:e170-e179.
5. Maisels MJ, Deridder JM, Kring EA, Balasubramaniam M. Routine transcutaneous bilirubin measurements combined with clinical risk factors improve the prediction of subsequent hyperbilirubinemia. *J Perinatol*. 2009;29:612-617.
6. Kaur S, Chawla D, Pathak U, Jain S. Predischarge non-invasive risk assessment for prediction of significant hyperbilirubinemia in term and late preterm neonates. *J Perinatol*. 2012;32:716-721.
7. Kaplan M, Hammerman C, Vreman HJ, Wong RJ, Stevenson DK. Hemolysis and hyperbilirubinemia in antiglobulin positive, direct ABO blood group heterospecific neonates. *J Pediatr*. 2010;157:772-777.
8. American Academy of Pediatrics, Subcommittee on Hyperbilirubinemia. Management of hyperbilirubinemia in the newborn infant 35 or more weeks of gestation. *Pediatrics*. 2004;114:297-316.

Dose-Response Relationship of Phototherapy for Hyperbilirubinemia

Vandborg PK, Hansen BM, Greisen G, et al (Aarhus Univ Hosp, Aalborg, Denmark; Copenhagen Univ Hosp, Rigshospitalet, Denmark)
Pediatrics 130:e352-e357, 2012

Background and Objective.—Using light-emitting diodes during conventional phototherapy, it is possible to reduce the distance from light source to infant, thus increasing light irradiance. The objective of this study was to search for a "saturation point" (ie, an irradiation level above which there is no further decrease in total serum bilirubin [TsB]). This was a prospective randomized study performed in the NICU of Aalborg Hospital, Denmark.

Methods.—One hundred fifty-one infants (gestational age ≥ 33 weeks) with uncomplicated hyperbilirubinemia were randomized to 1 of 4 distances from the phototherapy device to the mattress (20, 29, 38, and 47 cm). TsB was measured before and after 24 hours of phototherapy and irradiance every eighth hour. Main outcome was 24-hour decrease of TsB expressed in percent, (Δ TsB$_{0-24}$, difference between TsB$_0$ and TsB$_{24}$ [%]).

Results.—A highly significant linear relation was seen between light irradiance and Δ TsB$_{0-24}$ (%) ($P < .001$): when the irradiance increased from 20 to 55 μW/cm^2/nm, Δ TsB$_{0-24}$ (%) increased from approximately 30% to 50%. In addition, smooth regression showed no tendency for Δ TsB$_{0-24}$ (%) to level off as irradiance increased. Δ TsB$_{0-24}$ (%) was negatively correlated to birth weight and positively to formula volume. Average weight gain during phototherapy was 1%, independent of light irradiance.

Conclusions.—By using light-emitting diodes, we found a linear relation between light irradiance in the range of 20 to 55 μW/cm^2/nm and a decrease in TsB after 24 hours of therapy, with no evidence of a saturation point.

▶ These authors have addressed an unresolved question regarding the efficacy of phototherapy, a question that has always bothered me. We know that irradiance is a critical variable that affects the efficacy of phototherapy. Irradiance is the radiant power incident on a surface, per unit area of the surface, and the spectral irradiance is the irradiance in a specific wavelength band and is expressed as $\mu W/cm^2/nm$. Although there is a direct relationship between the irradiance and the efficacy of phototherapy, the concentration of plasma bilirubin at any given time depends on a number of complex kinetic factors: the rate of formation of bilirubin, the rate of elimination of the photoisomers, the rates of migration of bilirubin and the individual photoisomers into and out of the blood, and the rate of reabsorption of bilirubin from the intestine into the blood. Clearly, some of these rates are independent of the irradiance.

Nevertheless, there are good data documenting a strong relationship between the irradiance and the rate of decline in the serum bilirubin level. The most frequently quoted study of this relationship is that of Tan,[1] whose data suggest that there was a saturation point beyond which an increase in irradiance produced no added efficacy. But these data were troubling because the conversion of bilirubin to excretable products such as lumirubin is irreversible and follows first-order kinetics, suggesting there may not be a saturation point.

As demonstrated in this article, there was a highly significant and linear relation between the irradiance (as it increased from 20 to 55 $\mu w/cm^2/nm$) and the decrease in the bilirubin level. In addition, there was no tendency for the rate of decline in the bilirubin to level off as the irradiance increased. Of course, demonstrating that an irradiance of 55 $\mu W/cm^2/nm$ is effective does not mean it is safe, and we lack the data to address this. Nevertheless, when confronted with a late preterm or term infant with a bilirubin level of 25 mg/dL or more, I would not hesitate to use this level of irradiance to lower the bilirubin as quickly as possible. By contrast, I cannot envisage a scenario where such levels would be necessary in a small preterm infant, and, in that population, there are some data to suggest these levels could be quite harmful.[2]

M. J. Maisels, MB, BCh, DSc

References

1. Tan KL. The nature of the dose-response relationship of phototherapy for neonatal hyperbilirubinemia. *J Pediatr.* 1977;90:448-452.
2. Morris BH, Oh W, Tyson JE, et al. Aggressive vs. conservative phototherapy for infants with extremely low birth weight. *N Engl J Med.* 2008;359:1885-1896.

Neonatal Hyperbilirubinemia in the Low-Intermediate–Risk Category on the Bilirubin Nomogram
Bromiker R, Bin-Nun A, Schimmel MS, et al (Faculty of Medicine of the Hebrew Univ, Jerusalem, Israel)
Pediatrics 130:e470-e475, 2012

Objective.—Predischarge bilirubin screening predicts neonatal hyperbilirubinemia. We evaluated the incidence of false-negative bilirubin screening among readmissions for hyperbilirubinemia.

Methods.—In healthy term and late preterm, predominantly breastfeeding newborns, predischarge transcutaneous bilirubin values were plotted on the hour of life–specific bilirubin nomogram and confirmed with plasma total bilirubin in those with a transcutaneous reading ≥75th percentile, or between the 41st and 75th percentiles in the presence of predictive icterogenic risk factors. False-negative bilirubin screen was defined as a predischarge bilirubin value ≤75th percentile in a newborn who was subsequently readmitted for phototherapy.

Results.—Of a total of 25 439 neonates born between 2008 and 2009, 143 (0.56%) were readmitted with a mean plasma total bilirubin of 18.7 ± 1.7 mg/dL at 125 6 54 hours. False-negative predischarge bilirubin screen was identified in 46 (32.2%). Of these, 6 (4.2%) were in the low-risk zone (≤40th percentile, relative risk [RR] = 1) and 40 (28%) in the intermediate-low–risk zone (41st–75th percentile, RR 7.62 [95% confidence interval 3.23–17.96]). Of those in the high-risk zones, 76 (53.1%) were in the intermediate-high–risk zone (76th–95th percentile, RR 25.32 [11.03–58.10]) and 21 (14.7%) in the high-risk zone (>95th percentile, RR 27.78 [11.23–68.70]).

Conclusions.—Predischarge bilirubin levels in newborns classified as low risk did not eliminate the risk of readmission for hyperbilirubinemia. All newborns including those at low risk must be vigilantly observed for subsequent hyperbilirubinemia.

▶ There is no such thing in medicine as a zero risk, and these authors confirm what has been observed before with regard to the predictive value of predischarge bilirubin levels.[1,2] They used transcutaneous bilirubin (TcB) levels, measured on the morning of discharge and plotted on the Bhutani nomogram,[3] as their risk assessment tool. They found that 2.4 of 1000 infants whose predischarge TcB levels were below the 75th percentile were nevertheless readmitted for phototherapy. Keren et al[2] found a similar risk of 2 of 1000 for infants who were at least 38 weeks' gestation, while for those who were 35 to 37 weeks' gestation, the risk was 20-fold greater (40 of 1000), an important reminder of the dramatic effect of decreasing gestation on the risk of hyperbilirubinemia. In Maisels et al,[1] if the TcB was below the 50th percentile, the risk of subsequently developing a total serum bilirubin (TSB) of 17 mg/dL was only 5 of 10 000, but if the TSB was between the 50th and 75th percentile, the risk was 7 of 1000.

The nomogram that we use is one that we developed in our own population using TcB measurements,[1] and it is much closer to the natural history of neonatal bilirubinemia than the Bhutani nomogram.[3] This does not mean that the Bhutani nomogram is not an effective way of predicting risk, but it is important to understand that the 75th and 40th percentiles in this nomogram, particularly after 48 to 72 hours, do not describe the natural history of neonatal bilirubinemia. Because of sampling bias, these lower zones are spuriously elevated. For example, at 60 hours the 50th and 75th percentiles in the TcB nomogram currently used at the Beaumont Children's Hospital are values of about 8.4 and 9.8 mg/dL, respectively, while the values on the Bhutani nomogram at that age are about 9.5 for the 40th percentile and 12.7 for the 75th percentile. Thus, the TSB values in these lower-risk zones are not that low.

It is important to recognize that if the predischarge TcB is in a lower risk zone, the risk of developing significant hyperbilirubinemia is really quite low, and none of the infants in any of these studies developed truly dangerous TSB levels. Nevertheless, it is also useful to remember that even those with low TcB or TSB levels prior to discharge are not in a zero risk category, and this is particularly important in those infants who belong to ethnic groups in which glucose-6-phosphate dehydrogenase deficiency is prevalent.[4-6]

M. J. Maisels, MB, BCh

References

1. Maisels MJ, DeRidder JM, Kring EA, Balasubramaniam M. Routine transcutaneous bilirubin measurements combined with clinical risk factors improve the prediction of subsequent hyperbilirubinemia. *J Perinatol.* 2009;29:612-617.
2. Keren R, Luan X, Friedman S, Saddlemire S, Cnaan A, Bhutani V. A comparison of alternative risk-assessment strategies for predicting significant neonatal hyperbilirubinemia in term and near-term infants. *Pediatrics.* 2008;121:e170-e179.
3. Bhutani VK, Johnson L, Sivieri EM. Predictive ability of a predischarge hour-specific serum bilirubin for subsequent significant hyperbilirubinemia in healthy-term and near-term newborns. *Pediatrics.* 1999;103:6-14.
4. Johnson L, Bhutani VK, Karp K, Sivieri EM, Shapiro SM. Clinical report from the pilot USA Kernicterus Registry (1992 to 2004). *J Perinatol.* 2009;29:S25-S45.
5. Sgro M, Campbell DM, Kandasamy S, Shah V. Incidence of chronic bilirubin encephalopathy in Canada, 2007-2008. *Pediatrics.* 2012;130:e886-e890.
6. Kaplan M, Hammerman C. Glucose-6-phosphate dehydrogenase deficiency: a potential source of severe neonatal hyperbilirubinaemia and kernicterus. *Semin Neonatol.* 2002;7:121-128.

12 Renal, Metabolism, and Endocrine Disorders

Defining reduced urine output in neonatal ICU: importance for mortality and acute kidney injury classification
de Melo Bezerra CT, Vaz Cunha LC, Libório AB (Univ of Fortaleza, Ceará, Brazil; Universidade Federal Do Ceará, Fortaleza, Brazil)
Nephrol Dial Transplant 28:901-909, 2013

Background.—Acute kidney injury (AKI) is an independent risk factor for mortality in adults and children. Generally, urine output (UO) <1 mL/kg/h is accepted as oliguria in neonates, although it has not been systematically studied. pRIFLE criteria suggest UO cut-offs similar to those of the adult population (0.3 and 0.5 mL/kg/h). The aim of the present study was to investigate UO in correlation with mortality in critically ill neonates and suggest changes in the pRIFLE definition of reduced diuresis.

Methods.—A retrospective cohort study was performed in an eight-bed neonatal intensive care unit (NICU). UO was systematically measured by diaper weight each 3 h. Discriminatory capacity to predict mortality of UO was measured and patients were divided according to UO ranges: G1 >1.5 mL/kg/h; G2 1.0–1.5 mL/kg/h; G3 0.7–1.0 mL/kg/h and G4 <0.7 mL/kg/h. These ranges were incorporated to pRIFLE$_{GFR}$ criteria and its performance was evaluated.

Results.—Of 384 patients admitted at the NICU during the study period, 72 were excluded and overall mortality was 12.8%. UO showed good performance for mortality prediction (area under the curve 0.789, $P < 0.001$). There was a stepwise increase in hospital mortality according to UO groups after controlling for SNAPPE-II and diuretic use. Using these UO ranges with pRIFLE improves its discriminatory capacity (area under the receiver operating characteristic curve 0.882 versus 0.693, $P < 0.05$).

Conclusions.—UO is a predictor of mortality in NICU. An association between a UO threshold <1.5 mL/kg/h and mortality was observed, which is higher than the previously published pRIFLE thresholds. Adopting higher values of UO in pRIFLE criteria can improve its capacity to detect AKI severity in neonates.

▶ Acute kidney injury (AKI), formerly referred to as *acute renal failure*, is a common event even in the neonatal period.[1] The AKI definition was broad and largely different, making it difficult to compare study results. Recently, Akcan-Arikan et al[2] adopted and validated RIFLE (Risk, Injury, Failure, Loss and End-stage renal disease) criteria for critically ill children—pRIFLE. In this study, the authors have adapted glomerular filtration rate decline criteria from adults and maintained the same urinary output definition. However, before this report, the criteria had not been validated in neonates. The authors are to be complimented on the meticulous collection of output data and for performing the first study to evaluate pRIFLE criteria in a general neonatal intensive care unit. They found an excellent correlation between illness severity and decreased urine output. Urine output was low in asphyxiated infants, those with septic shock, those with low 5-min Apgar scores, and infants with low birth weight. Mortality was associated with asphyxia, septic shock, decreased urine output, and low platelets (Table 5 in the original article). There was a direct relationship between urine output and mortality, and Fig 3 in the original article shows the clear separation in mortality for babies with an output of less than 1.5 mL/h. The infants with reduced output also had other criteria of AKI, including hyperkalemia and metabolic acidosis.

Askenazi et al[3] have reported that urine biomarkers can predict AKI in newborns. Compared with the infants without AKI, those with AKI had higher levels of urine cystatin C, lower levels of UMOD, and lower levels of epithelial growth factor. Although the differences were not statistically significant, levels of urine neutrophil gelatinase-associated lipocalin (NGAL) kidney injury molecule 1, and osteopontin trended higher in infants with AKI. Safrides et al[4] have confirmed these findings, noting that serum and urinary NGAL as well as urinary cystatin C are sensitive early biomarkers that increase significantly in asphyxiated neonates, even those not fulfilling AKI criteria.

Jetton and Askenazi[5] note that increased attention is focused on the recognition and treatment of AKI. Clinicians should be alerted to this condition because it is associated with a high mortality rate. Early recognition and appropriate intervention may reduce this mortality.

A. A. Fanaroff, MBBCh, FRCPE

References

1. Koralkar R, Ambalavanan N, Levitan EB, et al. Acute kidney injury reduces survival in very low birth weight infants. *Pediatr Res.* 2011;69:354-358.
2. Akcan-Arikan A, Zappitelli M, Loftis LL, Washburn KK, Jefferson LS, Goldstein SL. Modified RIFLE criteria in critically ill children with acute kidney injury. *Kidney Int.* 2007;71:1028-1035.
3. Askenazi DJ, Koralkar R, Hundley HE, et al. Urine biomarkers predict acute kidney injury in newborns. *J Pediatr.* 2012;161:270-275.e1.
4. Sarafudis S, Tsepkenski E, Agakidou E, et al. Serum and urine acute kidney injury biomarkers in asphyxiated neonates. *Pediatr Nephrol.* 2012;27:1575-1582.
5. Jetton JG, Askenazi DJ. Update on acute kidney injury in the neonate. *Curr Opin Pediatr.* 2012;24:191-196.

Management of renal dysfunction following term perinatal hypoxia-ischaemia
Sweetman DU, Riordan M, Molloy EJ (Natl Maternity Hosp, Dublin, Ireland; Our Lady's Children's Hosp, Crumlin, Dublin, Ireland)
Acta Paediatr 102:233-241, 2013

Acute kidney injury frequently develops following the term perinatal hypoxia-ischaemia. Quantifying the degree of acute kidney injury is difficult, however, as the methods currently in use are suboptimal. Acute kidney injury management is largely supportive with little evidence basis for many interventions. This review discusses management strategies and novel biomarkers that may improve diagnosis and management of renal injury following perinatal hypoxia-ischaemia.

Conclusion.—Following perinatal hypoxia-ischaemia, acute kidney injury is common. Management of neonatal acute kidney injury is largely supportive. Novel acute kidney injury biomarkers may play a role in optimizing new categorical definitions of renal injury. Studies are needed to investigate the impact of neonatal acute kidney injury on long-term outcome.

▶ Renal injury is a frequent accompaniment of the multiorgan, multisystem dysfunction after intrapartum asphyxia. This interesting article thoroughly reviewed the pathophysiology and management of acute renal injury after perinatal hypoxic-ischemic insult in the term infant. As the authors indicate, most current management is not evidence based but stems from expert advice or personal experience. Some strategies, such as fluid restriction or sodium bicarbonate therapy, may do more harm than good.

The authors remind us that elevated serum creatinine, decreased glomerular filtration rate, and oliguria are imprecise measures of renal injury and that certain biomarkers (cystatin C, neutrophil gelatinase—associated lipocalin, liver-type fatty acid-binding protein, interleukin-18 and kidney injury molecule-1) may be more sensitive and specific.

A scheme of management is suggested, including diagnostic and therapeutic strategies, which is very helpful, but the true value of the report is to remind us of the limitations of our current knowledge and the need for continued investigation.

S. M. Donn, MD

The Role of Novel Biomarkers in Early Diagnosis and Prognosis of Acute Kidney Injury in Newborns
Argyri I, Xanthos T, Varsami M, et al (Natl and Kapodistrian Univ of Athens, Greece; et al)
Am J Perinatol 30:347-352, 2013

Acute kidney injury (AKI) refers to the rapid loss of renal function. In clinical practice, AKI is common among hospitalized patients of all age groups including neonates and remains an important cause of morbidity and mortality due to its late diagnosis and therefore delayed therapeutic intervention. Although the precise incidence of AKI in newborn is unknown, several studies have reported that 8 to 24% of all critically ill newborns in neonatal intensive care units may develop the condition. We aim at reviewing the existing literature on novel serum and urinary biomarkers and discuss their role in the early diagnosis and prognosis of AKI in newborns. Specifically, this review will focus on cystatin C (CysC), neutrophil gelatinase-associated lipocalin (NGAL) and interleukin-18 (IL-18) in serum and on CysC, NGAL, kidney injury molecule-1, and IL-18 in urine.

▶ I found this article to be very informative and useful. The diagnosis and treatment of acute kidney injury is a common challenge in the neonatal intensive care unit. Our traditional approach has been to examine markers of renal function—serum creatinine, blood urea nitrogen, and urine output. The first 2 seldom increase until after injury has occurred, and urine production can be extremely variable in the first 24 hours of life.

In this article, the authors describe the use of 3 novel biomarkers to diagnose and follow acute kidney injury in neonatal patients. As they suggest, earlier diagnosis would indeed be beneficial, not only in prognosis, but in actual management, given the large number of potentially nephrotoxic pharmaceuticals to which newborns are exposed. Although more investigation needs to occur, especially looking at subgroups and the relationship between the concentrations of biomarkers in blood/serum and urine, this is a new approach to acute kidney injury, which holds the promise of better care for affected infants.

S. M. Donn, MD

Antibiotic Prophylaxis for Urinary Tract Infections in Antenatal Hydronephrosis
Braga LH, Mijovic H, Farrokhyar F, et al (McMaster Univ, Hamilton, Ontario, Canada; et al)
Pediatrics 131:e251-e261, 2013

Background and Objective.—Continuous antibiotic prophylaxis (CAP) is recommended to prevent urinary tract infections (UTIs) in newborns with antenatal hydronephrosis (HN). However, there is a paucity of high-level evidence supporting this practice. The goal of this study was to conduct a systematic evaluation to determine the value of CAP in reducing the rate of UTIs in this patient population.

Methods.—Pertinent articles and abstracts from 4 electronic databases and gray literature, spanning publication dates between 1990 and 2010, were included. Eligibility criteria included studies of children <2 years old with antenatal HN, receiving either CAP or not, and reporting on development of UTIs, capturing information on voiding cystourethrogram (VCUG) result and HN grade. Full-text screening and quality appraisal were conducted by 2 independent reviewers.

Results.—Of 1681 citations, 21 were included in the final analysis ($N = 3876$ infants). Of these, 76% were of moderate or low quality. Pooled UTI rates in patients with low-grade HN were similar regardless of CAP status: 2.2% on prophylaxis versus 2.8% not receiving prophylaxis. In children with high-grade HN, patients receiving CAP had a significantly lower UTI rate versus those not receiving CAP (14.6% [95% confidence interval: 9.3–22.0] vs 28.9% [95% confidence interval: 24.6–33.6], $P < 01$). The estimated number needed to treat to prevent 1 UTI in patients with high-grade HN was 7.

Conclusions.—This systematic review suggests value in offering CAP to infants with high-grade HN, however the impact of important variables (eg, gender, reflux, circumcision status) could not be assessed. The overall level of evidence of available data is unfortunately moderate to low.

▶ It is not uncommon to detect renal abnormalities antenatally. Most would agree that all infants with abnormalities on antenatal sonogram should undergo postnatal evaluation with a sonogram shortly after birth and at 4 to 6 weeks of age. Becker[1] noted: "Recommended postnatal evaluation of these infants has evolved to minimize invasive testing while maximizing detection of significant abnormalities." The debate is whether to use prophylactic antibiotics for antenatally detected hydronephrosis.

Yiee et al[2] surveyed 461 pediatricians because they, rather than pediatric urologists, are the primary gatekeepers who initiate therapy for antenatally diagnosed hydronephrosis; 244 (53%) responded. Of the respondents, 56% routinely prescribed antibiotics for prenatally detected hydronephrosis and 57% performed the postnatal workup themselves. Of these, 98% routinely ordered ultrasound scans and 40% routinely ordered voiding cystourethrograms. Despite urology consultation being readily available for 94% of the respondents, only 41% were always referred to a specialist. The pediatricians who believe prophylactic antibiotics to be beneficial were significantly more likely to prescribe antibiotics than those who had not read the published data (odds ratio [OR] 6.1; 95% confidence interval [CI], 2 to 15). Those without specialist consultation readily available had an increased odds of starting prophylactic antibiotics compared with those who had consultation available (OR 7.2; 95% CI, 1.3 to 39).

Merguerian et al[3] created a survey questionnaire for pediatric urologists both in the United States and Europe to ascertain (1) which prenatal parameters trigger postnatal evaluation, (2) how pediatric urologists manage prenatal hydronephrosis, and (3) what their recommendations for antibiotic prophylaxis are. It should come as no great surprise that there was significant response variability to all of the questions answered, with no question achieving a consensus of more than 50%. Although European and US urologists were equally experienced overall, there was wide variability in the parameters triggering intervention and in the use of prophylactic antibiotics. Pediatric urologists in practice more than 15 years were less likely to prescribe antibiotic prophylaxis at birth than those in practice less than 15 years. Variation also existed by geographic region, with US physicians more likely to prescribe antibiotics for any prenatal hydronephrosis compared with their European counterparts (77% vs 40%,

P < .005), but these differences were less significant with high-grade hydronephrosis.

So we turn to these authors for the definitive answers. Starting with over 1600 articles, the final analysis included only 21 (N = 3876 infants). Of these, 76% were of moderate or low quality. After analyzing the data every way they could, they also concluded that continuous antibiotic prophylaxis was of value only in high-grade hydronephrosis. I doubt whether this will stop pediatricians from prescribing continuous antibiotics for all grades of hydronephrosis. It is important that this information be disseminated to pediatricians.

A. A. Fanaroff, MBBCh, FRCPE

References

1. Becker AM. Postnatal evaluation of infants with an abnormal antenatal renal sonogram. *Curr Opin Pediatr.* 2009;21:207-213.
2. Yiee JH, Tasian GE, Copp HL. Management trends in prenatally detected hydronephrosis: national survey of pediatrician practice patterns and antibiotic use. *Urology.* 2011;78:895-901.
3. Merguerian PA, Herz D, McQuiston L, Van Bibber M. Variation among pediatric urologists and across 2 continents in antibiotic prophylaxis and evaluation for prenatally detected hydronephrosis: a survey of American and European pediatric urologists. *J Urol.* 2010;184:1710-1715.

Hypoglycemia is Associated with Increased Risk for Brain Injury and Adverse Neurodevelopmental Outcome in Neonates at Risk for Encephalopathy

Tam EWY, Haeusslein LA, Bonifacio SL, et al (Univ of California San Francisco)
J Pediatr 161:88-93, 2012

Objective.—To investigate the contribution of hypoglycemia in the first 24 hours after birth to brain injury in term newborns at risk for neonatal encephalopathy.

Study Design.—A prospective cohort of 94 term neonates born between 1994 and 2010 with early postnatal brain magnetic resonance imaging studies were analyzed for regions of brain injury. Neurodevelopmental outcome was assessed at 1 year of age.

Results.—Hypoglycemia (glucose <46 mg/dL) in the first 24 hours after birth was detected in 16% of the cohort. Adjusting for potential confounders of early perinatal distress and need for resuscitation, neonatal hypoglycemia was associated with a 3.72-fold increased odds of corticospinal tract injury (*P* =.047). Hypoglycemia was also associated with 4.82-fold increased odds of 1-point worsened neuromotor score (*P* =.038) and a 15-point lower cognitive and language score on the Bayley Scales of Infant Development (*P* =.015).

Conclusion.—Neonatal hypoglycemia is associated with additional risks in the setting of neonatal encephalopathy with increased corticospinal tract injury and adverse motor and cognitive outcomes.

▶ Hypoxia-ischemia is the most common cause of neonatal encephalopathy. However, the etiologies can be varied and, in some instances, may include more than 1 factor. Animal model studies suggest that when neonatal hypoglycemia occurs in combination with perinatal hypoxia-ischemia, the outcome is worse.

The data in this article indicate that newborns who have evidence of hypoglycemia in the 24 hours after birth and who are at risk for hypoxic-ischemic encephalopathy (HIE) have increased odds of both corticospinal tract injury on magnetic resonance imaging (MRI) and motor and cognitive impairment at 1 year of age. At risk for HIE was defined as an umbilical artery pH less than 7.1, umbilical artery base deficit greater than 10, or a 5-minute Apgar score of 5 or lower.

The conclusion in the abstract is somewhat misleading. Although it is true that neonatal hypoglycemia was associated with additional risks in the setting of HIE, what is not evident from the abstract is that there was no correlation between cognitive impairment and the presence of corticospinal tract injury on MRI and that the 1-point difference in motor scores, while statistically significant, most likely was not clinically significant.

L. A. Papile, MD

Hypoglycemia is Associated with Increased Risk for Brain Injury and Adverse Neurodevelopmental Outcome in Neonates at Risk for Encephalopathy

Tam EWY, Haeusslein LA, Bonifacio SL, et al (Univ of California San Francisco)
J Pediatr 161:88-93, 2012

Objective.—To investigate the contribution of hypoglycemia in the first 24 hours after birth to brain injury in term newborns at risk for neonatal encephalopathy.

Study Design.—A prospective cohort of 94 term neonates born between 1994 and 2010 with early postnatal brain magnetic resonance imaging studies were analyzed for regions of brain injury. Neurodevelopmental outcome was assessed at 1 year of age.

Results.—Hypoglycemia (glucose <46 mg/dL) in the first 24 hours after birth was detected in 16% of the cohort. Adjusting for potential confounders of early perinatal distress and need for resuscitation, neonatal hypoglycemia was associated with a 3.72-fold increased odds of corticospinal tract injury $(P = .047)$. Hypoglycemia was also associated with 4.82-fold increased odds of 1-point worsened neuromotor score $(P = .038)$ and a 15-point lower cognitive and language score on the Bayley Scales of Infant Development $(P = .015)$.

Conclusion.—Neonatal hypoglycemia is associated with additional risks in the setting of neonatal encephalopathy with increased corticospinal tract injury and adverse motor and cognitive outcomes.

▶ Hypoglycemia is one of the common metabolic problems in neonatal medicine,[1] and although frequently observed low blood glucose levels in the majority of healthy newborn infants are the reflections of normal metabolic adaptation to extrauterine life, there has been a genuine concern that prolonged or recurrent low blood glucose levels may result in acute systemic effects and long-term neurological consequences.[2,3]

Important observational data from babies with birth weight < 1850 g reported in 1988 that the number of days on which moderate hypoglycemia (glucose concentration < 46 mg/dL) occurred was strongly related to reduced mental and motor development at 18 months of age, even after adjustment for a wide range of factors known to influence development.[4] These findings have had a profound influence in defining neonatal hypoglycemia ever since, and it was not long before clinicians were extrapolating from this observational study on preterm babies, and assuming that all newborn babies could be equally at risk from similar blood glucose levels, even when they seemed normal on clinical examinations.[5] Systematic review in 2006 of all the available data[6] concluded that none of the 18 eligible studies identified provided a valid estimate of the effect of neonatal hypoglycemia on neurodevelopment, and recently published data from a 15-year follow-up cohort found no evidence to support the belief that recurrent low blood glucose levels of < 46 mg/dL posed a hazard to preterm babies.[7]

It has been known that newborns with perinatal hypoxia—ischemia are at risk for hypoglycemia. However, attempts to look at the implications of neonatal hypoglycemia on brain injury in newborns with encephalopathy have come up with conflicting findings.[8-10] A prospective cohort study by Tam et al[11] has systematically examined the patterns of brain injury associated with hypoglycemia in the context of neonatal encephalopathy, and it has also provided additional information on associations between hypoglycemia in the first 24 hours with higher risk of adverse neurodevelopmental outcomes at 12 months of age. The authors of this study emphasized the lack of standardization of the frequency of blood glucose measurements in observational studies that might lead to a sampling bias or underrepresentation of the true degree of hypoglycemia. They also highlighted the challenges of statistical adjustments for important confounding factors and the difficulty of proving causation when an observational approach is used.

Much progress has been made over the years in our understanding of the mechanisms of glucose homeostasis in early postnatal life. However, the threshold values of blood glucose concentrations below which may cause acute systemic effects and long-term neurological consequences remain unknown. It is most important that we accept the knowledge gaps and address the research needs for understanding and treating neonatal hypoglycemia.[12]

W. Tin, MD, FRCPCH

References

1. Cornblath M. Neonatal hypoglycemia 30 years later: does it injure the brain? Historical summary and present challenges. *Acta Paediatr Jpn.* 1997;39:S7-11.
2. Pildes R, Cornblath M, Warren I, et al. A prospective controlled study of neonatal hypoglycemia. *Pediatrics.* 1974;54:5-14.
3. Anderson JM, Milner RDG, Strich SJ. Effects of neonatal hypoglycemia on the nervous system: a pathological study. *J Neurol Neurosurg Psychiatry.* 1967;30: 295-310.
4. Lucas A, Morley R, Cole TJ. Adverse neurodevelopmental outcome of moderate neonatal hypoglycaemia. *BMJ.* 1988;317:1481-1487.
5. Cornblath M, Schwartz R, Aynsley-Green A, et al. Hypoglycemia in infancy: the need for rational definition. A Ciba Foundation discussion meeting. *Pediatrics.* 1990;85:834-837.
6. Boyult N, van Kempen A, Offringa M. Neurodevelopment after neonatal hypoglycemia: a systematic review and design of an optimal future study. *Pediatrics.* 2006;117:2231-2243.
7. Tin W, Brunskill G, Kelly T, et al. 15-year follow-up of recurrent "hypoglycemia" in preterm infants. *Pediatrics.* 2012;130:e1497-e1503.
8. Salhab WA, Wyckoff MH, Laptook AR, et al. Initial hypoglycemia and neonatal brain injury in term infants with severe fetal acidemia. *Pediatrics.* 2004;114: 361-366.
9. Basu P, Som S, Chouduri N, et al. Contribution of the blood glucose level in perinatal asphyxia. *Eur J Pediatr.* 2009;168:833-838.
10. Nadeem M, Murray DM, Boylan GB, et al. Early blood glucose profile and neurodevelopmental outcome at two years in neonatal hypoxic-ischaemic encephalopathy. *BMC Pediatr.* 2011;11:10.
11. Tam EWY, Haeusslein LA, Bonifacio SL, et al. Hypoglycemia is associated with increased risk for brain injury and adverse neurodevelopmental outcome in neonates at risk for encephalopathy. *J Pediatr.* 2012;161:88-93.
12. Hay WW, Raju TNK, Higgins RD, et al. Knowledge gaps and research needs for understanding and treating neonatal hypoglycemia: workshop report from Eunice Kennedy Shriver National Institute of Child Health and Human Development. *J Pediatr.* 2009;155:612-617.

15-Year Follow-Up of Recurrent "Hypoglycemia" in Preterm Infants

Tin W, Brunskill G, Kelly T, et al (James Cook Univ Hosp, Middlesbrough, UK; Newcastle General Hosp, Newcastle upon Tyne, UK; et al)
Pediatrics 130:e1497-e1503, 2012

Background.—Observational study of 543 infants who weighed <1850 g, published in 1988 reported seriously impaired motor and cognitive development at 18 months in those with recurrent, asymptomatic hypoglycemia (plasma glucose level ≤2.5 mmol/L on ≥3 days). No study has yet replicated this observation.

Aim.—To quantify disability in a similar cohort of children followed up throughout childhood.

Population.—All children born at <32 weeks' gestation in the north of England in 1990−1991 and had laboratory blood glucose levels measured daily for the first 10 days of life.

Results.—Forty-seven index children of the 566 who survived to 2 years had a blood glucose level of ≤2.5 mmol/L on ≥3 days. All of these children and hypoglycemia-free controls, matched for hospital of care, gestation, and birth weight, were assessed at age 2. No differences in developmental progress or physical disability were detected. The families were seen again when the children were 15 years old, and 38 of the index children (81%) and matched controls agreed to detailed psychometric assessment. Findings in the 2 groups were nearly identical (mean full-scale IQ: 80.7 vs 81.2). Findings in the 21 children with a level of ≤2.5 mmol/L on ≥4 days, 7 children with a level this low on 5 days, and 11 children with a level of <2.0 mmol/L on 3 different days did not alter these conclusions.

Conclusions.—This study found no evidence to support the belief that recurrent low blood glucose levels (≤2.5 mmol/L) in the first 10 days of life usually pose a hazard to preterm infants.

▶ Sometimes it seems that the more we learn, the less we know. A few decades ago, it was accepted that low blood glucose levels in preterm infants, being common, were normal and did not require corrective intervention. Consequently, blood glucose levels as low as 20 to 25 mg/dL (1.1–1.3 mmol/L) were tolerated without concern in many quarters, but questions were raised about the wisdom of this sanguine attitude. In this context, a study reported by Lucas et al in 1988 provided data that proved influential for subsequent practice.[1] Based on observational data from 661 infants with birth weights less than 1850 g, they reported an increased risk of neurodevelopmental impairment (cerebral palsy or developmental delay at 18 months of age) among those whose blood glucose levels were less than 47 mg/dL (2.6 mmol/L) on multiple (3 to 7) days. While emphasizing that "the association between modest hypoglycemia and poor neurodevelopment… might not be causal and might reflect… failure to adjust adequately for confounding factors," they concluded that "it would be wise not to allow plasma glucose concentrations in preterm, and perhaps full term, infants to remain below 2.6 mmol/L." (It is notable that infants with subsequent neurodevelopmental impairment were also more likely to have been on assisted ventilation for more than 6 days, to have had persistent apnea for more than 6 days, to have undergone exchange transfusion, and to have had blood culture–proven bacterial infection.) To a large extent, these data have governed practice for the past 25 years. Now this large, population-based, long-term, prospective, observational study provides evidence that challenges the conclusion that the previously observed association is causal and suggests that an aggressive approach to maintenance of serum glucose levels greater than 45 mg/dL (2.5 mmol/L) is not necessary. In this prospectively identified cohort, including all 566 infants born before 32 weeks of gestation in the North of England in 1990 and 1991, serial blood glucose levels were systematically monitored daily for the first 10 postnatal days. Forty-seven infants who had glucose levels ≤45 mg/dL on 3 or more days were prospectively matched with control infants who did not have low glucose levels. Neurodevelopmental outcomes at 18 months and 15 years were essentially identical, and no gradient of risk with increasing severity of hypoglycemia was evident. Their conclusion that they "found no evidence… that recurrent low blood glucose levels of ≤2.5 mmol/L

(45 mg/dL) pose a hazard to preterm infants" should provide reassurance to those of us who must treat infants in whom that goal may be difficult to achieve. The authors provide an important caution regarding the limitations of this conclusion, however: "It would be unwise to assume that low blood glucose levels cannot be damaging in the preterm infant even in the absence of overt recognizable signs, simply because this study has failed to replicate the earlier study from Cambridge. All that the current study can do is show that the danger threshold must be lower than many had come to think it was." Similarly, it would not be wise to extrapolate these observations to infants with hyperinsulinemic hypoglycemia, in whom the physiologic circumstances and mechanisms of brain injury may be distinct from those in the otherwise uncomplicated preterm infant.

W. E. Benitz, MD

Reference

1. Lucas A, Morley R, Cole TJ. Adverse neurodevelopmental outcome of moderate neonatal hypoglycaemia. *BMJ.* 1988;297:1304-1308.

Limited response to CRH stimulation tests at 2 weeks of age in preterm infants born at less than 30 weeks of gestational age
Niwa F, Kawai M, Kanazawa H, et al (Kyoto Univ, Japan)
Clin Endocrinol 78:724-729, 2013

Background.—The high incidence of glucocorticoid-responsive complications in extremely preterm infants suggests the immaturity of their adrenal function; however, knowledge of the hypothalamus—pituitary—adrenal (HPA) axis in extremely preterm infants is limited.

Methods.—To clarify the characteristics of the HPA axis in preterm very low birthweight (VLBW) infants, we performed CRH tests repeatedly: at about 2 weeks of age and at term (37—41 weeks of postmenstrual age) for 21 VLBW infants with a gestational age (GA) < 30 weeks at birth.

Results.—Basal cortisol values at 2 weeks of age were significantly higher than those at term in VLBW infants < 30 weeks of gestation at birth (304·1 ± 146·3 nmol/l *vs* 184·7 ± 108·2 nmol/l). Response to corticotropin-releasing hormone (CRH) stimulation tests at 2 weeks of age was significantly lower than at term (delta cortisol 148·3 ± 90·7 nmol/l *vs* 271·8 ± 167·0 nmol/l, delta ACTH 3·9 ± 3·2 pmol/l *vs* 12·3 ± 9·2 pmol/l, respectively). We found that earlier GA contributed to the higher basal cortisol values, and antenatal glucocorticoid (AG) contributed to the lower response of cortisol to CRH tests at 2 weeks of age.

Conclusions.—VLBW infants showed a characteristic pattern in the HPA axis at 2 weeks of age: higher basal cortisol values and lower response to CRH tests. This study suggested that AG was related to the lower response to CRH tests, at least partly.

▶ Relative deficiency of cortisol seems to be an endemic feature of extreme prematurity. Extremely-low-birth-weight (ELBW) babies often exhibit hypotension that responds to cortisol replacement, either in the first few days after birth or as late-onset circulatory collapse in the second or third week. Low cortisol levels are associated with an increased risk of bronchopulmonary dysplasia (which is not altered by cortisol replacement) but are not predictive of hypotension or vasopressor drug requirements. The most severe complications of extreme prematurity (death, intraventricular hemorrhage, bowel perforation) are associated with high cortisol levels during the first 2 days after birth. The relationship between cortisol levels and hemodynamic compromise, therefore, remains uncertain.

Clinical observations show that hypotensive ELBW infants may have low basal cortisol levels but respond nicely to corticotropin stimulation, indicating that they can produce cortisol but choose not to. This article provides some insight into why. Examining the other end of the hypothalamic-pituitary-adrenal (HPA) axis in infants born at less than 30 weeks' gestation, these investigators from Kyoto found that stimulation of the HPA axis with corticotropin-releasing hormone (CRH) produced substantially smaller increments in cortisol and corticotropin levels and lower peak corticotropin levels at 2 weeks of age than upon retesting at the equivalent of term. Antenatal glucocorticoid treatment accounted for only part of this difference. These results imply that failure to mount a proportionate glucocorticoid response to stress in these ELBW infants may be regulated centrally, at least partly through blunted hypothalamic responsiveness to CRH. If this is so, corticotropin stimulation test results (ie, serum cortisol levels before and after administration of a corticotropin dose) are likely to be poor predictors of the need for or response to hydrocortisone supplementation in this population. We are in great need of additional data to characterize the function of the HPA axis in this unique population, particularly at earlier ages than were studied in this important article.

W. E. Benitz, MD

Clinical Outcomes of Neonatal Onset Proximal versus Distal Urea Cycle Disorders Do Not Differ
Ah Mew N, on behalf of the Urea Cycle Disorders Consortium of the Rare Diseases Clinical Research Network (Children's Natl Med Ctr, Washington, DC; et al)
J Pediatr 162:324-329.e1, 2013

Objective.—To compare the clinical course and outcome of patients diagnosed with one of 4 neonatal-onset urea cycle disorders (UCDs): deficiency of carbamyl phosphate synthase 1 (CPSD), ornithine transcarbamylase (OTCD), argininosuccinate synthase (ASD), or argininosuccinate lyase (ALD).

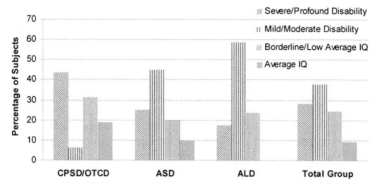

FIGURE 1.—Neurodevelopmental outcome of subjects age 4 years and older by diagnosis. Each diagnostic cohort—proximal UCD (CPSD/OTCD), ASD, and ALD—as well as the total neonatal UCD cohort, is stratified by neurodevelopmental outcome. When no FSIQ was available, Verbal IQ or Performance IQ was used to determine categorization. *Profound/severe range of disability,* Subject was not testable by traditional IQ testing for their age range Bayley Scales were instead administered to derive a DQ; *Mild-moderate range of disability,* FSIQ score of 45-69. *Low average/borderline functioning,* FSIQ score of 70-89; *Broadly average,* FSIQ score 90-109; *Above average,* FSIQ score ≥110 (No subject met this criterion). (Reprinted from Journal Pediatrics. Ah Mew N, on behalf of the Urea Cycle Disorders Consortium of the Rare Diseases Clinical Research Network. Clinical outcomes of neonatal onset proximal versus distal urea cycle disorders do not differ. *J Pediatr.* 2013;162:324-329.e1, Copyright 2013, with permission from Elsevier.)

Study Design.—Clinical, biochemical, and neuropsychological data from 103 subjects with neonatal-onset UCDs were derived from the Longitudinal Study of Urea Cycle Disorders, an observational protocol of the Urea Cycle Disorders Consortium, one of the Rare Disease Clinical Research Networks.

Results.—Some 88% of the subjects presented clinically by age 7 days. Peak ammonia level was 963 μM in patients with proximal UCDs (CPSD or OTCD), compared with 589 μM in ASD and 573 μM in ALD. Roughly 25% of subjects with CPSD or OTCD, 18% of those with ASD, and 67% of those with ALD had a "honeymoon period," defined as the time interval from discharge from initial admission to subsequent admission for hyperammonemia, greater than 1 year. The proportion of patients with a poor outcome (IQ/Developmental Quotient <70) was greatest in ALD (68%), followed by ASD (54%) and CPSD/OTCD (47%). This trend was not significant, but was observed in both patients aged <4 years and those aged ≥4 years. Poor cognitive outcome was not correlated with peak ammonia level or duration of initial admission.

Conclusion.—Neurocognitive outcomes do not differ between patients with proximal UCDs and those with distal UCDs. Factors other than hyperammonemia may contribute to poor neurocognitive outcome in the distal UCDs (Fig 1).

▶ This study describes a cohort of 103 subjects from the Urea Cycle Consortium of the Rare Diseases Clinical Research Network, a group comprising 14 research sites at academic centers in the United States, Canada, and Europe. The purpose was to compare the clinical course and outcome of patients who had one of

4 neonatal-onset urea cycle disorders. These included carbamyl phosphate synthase 1 (CPSD), ornithine transcarbamylase (OTCD), argininosuccinate synthase (ASD), and argininosuccinate lyase (ALD) deficiencies. The first 2 were categorized as proximal urea cycle disorders and the second 2 as distal urea cycle disorders. This was a complex study because many of these infants underwent significant interventions during the course of their disease, including many who had liver transplantation. Of major interest was that the mortality of these patients was low (only 4 deaths) despite their severe illness. Most of these infants presented with symptoms in the first week after birth, with the proximal deficiency diseases presenting a bit earlier than the distal. Mean Bayley Cognitive scores in those less than 4 years of age were in the 70s in all groups without a clear difference. After 4 years of age, poor cognitive outcomes appeared slightly worse (not statistically significant) in the ALD group, but of interest was the finding that some children in the CPSD/OTCD and ASD groups had average IQs but none in the ALD group (Fig 1). Hyperammonemia shortly after birth was highest in the proximal group, but this did not correlate with subsequent neurodevelopmental outcome.

I really like this study because it accumulated and summarized much data from different centers in a useful manner that can be used by clinicians caring for these children as well as the children's families.

J. Neu, MD

13 Miscellaneous

Mortality and Neonatal Morbidity Among Infants 501 to 1500 Grams From 2000 to 2009

Horbar JD, Carpenter JH, Badger GJ, et al (Univ of Vermont, Burlington)

Pediatrics 129:1019-1026, 2012

Objective.—To identify changes in mortality and neonatal morbidities for infants with birth weight 501 to 1500 g born from 2000 to 2009.

Methods.—There were 355806 infants weighing 501 to 1500 g who were born in 2000–2009. Mortality during initial hospitalization and major neonatal morbidity in survivors (early and late infection, chronic lung disease, necrotizing enterocolitis, severe retinopathy of prematurity, severe intraventricular hemorrhage, and periventricular leukomalacia) were assessed by using data from 669 North American hospitals in the Vermont Oxford Network.

Results.—From 2000 to 2009, mortality for infants weighing 501 to 1500 g decreased from 14.3% to 12.4% (difference, -1.9%; 95% confidence interval, -2.3% to -1.5%). Major morbidity in survivors decreased from 46.4% to 41.4% (difference, -4.9%; 95% confidence interval, -5.6% to -4.2%). In 2009, mortality ranged from 36.6% for infants 501 to 750 g to 3.5% for infants 1251 to 1500 g, whereas major morbidity in survivors ranged from 82.7% to 18.7%. In 2009, 49.2% of all very low birth weight infants and 89.2% of infants 501 to 750 g either died or survived with a major neonatal morbidity.

Conclusions.—Mortality and major neonatal morbidity in survivors decreased for infants with birth weight 501 to 1500 g between 2000 and 2009. However, at the end of the decade, a high proportion of these infants still either died or survived after experiencing ≥ 1 major neonatal morbidity known to be associated with both short- and long-term adverse consequences (Fig 1).

▶ This series of analyses of Vermont Oxford Network data by Horbar et al shows modest but steady improvement in neonatal intensive care unit mortality and morbidity among infants born 155 to 501 g over the period from 2000 through 2009. Mortality rate decreased among the overall group from 14.3% to 12.4% and was modestly but consistently lower across all birth weight subgroups. The risk of any major morbidity in the overall group decreased from 45.8% to 41.4%, with rates showing the greatest declines among infants born at 751 g or greater. Specific morbidities showing a significant decline included late bacterial infection, necrotizing enterocolitis, chronic lung disease, severe intraventricular

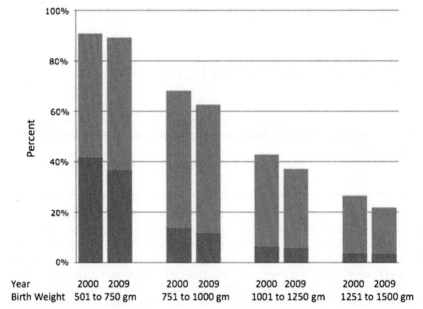

FIGURE 1.—Mortality and major neonatal morbidity in survivors in 2009 compared with 2000 by birth weight category for infants 501 to 1500 g. Mortality (red bar) and major neonatal morbidity in survivors (blue bar) by 250-g birth weight category in 2000 and 2009. The total height of the bar represents the percentage of infants who either died or survived with ≥1 more major neonatal morbidity. For interpretation of the references to color in this figure legend, the reader is referred to web version of this article. (Reproduced with permission from Pediatrics. Horbar JD, Carpenter JH, Badger GJ, et al. Mortality and neonatal morbidity among infants 501 to 1500 grams from 2000 to 2009. *Pediatrics*. 2012;129:1019-1026, Copyright 2012, by the American Academy of Pediatrics.)

hemorrhage, periventricular leukomalacia, and severe retinopathy of prematurity. The sad news is that the rates of morbidity remain unacceptably high, especially among the lowest birth weight babies, with 82.7% of infants born 501 to 750 g and 57% of infants born 751 to 1000 g experiencing at least one major morbidity. An accompanying editorial[1] focused mainly on neurologic outcomes; former Pediatrics editor Dr Jerold Lucey claims, "we can do better"—indeed must do better—an outcome that only can be accomplished through redoubled efforts to form productive international research consortia that foster more rapid completion of clinical trials of potential new interventions. Dr Lucey is so right.

L. J. Van Marter, MD, MPH

Reference

1. Lucey J. A new era in neonatology brain care: we can do better. *Pediatrics*. 2012; 129:1164-1165.

Mortality and Neonatal Morbidity Among Infants 501 to 1500 Grams From 2000 to 2009

Horbar JD, Carpenter JH, Badger GJ, et al (Univ of Vermont, Burlington; Vermont Oxford Network, Burlington)
Pediatrics 129:1019-1026, 2012

Objective.—To identify changes in mortality and neonatal morbidities for infants with birth weight 501 to 1500 g born from 2000 to 2009.

Methods.—There were 355 806 infants weighing 501 to 1500 g who were born in 2000–2009. Mortality during initial hospitalization and major neonatal morbidity in survivors (early and late infection, chronic lung disease, necrotizing enterocolitis, severe retinopathy of prematurity, severe intraventricular hemorrhage, and periventricular leukomalacia) were assessed by using data from 669 North American hospitals in the Vermont Oxford Network.

Results.—From 2000 to 2009, mortality for infants weighing 501 to 1500 g decreased from 14.3% to 12.4% (difference, -1.9%; 95% confidence interval, -2.3% to -1.5%). Major morbidity in survivors decreased from 46.4% to 41.4% (difference, -4.9%; 95% confidence interval, -5.6% to -4.2%). In 2009, mortality ranged from 36.6% for infants 501 to 750 g to 3.5% for infants 1251 to 1500 g, whereas major morbidity in survivors ranged from 82.7% to 18.7%. In 2009, 49.2% of all very low birth weight infants and 89.2% of infants 501 to 750 g either died or survived with a major neonatal morbidity.

Conclusions.—Mortality and major neonatal morbidity in survivors decreased for infants with birth weight 501 to 1500 g between 2000 and 2009. However, at the end of the decade, a high proportion of these infants still either died or survived after experiencing ≥ 1 major neonatal morbidity known to be associated with both short- and long-term adverse consequences.

▶ There is beauty in being able to work with reliable, large datasets, incorporating many units from different countries and, thus, generating data that may be generalizable. These authors and the Vermont Oxford Network members are to be congratulated for this excellent dataset. However, the manner in which you interpret the numbers depends on whether you are an optimist or a pessimist. The optimist will point to the increased survival of infants between 501 and 1500 g between 2000 and 2009. The pessimist will draw your attention to the fact that many more of these infants died, when compared with their term peers, and they also incurred significant neonatal morbidity. In any event, the gains in survival are occurring at a glacial pace, and for infants with a birth weight of 501 to 750 g, almost 90% died or survived with a major neonatal morbidity.

Since the widespread use of antenatal corticosteroids and the introduction of surfactant, there have been no major breakthroughs (magic bullets) for this cohort of infants. True, nutritional support has improved, nosocomial infections have been reduced, and chronic lung disease and severe retinopathy have decreased. Nevertheless, more infants required operative intervention for retinopathy. The long-term follow-up until school age will expand the report card on this cohort, but there is little reason to suspect that their outcomes will be any better than those for preceding cohorts.

Greater efforts need to be extended to decrease the prevalence of prematurity and to minimize the center-to-center variation in short-term and long-term outcomes. The expanded use of multicenter and statewide quality improvement initiatives addressing the major neonatal morbidities may eventually accomplish this. So I am looking at this dataset as a realist but leaning to the side of optimism.

A. A. Fanaroff, MBBCh, FRCPE

Potential Sources of Bisphenol A in the Neonatal Intensive Care Unit

Duty SM, Mendonca K, Hauser R, et al (Simmons College, Boston, MA; Harvard School of Public Health, Boston, MA; et al)
Pediatrics 131:483-489, 2013

Objectives.—To determine whether nutritional intake and medical devices are bisphenol A (BPA) exposure sources among premature infants in the NICU.

Methods.—Mothers and their premature infants cared for in the NICU for the past 3 days were recruited for this exposure assessment study. Forty-three mothers contributed 1 nutrition sample (breast milk or formula) to characterize the infant's intake. Two urine samples (before and after feeding) were collected from each of 55 infants. Medical device use was categorized as "low" or "high" based on the number and invasiveness of devices used. BPA urinary concentrations used as a biomarker to estimate BPA exposure were measured by online solid-phase extraction, high-performance liquid chromatography, isotope dilution, tandem mass spectrometry. Nonparametric equivalence tests, intraclass correlations, and hierarchical linear mixed-effects models were conducted.

Results.—Breast milk and formula samples did not differ in total BPA concentration nor did infants' median urinary concentration of total BPA before or after feedings. However, the median urinary total BPA concentration among infants who required the use of 4 or more medical devices in the past 3 days was significantly higher (36.6 µg/L) than among infants who required the use of 0 to 3 devices (13.9 μg/L). The calculated BPA exposures are lower than the US Environmental Protection Agency reference dose, but considerably higher (16- to 32-fold) than among infants or children from the general population.

Conclusions.—The number of medical devices used in the past 3 days, but not nutritional intake, was positively associated with exposure to BPA.

▶ Medical technology and devices enable survival of extremely preterm infants. Exposures to toxins associated with such materials may be unavoidable, but data to characterize such exposures are largely lacking. This study of relatively stable infants in a neonatal intensive care unit examines urinary bisphenol-A (BPA) levels from 55 infants. The authors studied whether feeding type (breast milk or formula) or medical technology dependence (nasogastric tube, nasal cannula, continuous positive airway pressure or intravenous lines) were associated with BPA concentration in the urine. They found that infants requiring 4 or more devices in the 3 days before obtaining the urine sample had higher BPA levels (36.6 µg/L) compared with those exposed to 3 devices or fewer (13.9 µg/L). Additionally, the BPA levels obtained from these infants were considerably higher than those in children in the general population (16- to 32-fold). The authors do not state whether such exposures are associated with later morbidities. However, future inquiry into this issue is warranted given the endocrine-disrupting qualities of this chemical.

L. J. Van Marter, MD, MPH

H. Burris, MD

Radiation exposure from CT scans in childhood and subsequent risk of leukaemia and brain tumours: a retrospective cohort study
Pearce MS, Salotti JA, Little MP, et al (Newcastle Univ, Newcastle Upon Tyne, UK; Natl Cancer Inst, Bethesda, MD; et al)
Lancet 380:499-505, 2012

Background.—Although CT scans are very useful clinically, potential cancer risks exist from associated ionising radiation, in particular for children who are more radiosensitive than adults. We aimed to assess the excess risk of leukaemia and brain tumours after CT scans in a cohort of children and young adults.

Methods.—In our retrospective cohort study, we included patients without previous cancer diagnoses who were first examined with CT in National Health Service (NHS) centres in England, Wales, or Scotland (Great Britain) between 1985 and 2002, when they were younger than 22 years of age. We obtained data for cancer incidence, mortality, and loss to follow-up from the NHS Central Registry from Jan 1, 1985, to Dec 31, 2008. We estimated absorbed brain and red bone marrow doses per CT scan in mGy and assessed excess incidence of leukaemia and brain tumours cancer with Poisson relative risk models. To avoid inclusion of CT scans related to cancer diagnosis, follow-up for leukaemia began 2 years after the first CT and for brain tumours 5 years after the first CT.

Findings.—During follow-up, 74 of 178 604 patients were diagnosed with leukaemia and 135 of 176 587 patients were diagnosed with brain tumours. We noted a positive association between radiation dose from CT scans and leukaemia (excess relative risk [ERR] per mGy $0·036$, 95% CI $0·005-0·120$; $p = 0·0097$) and brain tumours ($0·023$, $0·010-0·049$; $p < 0·0001$). Compared with patients who received a dose of less than 5 mGy, the relative risk of leukaemia for patients who received a cumulative dose of at least 30 mGy (mean dose $51·13$ mGy) was $3·18$ (95% CI $1·46-6·94$) and the relative risk of brain cancer for patients who received a cumulative dose of 50–74 mGy (mean dose 60·42 mGy) was 2·82 (1·33–6·03).

Interpretation.—Use of CT scans in children to deliver cumulative doses of about 50 mGy might almost triple the risk of leukaemia and doses of about 60 mGy might triple the risk of brain cancer. Because these cancers are relatively rare, the cumulative absolute risks are small: in the 10 years after the first scan for patients younger than 10 years, one excess case of leukaemia and one excess case of brain tumour per 10 000 head CT scans is estimated to occur. Nevertheless, although clinical benefits should outweigh the small absolute risks, radiation doses from CT scans ought to be kept as low as possible and alternative procedures, which do not involve ionising radiation, should be considered if appropriate.

▶ The importance of this study cannot be overstated, and its relatively sudden impact on perinatal imaging has been dramatic. Prior to relatively recent concerns about the cumulative risk of radiation, most premature newborns had frequent, often daily, radiographs to confirm adequate positioning of lines and tubes and stability of pulmonary or abdominal status, given risks of long-term intubation and the high risk for necrotizing enterocolitis. Individual radiographs, though individually relatively low in radiation dose, added up to a fairly high dose in a premature infant when viewed together over weeks and months of hospitalization. Until very recently, and perhaps not until this study was published and thus could not be ignored, the workup of the asphyxiated, seizing newborn relied on urgent computed tomography of the brain, given the previous relative unavailability of urgent off-hours neonatal brain magnetic resonance and the difficulty of safely imaging and monitoring an intubated, ventilated premature infant in a magnetic resonance scanner. Even before its publication, but certainly since, there has been a concerted effort from the governance of the pediatric imaging societies, such as the Society for Pediatric Radiology, to "Image Gently" and to reduce radiation in children of all ages, at all times, following the ALARA principle to keep radiation dose as low as is reasonably achievable.

J. Estroff, MD

Imaging, radiation exposure, and attributable cancer risk for neonates with necrotizing enterocolitis
Baird R, Tessier R, Guilbault MP, et al (McGill Univ, Montreal, Quebec, Canada)
J Pediatr Surg 48:1000-1005, 2013

Purpose.—Neonates with necrotizing enterocolitis (NEC) receive numerous radiologic investigations that potentially increase their lifetime cancer mortality risk. We evaluated our radiologic practice pattern for patients with NEC and estimated cumulative radiation exposure and lifetime cancer risk.

Methods.—Infants with NEC in a tertiary care NICU had patient demographics, imaging, treatments/interventions, and outcomes analyzed over 3 years. The number and type of imaging were recorded, including NEC-related imaging (thoraco-abdominal "babygrams" and abdominal radiographs), and all other imaging modalities. Patients were stratified by birth weight: group 1 (<750 g); group 2 (751—1500 g); and group 3 (>1501 g). Pre-existing normative data were used to calculate radiation exposure, absorption, and attributable cancer risk from NEC-related imaging.

Results.—Sixty-four neonates with 72 episodes of NEC were identified. Overall survival was 75.0%. When stratified by birth weight, mean abdominal radiographs and babygrams comprised 51%, 60%, and 74% of total imaging, giving median mGy doses of 2.1, 0.4, and 0.2, respectively. Compared to normative data, radiation dosing, and median cumulative cancer lifetime mortality risk increased by an average of 4.3× from baseline, with two cases documenting a 20-fold increase.

Conclusion.—Neonates with NEC are exposed to significant amounts of radiation directly attributable to disease surveillance. Non-radiologic surveillance methods could significantly reduce radiation exposure and cancer risk in these infants.

▶ Radiologic surveillance with serial abdominal imaging is used to guide clinical management and treatment of infants with necrotizing enterocolitis (NEC). In the above study, the authors sought to quantitate the cumulative radiation exposure and lifetime cancer risk during an episode of NEC for infants admitted to their center's neonatal intensive care unit between October 2007 and February 2011. An episode of NEC was defined as the first documentation of the disease until resumption of oral intake. There was no protocol in place specifying the frequency and type of imaging for infants with NEC. When images were stratified by the severity of NEC (Bell grade I—III) there was no significant difference; during the episode of NEC, abdominal radiographs and babygrams (thoraco-abdominal radiographs) accounted for approximately 60% of the images for each stage of NEC. The highest number of NEC-related images was 72. The median cancer lifetime mortality risk attributable to NEC-related imaging ranged from a 3-fold increase for infants with a birth weight of 750 to 1500 g to a 5.5-fold increase in the less-than-750-g birth weight group. Because imaging directly attributable to NEC surveillance represented only 50% of all radiographs for the less-than-750-g cohort, the risk is most likely higher for this group. The results of this observational study are sobering and should provide impetus for continued evaluation of novel tools for NEC surveillance, such as Doppler ultrasound scan and clinical scoring systems, to reduce the need for frequent radiologic examinations.[1,2]

L. A. Papile, MD

References

1. Faingold R, Daneman A, Tomlinson G, et al. Necrotizing enterocolitis: assessment of bowel viability with color Doppler US. *Radiolgoy.* 2005;235:587-594.

2. Tepas JJ 3rd, Leaphart C, Plumley D. Trajectory of metabolic derangement in infants with necrotizing enterocolitis should drive timing and technique of surgical intervention. *J Am Coll Surg.* 2010;210:847-852.

Factors Associated With Developmental Concern and Intent to Access Therapy Following Discharge From the NICU

Pineda RG, Castellano A, Rogers C, et al (Washington Univ School of Medicine, St Louis, MO)
Pediatr Phys Ther 25:62-69, 2013

Purpose.—To determine factors associated with mothers' concern about infant development and intent to access therapy services following neonatal intensive care unit (NICU) discharge.

Methods.—Infant medical factors, magnetic resonance imaging results, neurobehavior at term, maternal factors, and maternal perceptions about developmental concern and intent to access therapy at NICU discharge were prospectively collected in 84 infants born premature (<30 weeks gestation). Regression was used to determine factors associated with developmental concern and intent to access therapy at NICU discharge.

Results.—Decreased developmental concern was reported by mothers with more children ($P = .007$). Infant stress signs ($P = .038$), higher maternal education ($P = .047$), reading books ($P = .030$), and maternal depression ($P = .018$) were associated with increased developmental concern. More maternal education was associated with more intent to access services ($P = .040$).

Conclusion.—Maternal factors, rather than infant factors, had important associations with caregiver concern. In contrast, abnormal term neurobehavior and/or the presence of cerebral injury were not associated with caregiver concern about development.

▶ Early intervention therapy services are often recommended at discharge from the neonatal intensive care unit (NICU). Although many infants are referred for early intervention services, it is apparent from the literature that there is a gap between the developmental needs and the use of services for infants at high risk. One potential barrier to assessing follow-up services may be parental perception of the severity of their infant's neurologic impairment. The above observational study explored factors related to maternal perceptions of developmental concern and intent to access interventional therapies.

Immediately before or after NICU discharge, mothers completed an extensive questionnaire aimed at identifying family traits and perceptions. The questionnaire contained standardized measures of anxiety (State Trait Anxiety Inventory), depression (Edinburgh Postnatal Depression Scale), coping style (Coping Inventory for Stressful Situations), and stress (Life Stress Subscale of the Parenting Stress Index) as well as demographic data. Infant factors included in the analyses were medical data, extent of brain injury noted on magnetic resonance imaging at term-equivalent age, measured neurobehavioral outcome determined between

37 and 42 weeks of postmenstrual age (NICU Network Neurobehavioral Scale, Dubowitz Neurological Examination), and infant feeding performance (Oral Motor Assessment Scale).

The mean gestational age of the infants included in the study was 26.92 weeks. Despite this, only 61% of mothers indicated that they were concerned about their infants' development. Interestingly, the reason for their concern was not related to the severity of their infants' medical condition, the presence/extent of brain injury, or abnormal neurologic findings but rather to signs of stress, suggesting that parental perceptions about early development correspond with behavior and not objective information.

L. A. Papile, MD

Care of the newborn with ichthyosis
Dyer JA, Spraker M, Williams M (Univ of Missouri, Columbia)
Dermatol Ther 26:1-15, 2013

Mendelian disorders of cornification (ichthyosis; MeDOC) often present in the neonatal period with little warning to providers or parents. This report reviews the majority of ichthyoses with congenital findings. The neonatal presentation of many MeDOC often differs from the later phenotype because of the changes in the skin that occur with transition from an intrauterine to extrauterine environment. While differentiation of ichthyosis subtypes in the neonatal period is difficult, there are certain phenotypic groups within which these neonates fall, recognition of which can guide initial work up and treatment. For this report, these are categorized as: exuberant vernix; collodion baby/harlequin ichthyosis (HI); ichthyosiform erythroderma; blistering; and normal skin/xerosis phenotypes (Fig).

▶ This is a useful and informative review of the Mendelian disorders of cornification, better known as *ichthyosis* (Fig). Although some of the variants of

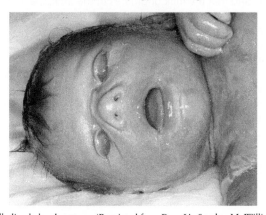

FIGURE.—Collodion baby phenotype. (Reprinted from Dyer JA, Spraker M, Williams M. Care of the newborn with ichthyosis. *Dermatol Ther.* 2013;26:1-15, with permission from Wiley Periodicals, Inc.)

these disorders first present well after birth, at least 7 of them described in detail in this article may present at birth, most often without warning, as this is not readily detectable by ultrasound scan or other forms of prenatal testing. These are organized as exuberant vernix, collodion baby/harlequin ichthyosis, ichthyosiform erythroderma, blistering, and normal skin/xerosis phenotypes. Some of these are relatively mild, such as the normal skin/xerosis phenotype, whereas others, such as the classic harlequin baby, can be life threatening and present a major challenge in terms of treatment. This review presents the clinical presentation of each of these phenotypes as well as treatment. The authors discuss the importance of a multidisciplinary team approach, including neonatology, dermatology, and genetics, with the addition of other specialists, such as ophthalmology, otolaryngology, and plastic surgery in individual cases.

J. Neu, MD

Bad milk, part 1: antique doctrines that impeded breastfeeding
Obladen M (Charité Univ Medicine, Berlin, Germany)
Acta Paediatr 101:1102-1104, 2012

Even though philosophical and medical authorities explicitly promoted breastfeeding, a large proportion of infants were not breastfed by their mother. Infants not breastfed by their own mothers had diminished chances to survive. This was even more true longer ago (1), especially in summer, when bacterial growth was rapid in unrefrigerated milk.

▶ This is a set of reports (see also part 2, reference 1) that discuss antique (part 1) and new age (part 2) doctrines that have impeded breastfeeding. Several salient historical issues are presented, and a few of them will be mentioned here just as a teaser for Dr Obladen's fascinating review:

1. Greek scholars imagined a physical connection to transfer menstrual blood to the breasts and that the milk originates in the uterus, and these teachings were propagated through history and through this classical theory: scientists prohibited intercourse during lactation. In Galen's words: "I order all women who are nursing babies to abstain completely from sex relations. For menstruation is provoked by intercourse, and the milk no longer remains sweet." Practically all authors from the 15th to the 18th century reiterated the intercourse ban during lactation. According to Obladen, "This ban isolated the mother, provided an alibi for paternal infidelity and made the infant its own father's rival."

2. Breastfeeding should be delayed because colostrum was poisonous to the infant.

3. Breastfeeding destroys maternal health and beauty.

This is excellent reading to provide perspective for all pediatricians.

J. Neu, MD

Is Breast Always Best?: A Personal Reflection on the Challenges of Breastfeeding

Shah DK (Univ of Iowa Hosps and Clinics)
Obstet Gynecol 121:869-871, 2013

Background.—The American Academy of Pediatrics, the American College of Obstetricians and Gynecologists, the World Health Organization, and the United Nations Children's Fund have programs that actively affirm breastfeeding as the best choice for new mothers. The lay press includes many articles touting the benefits of breastfeeding for both mother and child. On the other side, Michael Bloomberg's Latch On NYC initiative instructs labor and delivery staff to restrict access and track the distribution of formula and have mothers who use formula listen to a mandatory speech about why breastfeeding is the best choice. Cans of formula carry a label stating the breastfeeding is recommended. The current message denigrates any woman who tries but is unable to breastfeed, making her feel that she is deliberately choosing an inferior option to meet her needs rather than considering those of her infant. Medical professionals dealing with new mothers must offer support for both those who breastfeed and those who do not.

Obstacles to Breastfeeding.—Despite motivation, persistence, and the use of all available resources, some women are unable to breastfeed. Many of these women are already feeling guilty and/or inadequate and under the condemnation of family and friends. This emotional burden is on top of the anxiety, guilt, and inadequacy that new mothers inevitably feel. A 2011 study of 2586 breastfeeding women found that negative early breastfeeding experiences are important predictors of postpartum depression and recommended screening women who experience difficulty breastfeeding for depressive symptoms. Those women who cannot breastfeed are being isolated, which increases their negative experience.

Conclusions.—Medical professionals should adopt a more balanced, reassuring role in helping women who cannot breastfeed for months after the birth of their children. These new mothers should be relieved of their guilt and helped to release this perceived failure and move on. They can be encouraged that their child will be fine. Difficulty with or an inability to breastfeed should be normalized. A holistic, family-friendly approach to both breastfeeding and postnatal care should be adopted that addresses the physical, mental, and emotional health of both mother and baby. There is no one path to successful parenting.

▶ This article is from a highly motivated, obviously intelligent and caring mother. She is a physician who experienced major challenges with breastfeeding her infant. The article details her personal reflections as well as experiences many mothers undergo while trying their best to breastfeed their infants and the personal anxiety, guilt, enhancement of postpartum depression, and feelings of inadequacy that these moms face when all does not go smoothly. Experiences like this should make us pause as we proceed with the "breast is best" and "baby-friendly" initiatives that are being supported by various groups, such as the American Academy of Pediatrics, World Health Organization, UNICEF, and American Congress of Obstetricians and Gynecologists. Are we going too far? In the battles against formula feeding, is there collateral damage to moms, babies, and families who really want to breastfeed but can't? The experiences of this author and many other mothers suggest that this is the case, and we may actually be doing some harm when it comes to an overly dogmatic approach where there is only one way—exclusive breastfeeding. Although there remains little question that breastfeeding should be supported whenever possible, an overly dogmatic approach to exclusive breastfeeding has the potential to cause harm. As this article clearly shows, the zeal to be baby friendly may have negative repercussions, and there is room for a pragmatic approach. Highly pertinent to this mother's experience, recent data from an Australian study suggest that in hospitals in which breastfeeding rates are already high, baby-friendly accreditation does not have a positive impact on short- and medium-term breastfeeding rates as initiation rates reach ceiling levels.[1]

J. Neu, MD

Reference

1. Brodribb W, Kruske S, Miller YD. Baby-friendly hospital accreditation, in-hospital care practices, and breastfeeding. *Pediatrics*. 2013;131:685-692.

14 Pharmacology

Erythropoietin for Neuroprotection in Neonatal Encephalopathy: Safety and Pharmacokinetics
Wu YW, Bauer LA, Ballard RA, et al (Univ of California, San Francisco; Univ of Washington, Seattle; et al)
Pediatrics 130:683-691, 2012

Objective.—To determine the safety and pharmacokinetics of erythropoietin (Epo) given in conjunction with hypothermia for hypoxic-ischemic encephalopathy (HIE). We hypothesized that high dose Epo would produce plasma concentrations that are neuroprotective in animal studies (ie, maximum concentration = 6000–10 000 U/L; area under the curve = 117 000–140 000 U*h/L).

Methods.—In this multicenter, open-label, dose-escalation, phase I study, we enrolled 24 newborns undergoing hypothermia for HIE. All patients had decreased consciousness and acidosis (pH <7.00 or base deficit ≥12), 10-minute Apgar score ≤5, or ongoing resuscitation at 10 minutes. Patients received 1 of 4 Epo doses intravenously: 250 (N = 3), 500 (N = 6), 1000 (N = 7), or 2500 U/kg per dose (N = 8). We gave up to 6 doses every 48 hours starting at <24 hours of age and performed pharmacokinetic and safety analyses.

Results.—Patients received mean 4.8 ± 1.2 Epo doses. Although Epo followed nonlinear pharmacokinetics, excessive accumulation did not occur during multiple dosing. At 500, 1000, and 2500 U/kg Epo, half-life was 7.2, 15.0, and 18.7 hours; maximum concentration was 7046, 13780, and 33 316 U/L, and total Epo exposure (area under the curve) was 50306, 131054, and 328 002 U*h/L, respectively. Drug clearance at a given dose was slower than reported in uncooled preterm infants. No deaths or serious adverse effects were seen.

Conclusions.—Epo 1000 U/kg per dose intravenously given in conjunction with hypothermia is well tolerated and produces plasma concentrations that are neuroprotective in animals. A large efficacy trial is needed to determine whether Epo add-on therapy further improves outcome in infants undergoing hypothermia for HIE.

▶ Although therapeutic hypothermia is an effective therapy for neonatal encephalopathy, it provides only modest improvements in outcome with more than 40% of treated infants either dying or exhibiting moderate-to-severe disabilities, including cerebral palsy, intellectual impairment, and epilepsy. In animal models of neonatal hypoxic-ischemic encephalopathy (HIE) several adjuvant therapies, including high doses of erythropoietin (epo), have proved to be more beneficial than hypothermia alone.[1]

Two published clinical trials suggest that infants with HIE treated with epo experienced improved neurologic outcomes.[2,3] However, dosing, dosing intervals, duration of dosing, and total amount of epo given differed in the 2 trials. More importantly, the safety of high-dose epo was not evaluated rigorously.

The above safety and pharmacokinetic study was done in preparation for designing a multicenter, randomized, clinical trial comparing the neuroprotective efficacy of high-dose epo, given as add-on therapy to hypothermia, with hypothermia alone. The results suggest that epo 1000 U/kg per dose would be a reasonable dose for evaluation.

L. A. Papile, MD

References

1. Spasojevic SD, Sojanovic VD, Barisic NA, Doronjski AR, Zikic DR, Babovic SM. Neuroprotective effects of hypothermia and erythropoietin after perinatal asphyxia in newborn rats. *J Matern Fetal Neonatal Med.* 2013 May 2 [Epub ahead of print].
2. Zhu C, Kang W, Xu F, et al. Erythropoietin improved neurologic outcomes in newborns with hypoxic-ischemic encephalopathy. *Pediatrics.* 2009;124. www.pediatrics.org/cgi/content/full/124/2/e218. Accessed July 1, 2013.
3. Elmahdy H, El-Mashad AR, El-Bahrawy H, El-Gohary T, El-Barbary A, Aly H. Human recombinant erythropoietin in asphyxia neonatorum: a pilot trial. *Pediatrics.* 2010;125. www.pediatrics.org/cgi/content/full/125/5/e1135. Accessed July 1, 2013.

The Effect of Prenatal Antidepressant Exposure on Neonatal Adaptation: A Systematic Review and Meta-Analysis

Grigoriadis S, VonderPorten EH, Mamisashvili L, et al (Women's College Hosp, Toronto, Ontario, Canada; et al)
J Clin Psychiatry 74:e309-e320, 2013

Objective.—Conflicting reports on potential risks of antidepressant exposure during gestation for the infant have been reported in the literature. This systematic review and meta-analysis on immediate neonatal outcomes were conducted to clarify what, if any, risks are faced by infants exposed to antidepressants in utero. Subanalyses address known methodological limitations in the field.

Data Sources.—MEDLINE, EMBASE, CINAHL, and PsycINFO were searched from their start dates to June 2010. Various combinations of keywords were utilized including, but not limited to, *depressive/mood disorder, pregnancy/pregnancy trimesters, antidepressant drugs,* and neonatal effects.

Study Selection.—English language and cohort and case-control studies reporting on a cluster of signs defined as poor neonatal adaptation syndrome (PNAS) or individual clinical signs (respiratory distress and tremors) associated with pharmacologic treatment were selected. Of 3,074 abstracts reviewed, 735 articles were retrieved and 12 were included in this analysis.

Data Extraction.—Two independent reviewers extracted data and assessed the quality of the articles.

Results.—Twelve studies were retrieved that examined PNAS or the signs of respiratory distress and tremors in the infant. There was a significant association between exposure to antidepressants during pregnancy and overall occurrence of PNAS (odds ratio [OR] = 5.07; 95% CI, 3.25–7.90; $P < .0001$). Respiratory distress (OR = 2.20; 95% CI, 1.81–2.66; $P < .0001$) and tremors (OR = 7.89; 95% CI, 3.33–18.73; $P < .0001$) were also significantly associated with antidepressant exposure. For the respiratory outcome, studies using convenience samples had significantly higher ORs ($Q_1 = 5.4$, $P = .020$). No differences were found in any other moderator analyses.

Conclusions.—An increased risk of PNAS exists in infants exposed to antidepressant medication during pregnancy; respiratory distress and tremors also show associations. Neonatologists need to be prepared and updated in their management, and clinicians must inform their patients of this risk.

▶ The frequent use of antidepressants during pregnancy, especially selective serotonin reuptake inhibitors, has led to numerous reports and prior meta-analyses of their potential effects on the newborn. The results have been inconclusive and even contradictory, not surprising in light of the methodologies.

In this latest meta-analysis, these authors analyzed 12 published studies that looked for poor neonatal adaptation syndrome (PNAS), defined as "transient short-term adverse neonatal or neurobehavioral effects observed in the neonate." They determined that exposed infants were more likely than nonexposed infants to display respiratory distress and tremors. They hypothesized that this may reflect a withdrawal or discontinuation syndrome, which certainly has a biological plausibility. They caution us to "inform and prepare pregnant women taking antidepressants during pregnancy that their infant may show signs of PNAS and, in case they occur, how they will be managed."

Although this study strengthens the association of antidepressant use in the mother and short-term (presumably self-limited and not life-threatening) effects on the newborn, it also demonstrates some of the limitations of meta-analysis. Of the 3074 publications screened, 2339 were excluded, and of the 735 full-text articles, they were left with only 12 that met their criteria. I am not convinced that selection bias was adequately considered.

We are still left with the same dilemma: Which is worse, maternal depression during pregnancy or its treatment? Until we know the true effects of maternal depression, we will not be able to construct a true risk-to-benefit ratio.

S. M. Donn, MD

Breastfeeding after anaesthesia: a review of the pharmacological impact on children

Chu TC, McCalum J, Yii MF (Wyong Hosp, New South Wales, Australia)
Anaesth Intensive Care 41:35-40, 2013

Post-anaesthetic advice imparted to breastfeeding mothers can vary. This is due in part to the differing information from published data, product information sheets and inevitably from the unhindered flow of opinions available on the internet. This literature review examined the evidence relating to drugs commonly used in the modern anaesthetic setting and their impact on breastfed children. It suggests that special precautions are rarely warranted in the post-anaesthetic care of breastfeeding patients (Table 1).

▶ Mothers who wish to breastfeed their babies often are exposed to anesthetic and analgesic agents, and the question often arises which of these might be unsafe for the infant who is breastfeeding. It is difficult to find good guidance because often the recommendations from pharmaceutical companies, from which much of the published data are available, is not derived from high-level evidence but rather consists of generic warnings that are more legal disclaimers than real advice. The authors have compiled a tabulated summary of current evidence for drugs used in anesthetic practice and their impact on children via breast milk (Table 1).

Many drugs do not cross into the lactating ducts in meaningful quantities. These include warfarin, an anticoagulant. Other drugs that are excreted in breast milk in doses that are too low to be clinically significant include heparin, thiopentone, propofol, midazolam, fentanyl, and paracetamol (acetaminophen).

Of the drugs that are known to be detectable in breast milk, many are still safe for the nursing infant. These included metronidazole, ampicillin, and gentamicin. Of the nonsteroidal anti-inflammatory drugs, only aspirin has been recorded as having an adverse effect on nursing infants. Caffeine usually has minimal effect, but high intakes by the mother have been associated with irritability in the infant.

Diazepam appears to be one of the drugs that should be avoided because it has been shown to cause sedation and feeding difficulties in some breastfed infants. Another drug of concern is codeine, largely because some mothers may be rapid metabolizers through their CYP2D6 genotype, and this rapid metabolism to morphine has been implicated in the death of one breastfed infant whose mother was prescribed codeine.

Overall, special precautions are rarely warranted in the postanesthetic care of breastfeeding patients. One point that is obvious from this report is that despite the authors' attempt to find good evidence based on high-level studies, very little is available, but they should be commended for tabulation of the information that is available.

J. Neu, MD

TABLE 1.—Categorised Summary of Drug Safety Associated with Breastfeeding in the Perioperative Setting

Proven to be Safe (Nil to Negligible Trace in Breastmilk)	Detectable in Breastmilk but no Known Adverse Effects	Potential or Mild Impact	Serious Adverse Reactions	No human data Available but no Reports of Adverse Effects on Breastfed Infants
Inhalational anaesthetics				
Isoflurane[12]	—	—	—	Sevoflurane[51]
Nitrous oxide[18]				Desflurane[51]
Xenon[2]				
Premedicant and induction drugs				
Thiopentone[12]	—	—	Diazepam[39-42] (esp. chronic use)	Dexmetomidine
Propofol[12,19]				Ketamine
Midazolam[19]				
Neuromuscular blocking and reversal drugs				
Neostigmine[7]	—	—	—	Succinylcholine
Glycopyrrolate[18]				Atropine[50]
Non-depolarisers[12] (quaternary ions unlikely to cross into milk ducts)				Sugammadex
Opioids				
Fentanyl[4,5,12,19,25] (parenteral and epidural)	Remifentanil[2] (in conjunction with xenon)	Pethidine (intravenous, multi-dose)[36]	Codeine[3,43-47] (use >4 days)	Alfentanil[51]
Tramadol[23]	Morphine[12,24,35]	Oxycodone[6,48,49] (esp. older children)		
	Methadone[36] (caution with abrupt withdrawal)[38]			
	Pethidine (single dose)[12,24]			
	Pethidine (epidural)[26]			
Local anaesthetic agents				
Lignocaine[21]	—	—	—	—
Bupivacaine[21,22]				
Ropivacaine[22]				
Other analgesics				
Paracetamol[12,24]	Parecoxib[30]	Aspirin[29]	—	—
NSAIDs[24]				

(Continued)

TABLE 1.—(Continued)

Proven to be Safe (Nil to Negligible Trace in Breastmilk)	Detectable in Breastmilk but no Known Adverse Effects	Potential or Mild Impact	Serious Adverse Reactions	No human data Available but no Reports of Adverse Effects on Breastfed Infants
Anticoagulants Heparin[17] Enoxaparin[20] Warfarin[13]	—	—	—	—
Anti-emetics Metoclopramide[14–16]	—	Droperidol[32]	—	Ondansetron Prochlorperazine Dexamethasone[53]
Antibiotics Metronidazole[8] Ampicillin[27] Gentamicin (single dose)[28,29]	—	—	—	Vancomycin Cephalothin[51]
Other Nicotine patch[31]	—	Caffeine[33,34]	—	—

Editor's Note: Please refer to original journal article for full references.
NSAID = nonsteroidal anti-inflammatory drugs.

Selective Serotonin Reuptake Inhibitors and Persistent Pulmonary Hypertension of the Newborn
Andrade C (Natl Inst of Mental Health and Neurosciences, Bangalore, India)
J Clin Psychiatry 73:e601-e605, 2012

■ Some studies have associated antenatal use of SSRIs with increased risk of a potentially fatal neonatal condition, persistent pulmonary hypertension of the newborn (PPHN).

■ This article reviews the findings for physicians and provides plain-language talking points that can be used to answer patients' questions and guide them in making informed decisions about treatment.

▶ The relationship of maternal selective serotonin reuptake inhibitor (SSRI) use during pregnancy to persistent pulmonary hypertension (PPHN) in the newborn has become a hot issue both medically and legally. The evidence supporting a cause-and-effect relationship is weak, at best, and prompted a recent Food and Drug Administration statement to that effect. This article, which actually is a summary of a review by Kieler et al,[1] offers practical advice to obstetricians managing pregnant patients with depression on how to counsel these patients regarding the risks and benefits of continuing SSRI treatment during gestation. Neonatologists who do prenatal consultation will find it helpful in addressing questions that are often raised by expectant mothers who were taking these drugs before or after conception.

The article also intrigued me from the epidemiologic perspective. Despite the large sample size of the Scandinavian study, it is hard to make valid conclusions when the incidence of the event of interest is so low. By the time corrections are made for confounders, the incidence in both groups (SSRI vs no SSRI) falls to a fraction of 1%. In this article, Andrade adroitly notes that the psychiatric illness itself (for which the SSRI was prescribed) may increase the risk of PPHN independent of the drug, and thus what we are left with is merely an association. The Kieler study also found that women with previous psychiatric hospitalizations, not treated with an SSRI, also had a higher incidence of PPHN in their offspring.

It is time for a prospective, randomized, masked clinical trial.

S. M. Donn, MD

Reference

1. Kieler H, Artama M, Engeland A, et al. Selective serotonin reuptake inhibitors during pregnancy and the risk of persistent pulmonary hypertension in the newborn: population based cohort study from the five Nordic countries. *BMJ*. 2012;344:d8012.

Whom are We Comforting? An Analysis of Comfort Medications Delivered to Dying Neonates

Janvier A, Meadow W, Leuthner SR, et al (Université de Montréal, Québec, Canada; Univ of Chicago, IL; Med College of Milwaukee, WI; et al)
J Pediatr 159:206-210, 2011

Objectives.—To clarify the use of end-of-life comfort medications or neuromuscular blockers (NMBs) in culturally different neonatal intensive care units (NICUs).

Study Design.—Review of medical files of newborns > 22 weeks gestation who died in the delivery room or the NICU during 12 months in four NICUs (Chicago, Milwaukee, Montreal, and Groningen). We compared use of end-of-life comfort medications and NMBs.

Results.—None of the babies who died in the delivery room received comfort medications. The use of opiods (77%) or benzodiazepines (41%) around death was similar in all NICUs. Increasing this medication around extubation occurred most often in Montreal, rarely in Milwaukee and Groningen, and never in Chicago. Comfort medications use had no significant impact on the time between extubation and death. NMBs were never used around death in Chicago, once in Montreal, and more frequently in Milwaukee and Groningen. Initiation of NMB after extubation occurred only in Groningen.

Conclusion.—Comfort medications were administered to almost all dying infants in each NICU. Some, but not all, centers were comfortable increasing these medications around or after extubation. In three centers, NMBs were at times present at the time of death. However, only in Holland were NMBs initiated after extubation.

▶ The authors of this study have divided the deaths of newborn infants into 4 categories: (1) those who die while getting active cardiopulmonary resuscitation (CPR); (2) those who die with CPR being withheld; (3) moribund babies who die after extubation; and (4) stable babies who are electively extubated, or other treatment is withheld where survival is considered possible but with a very poor neurodevelopmental outcome. This categorization was applied retrospectively in 4 neonatal intensive care units (NICUs) in 3 countries to examine the use of comfort medication in dying neonates and whether this was directed solely at the neonate or, at least in part, directed at the concerns of others—parents, nurses, and physicians.

Most dying babies received some comfort medication; opioids were used primarily, then benzodiazepines, and far lower use of neuromuscular blocker (NMB) agents. The review detected differences in the agents used and different approaches to increasing medication in the hour before or after extubation. (Interestingly, the increase in medications around extubation had no significant impact on the time between extubation and death, although how this was determined is unclear.) The prior-to-withdrawal use of NMBs was reversed in some babies but not all, as the babies were considered so unstable that they would have died while waiting for the paralysis to cease. In addition, in view of the desire to allow babies to die in their parents' arms, withdrawal without reversal of NMB occurred in a small number of babies, as this was considered less cruel than waiting for reversal. In Groningen, NMBs were used at the parents' request to prevent perceived infant suffering but always in conjunction with opioids and benzodiazepines. NMBs were never initiated after extubation other than in Groningen.

Thus, we see that most infants dying in the NICUs in 3 different countries received comfort medications during the 48 hours preceding their death, and this practice was continued after extubation. Different approaches were seen in the use of comfort medications to neonates in similar clinical dying circumstances. The use of these medications appears to depend more on the rationalization of the use of comfort measures; in some contexts the notion of hastening death precludes increasing dosages, whereas in others, hastening death prevents unnecessary suffering. With regard to the use of NMB agents in Groningen, the view was to alleviate parental distress around the infant's gasping, whereas in other units, gasping is likely regarded as an inherent part of the dying process with a tolerable amount of discomfort and with parents forewarned and prepared for this potential terminal event.

What there does seem to be agreement about is that we are likely treating more than the baby. An empirical study such as this exposes what is being done in these challenging circumstances. It cannot tell us what should be done, but certainly diminishing parental anguish and caregiver distress at this time must carry some moral weight to justify attention to the comfort of all, not only the baby. Of note is that the use of NMBs in Dutch NICUs is clearly a subject of intense debate. A recent study found great variability among the 14 neonatologists who agreed to be interviewed.[1]

J. Hellmann, MBBCh, FCP(SA), FRCPC, MHSc

Reference

1. Moratti S. Ethical and legal acceptability of the use of neuromuscular blockers (NMBs) in connection with abstention decisions in Dutch NICUs: interviews with neonatologists. *J Med Ethics*. 2011;37:29-33.

15 Postnatal Growth and Development/ Follow-up

Neurodevelopmental Outcomes in the Early CPAP and Pulse Oximetry Trial

Vaucher YE, for the SUPPORT Study Group of the Eunice Kennedy Shriver NICHD Neonatal Research Network (Univ of California at San Diego; et al)

N Engl J Med 367:2495-2504, 2012

Background.—Previous results from our trial of early treatment with continuous positive airway pressure (CPAP) versus early surfactant treatment in infants showed no significant difference in the outcome of death or bronchopulmonary dysplasia. A lower (vs. higher) target range of oxygen saturation was associated with a lower rate of severe retinopathy but higher mortality. We now report longer-term results from our prespecified hypotheses.

Methods.—Using a 2-by-2 factorial design, we randomly assigned infants born between 24 weeks 0 days and 27 weeks 6 days of gestation to early CPAP with a limited ventilation strategy or early surfactant administration and to lower or higher target ranges of oxygen saturation (85 to 89% or 91 to 95%). The primary composite outcome for the longer-term analysis was death before assessment at 18 to 22 months or neurodevelopmental impairment at 18 to 22 months of corrected age.

Results.—The primary outcome was determined for 1234 of 1316 enrolled infants (93.8%); 990 of the 1058 surviving infants (93.6%) were evaluated at 18 to 22 months of corrected age. Death or neurodevelopmental impairment occurred in 27.9% of the infants in the CPAP group (173 of 621 infants), versus 29.9% of those in the surfactant group (183 of 613) (relative risk, 0.93; 95% confidence interval [CI], 0.78 to 1.10; $P = 0.38$), and in 30.2% of the infants in the lower-oxygen-saturation group (185 of 612), versus 27.5% of those in the higher-oxygen-saturation group (171 of 622) (relative risk, 1.12; 95% CI, 0.94 to 1.32; $P = 0.21$). Mortality was increased with the lower-oxygen-saturation target (22.1%, vs. 18.2% with the higher-oxygen-saturation target; relative risk, 1.25; 95% CI, 1.00 to 1.55; $P = 0.046$).

Conclusions.—We found no significant differences in the composite outcome of death or neurodevelopmental impairment among extremely premature infants randomly assigned to early CPAP or early surfactant administration and to a lower or higher target range of oxygen saturation. (Funded by the Eunice Kennedy Shriver National Institute of Child Health and Human Development and the National Heart, Lung, and Blood Institute; SUPPORT ClinicalTrials.gov number, NCT00233324.)

▶ In their 2010 publication of the results of the SUPPORT trial—a 2 × 2 factorial design evaluating the effects of continuous positive airway pressure (CPAP) vs surfactant treatment and 2 levels of target oxygen saturation (Sao_2) among infants born between 24 and 27 6/7 weeks of gestation—the Eunice Kennedy Shriver National Institutes of Child Health and Human Development Neonatal Research Network shared important findings that raised concern within the neonatal community regarding the common practice of lowering target ranges of Sao_2 in an effort to reduce retinopathy of prematurity (ROP) among extremely preterm infants.

Although the SUPPORT study showed reduced severe ROP risk among survivors in the group randomly assigned to lower Sao_2, there was no difference in overall rates of ROP and increased risk of death before hospital discharge (19.9% vs 16.2%) among infants randomly assigned to the low Sao_2 (85%–89%) compared with the higher Sao_2 (91%–95%) group. This 2012 publication reports the results of analyses of the SUPPORT study primary outcome: death or neurodevelopmental impairment at 2 years of age. Among the 93.8% of the study population who were seen for detailed neurodevelopmental evaluation at approximately 2 years of age, analyses adjusted for gestational age group and study center showed no difference in the primary composite outcome (death or neurodevelopmental impairment) among children assigned to CPAP vs surfactant or lower vs higher Sao_2 targets. The increased risk of mortality associated with randomization to the lower Sao_2 group was confirmed (22.1% vs 18.2%; relative risk, 1.25; 95% confidence interval, 1.00–1.55), mainly reflecting neonatal (predischarge) mortality. In a brief 2011 report,[1] investigators in the United Kingdom, Australia, and New Zealand reported that another study of neonatal Sao_2 targets, the BOOST II study, was stopped early for similar findings; 2-year outcomes are awaited for this study as well as for the Canadian Oxygen Trial, a third study of target oxygenation, conducted at centers in Canada, the United States, Argentina, Finland, Germany, and Israel. Together these large and rigorously conducted trials will provide important and much-needed evidence on the merits and risks of lower vs higher Sao_2 targets that undoubtedly will have immediate impact on the care of extremely preterm infants.

L. J. Van Marter, MD, MPH

Reference

1. Stenson B, Brockelhurst P, Tarnow-Mordi W. Increased 36-week survival with high oxygen saturation target in extremely preterm infants. *N Engl J Med.* 2011;364: 1680-1682.

Congenital diaphragmatic hernia with(out) ECMO: impaired development at 8 years

Madderom MJ, Toussaint L, van der Cammen-van Zijp MH, et al (Erasmus Med Ctr-Sophia Children's Hosp, Rotterdam, The Netherlands)

Arch Dis Child Fetal Neonatal Ed 2012 [Epub ahead of print]

Objective.—To evaluate developmental and social-emotional outcomes at 8 years of age for children with congenital diaphragmatic hernia (CDH), treated with or without neonatal extracorporeal membrane oxygenation (ECMO) between January 1999 and December 2003.

Design.—Cohort study with structural prospective follow-up.

Setting.—Level III University Hospital.

Patients.—35 children (ECMO: n = 16; non-ECMO: n = 19) were assessed at 8 years of age.

Interventions.—None.

Main Outcome Measures.—Intelligence and motor function. Concentration, behaviour, school performance, competence and health status were also analysed.

Results.—Mean (SD) intelligence for the ECMO group was 91.7 (19.5) versus 111.6 (20.9) for the non-ECMO group ($p = 0.015$). Motor problems were apparent in 16% of all participants and differed significantly from the norm ($p = 0.015$) without differences between treatment groups. For all participants, problems with concentration (68%, $p < 0.001$) and with behavioural attention (33%, $p = 0.021$) occurred more frequently than in reference groups, with no difference between treatment groups. School performance and competence were not affected.

Conclusions.—Children with CDH—whether or not treated with neonatal ECMO—are at risk for long-term morbidity especially in the areas of motor function and concentration. Despite their impairment, children with CDH have a well-developed feeling of self-competence.

▶ It is presumed that infants with congenital diaphragmatic hernia (CDH) who require rescue with extracorporeal membrane oxygenation (ECMO) are at higher risk for poor neurodevelopmental outcome than infants who can be treated without ECMO. However, there are scant data to support this presumption. In the above observational study, the authors evaluated the intelligence and motor function of infants with CDH treated with or without ECMO at 8 years of age.

The abstract contains the mean intelligence scores of the ECMO and the non-ECMO cohorts; however, because intelligence quotient (IQ) scores are nonlinear, comparison of mean scores can be somewhat misleading. In fact, the frequency of IQ scores greater than one standard deviation below the mean (< 85) in the ECMO cohort was more than 6-fold higher than that of the non-ECMO group (54% vs 8%). In addition, motor problems are reported for the aggregate CDH cohort; however, abnormal motor function was 2-fold higher for the ECMO cohort (31% vs 16%). Overall, developmental impairment (IQ < 85 and poor motor function) was noted in 54% of the ECMO cohort compared with 15% in the non-ECMO group. Despite the marked differences in outcome, the percentage of children who were in special education classes or receiving extra support in school was similar (50% vs 42%).

L. A. Papile, MD

Psychiatric outcomes at age seven for very preterm children: rates and predictors
Treyvaud K, Ure A, Doyle LW, et al (Murdoch Childrens Res Inst, Victoria, Australia; et al)
J Child Psychol Psychiatry 54:772-779, 2013

Background.—Uncertainty remains about the rate of specific psychiatric disorders and associated predictive factors for very preterm (VPT) children. The aims of this study were to document rates of psychiatric disorders in VPT children aged 7 years compared with term born children, and to examine potential predictive factors for psychiatric diagnoses in VPT children.

Methods.—Participants were 177 VPT and 65 term born children. Perinatal medical data were collected, which included brain abnormalities detected using magnetic resonance imaging. The Infant-Toddler Social-Emotional Assessment (ITSEA) and Strengths and Difficulties Questionnaire (SDQ) were administered at 2 and 5 years respectively. At 7 years of age, the Developmental and Well-being Assessment (DAWBA) was used to indicate psychiatric diagnoses.

Results.—Compared with term born children, VPT children had three times the odds of meeting criteria for any psychiatric diagnosis at age 7 years (odds ratio 3.03; 95% confidence interval 1.23, 7.47, $p = .02$). The most common diagnoses were anxiety disorders (11% VPT, 8% term), attention-deficit/hyperactivity disorder (10% VPT, 3% term) and autism spectrum disorder (4.5% VPT, 0% term). For VPT children, those with severe global brain abnormalities ($p = .02$), those who displayed social-emotional problems at age 5 ($p = .000$) and those with higher social risk at age 7 ($p = .001$) were more likely to meet criteria for a psychiatric illness at age 7.

Conclusions.—Compared with term born children, VPT children have higher rates of psychiatric diagnoses at early school age, predicted by neonatal brain abnormalities, prior social-emotional problems and social factors.

▶ Preterm- compared with term-born children have a 2- to 6-fold higher reported risk of poor social-emotional outcomes. Factors that have been linked to psychiatric disorders among preterm children include cognitive impairment, serious functional disability, increased social risk, and male sex. In the above observational study, the authors sought to examine several factors that might be predictive of having a psychiatric disorder at 7 years of age, including brain abnormalities noted on magnetic resonance imaging (MRI) at term-equivalent age.

Overall, 24% of the very preterm group and 6% of their term counterparts had evidence of a psychiatric illness. The rates of attention-deficit/hyperactivity disorder, autism spectrum, and anxiety in very preterm born children in the report are consistent with what has been termed the "preterm behavioral phenotype."[1]

Similar to previous reports, preterm children who had a poor social environment and those who had social-emotional difficulties diagnosed before 7 years of age were more likely to fulfill the criteria for a psychiatric illness. However, global brain abnormalities on MRI did not place a child at risk for psychiatric illness unless the abnormality was severe, a condition noted in only 6% of the cohort studied. Even then, only 50% of children with severe brain abnormalities were noted to have a psychiatric illness. Thus, it would appear that detecting brain abnormalities on MRI at term-equivalent age is not very useful for the early identification of very preterm infants at risk for poor social-emotional outcomes.

L. A. Papile, MD

Reference

1. Johnson S, Marlow N. Preterm birth and childhood psychiatric disorders. *Pediatr Res.* 2011;69:11R-18R.

Postnatal corticosteroids and neurodevelopmental outcomes in extremely low birthweight or extremely preterm infants: 15-year experience in Victoria, Australia
Cheong JL, Victorian Infant Collaborative Study Group (Royal Women's Hosp, Parkville, Victoria, Australia)
Arch Dis Child Fetal Neonatal Ed 98:F32-F36, 2013

Objective.—Postnatal corticosteroids (PCS) are used to prevent or treat bronchopulmonary dysplasia (BPD) in extremely low birthweight (ELBW; <1000 g) or extremely preterm (EPT; <28 weeks) infants. In the early 2000s, concerns were raised about increased risks of cerebral palsy (CP) in association with PCS, which may have affected prescribing of PCS, and influenced rates of BPD, mortality or long-term neurosensory morbidity. Our aim was to determine the changes over time in the rates of PCS use and 2-year outcomes in ELBW/EPT infants in Victoria, Australia.

Design.—All ELBW or EPT infants born in Victoria, Australia in three distinct eras (1991—92, 1997 and 2005) who were alive at 7 days were included. Rates of PCS use, rates of BPD (oxygen dependency at 36 weeks' corrected age), death before 2 years of age, CP and major disability (any of moderate/severe CP, developmental quotient <−2 SD, blindness or deafness) were contrasted between cohorts.

Results.—The rate of PCS use and the dose prescribed diminished significantly in 2005 compared with earlier eras, but the rate of BPD rose. Nonsignificant changes in the rates of mortality over time were mirrored by non-significant changes in the rates of CP or major disability. Combined outcomes of mortality with either major disability or CP were similar over the three eras.

Conclusions.—PCS use decreased in 2005 compared with earlier eras, and was accompanied by a rise in BPD, with no significant changes in mortality or neurological morbidity.

▶ In 2002, the American Academy of Pediatrics published, and in 2010 updated, a consensus statement cautioning the use of postnatal corticosteroids to either treat or prevent bronchopulmonary dysplasia (BPD), as death rates were unchanged, and any benefit of a reduction in the rate of BPD was potentially offset by an increased risk of cerebral palsy (CP).[1,2] The publication of the 2002 statement led to a decrease in postnatal corticosteroid use worldwide. Several studies reported increased rates of BPD with the subsequent decrease in postnatal steroid use, whereas other publications reported rates of BPD that were unchanged despite a reduction in postnatal steroid use. However, in many cohorts, a reduction in the frequency, duration, and total dose of postnatal steroids was not accompanied by a change in neurodevelopmental morbidity and mortality.

Preliminary data indicate that the effect of postnatal corticosteroids on the combined outcome of death or CP varies with BPD risk, suggesting that babies at very high risk of BPD might benefit in the long term.[3] Given the lack of equipoise, it is unlikely that a randomized, controlled trial of dexamethasone compared with placebo for the treatment of BPD targeted at infants at high risk of BPD is possible in the near future. However, there may be a role for randomized, controlled trials of alternative postnatal steroids, such as hydrocortisone, compared with dexamethasone among infants at high risk of BPD in the efficacy of treatment or prevention of BPD as well as adverse neurodevelopmental effects.

L. A. Papile, MD

References

1. American Academy of Pediatrics, Committee on Fetus and Newborn and Canadian Paediatric Society, Fetus and Newborn Committee. Postnatal corticosteroids to treat or prevent chronic lung disease in preterm infants. *Pediatrics.* 2002;109:330-338.
2. Watterberg KL; American Academy of Pediatrics, Committee on Fetus and Newborn. Policy statement—postnatal corticosteroids to prevent or treat bronchopulmonary dysplasia. *Pediatrics.* 2010;126:800-808.
3. Doyle LW, Halliday HL, Ehrenkranz RA, Davis PG, Sinclair JC. Impact of postnatal systemic corticosteroids on mortality and cerebral palsy in preterm infants: effect modification by risk for chronic lung disease. *Pediatrics.* 2005;115:655-661.

Effect of inborn vs. outborn delivery on neurodevelopmental outcomes in infants with hypoxic–ischemic encephalopathy: secondary analyses of the NICHD whole-body cooling trial

Natarajan G, Pappas A, Shankaran S, et al (Wayne State Univ, Detroit, MI; et al)
Pediatr Res 72:414-419, 2012

Background.—The effect of birth location on hypothermia-related outcomes has not been rigorously examined in the literature. In this study, we determined whether birth location had an impact on the benefits of whole-body cooling to 33.5 °C for 72 h in term infants ($n = 208$) with hypoxic–ischemic encephalopathy (HIE) who participated in the Neonatal Research Network (NRN) randomized controlled trial.

Methods.—Heterogeneity by birth location was examined with respect to cooling treatment for the 18-mo primary outcomes (death, moderate disability, severe disability) and secondary outcomes (death, components of disability), and in-hospital organ dysfunction. Logistic regression models were used to generate adjusted odds ratios.

Results.—Infants born at a location other than an NRN center (outborn) ($n = 93$) experienced significant delays in initiation of therapy (mean (SD): 5.5 (1.1) vs. 4.4 (1.2) h), lower baseline temperatures (36.6 (1.2) vs. 37.1 (0.9) °C), and more severe HIE (43 vs. 29%) than infants born in an NRN center (inborn) ($n = 115$). Maternal education <12 y (50 vs. 14%) and African-American ethnicity (43 vs. 25%) were more common in the inborn group. When adjusted for NRN center and HIE severity, there were no significant differences in 18-mo outcomes or in-hospital organ dysfunction between inborn and outborn infants.

Conclusion.—Although limited by sample size and some differences in baseline characteristics, the study showed that birth location does not appear to modify the treatment effect of hypothermia after HIE.

▶ Meta-analyses of randomized, clinical trials of therapeutic hypothermia in newborns with hypoxic-ischemic encephalopathy (HIE) demonstrate a statistically and clinically important reduction in the combined outcome of death and major developmental disability in early childhood. There are scarce data on the outcomes of infants treated with hypothermia who are transferred to a cooling center compared with those born at the center.

This article, a secondary analysis of the Neonatal Research Network's randomized, controlled trial of systemic hypothermia, explored the interaction between hypothermia treatment and location of birth. The unadjusted rate of death or neurodevelopmental disability was higher in the outborn population as compared with the inborn population in both the hypothermia treated and control subgroups, but was no longer significant when the data were adjusted for the network center and severity of HIE. However, there were several significant differences between the groups that could have obscured an effect of location of birth on outcome. Significantly more mothers of infants in the inborn group had a maternal fever, and their infants had a significantly higher temperature at randomization. In addition, 50% of mothers of inborn infants had less than a high school education compared with 14% of mothers of the outborn cohort. Each of these factors may have adversely affected the outcome of the inborn cohort.

In addition, several factors related to the outborn group are notable. In general, a significantly greater proportion required continued resuscitation at 10 minutes of age, experienced onset of spontaneous respirations at greater than 10 minutes of age, and had severe, rather than moderate, HIE. Whether these differences related to the quality and effectiveness of resuscitation at the referring hospital or reflected a referral bias with the most severely HIE-affected infants being referred for cooling cannot be ascertained from the data presented.

L. A. Papile, MD

Childhood Outcomes after Hypothermia for Neonatal Encephalopathy

Shankaran S, for the Eunice Kennedy Shriver NICHD Neonatal Research Network (Wayne State Univ, Detroit, MI; et al)
N Engl J Med 366:2085-2092, 2012

Background.—We previously reported early results of a randomized trial of whole-body hypothermia for neonatal hypoxic—ischemic encephalopathy showing a significant reduction in the rate of death or moderate or severe disability at 18 to 22 months of age. Long-term outcomes are now available.

Methods.—In the original trial, we assigned infants with moderate or severe encephalopathy to usual care (the control group) or whole-body cooling to an esophageal temperature of 33.5°C for 72 hours, followed by slow rewarming (the hypothermia group). We evaluated cognitive, attention and executive, and visuospatial function; neurologic outcomes; and physical and psychosocial health among participants at 6 to 7 years of age. The primary outcome of the present analyses was death or an IQ score below 70.

Results.—Of the 208 trial participants, primary outcome data were available for 190. Of the 97 children in the hypothermia group and the 93 children in the control group, death or an IQ score below 70 occurred in 46 (47%) and 58 (62%), respectively ($P = 0.06$); death occurred in 27 (28%) and 41 (44%) ($P = 0.04$); and death or severe disability occurred in 38 (41%) and 53 (60%) ($P = 0.03$). Other outcome data were available for the 122 surviving children, 70 in the hypothermia group and 52 in the control group. Moderate or severe disability occurred in 24 of 69 children (35%) and 19 of 50 children (38%), respectively ($P = 0.87$). Attention—executive dysfunction occurred in 4% and 13%, respectively, of children receiving hypothermia and those receiving usual care ($P = 0.19$), and visuospatial dysfunction occurred in 4% and 3% ($P = 0.80$).

Conclusions.—The rate of the combined end point of death or an IQ score of less than 70 at 6 to 7 years of age was lower among children undergoing whole-body hypothermia than among those undergoing usual care, but the differences were not significant. However, hypothermia resulted in lower death rates and did not increase rates of severe disability among survivors. (Funded by the National Institutes of Health and the Eunice Kennedy Shriver NICHD Neonatal Research Network; ClinicalTrials.gov number, NCT00005772.)

▶ Seventy-two hours of therapeutic hypothermia (TH), beginning within 6 hours of birth, reduces the risk of death and moderate or severe disability at 18 to 22 months of age among newborns with hypoxic-ischemic encephalopathy (HIE).[1] The current publication describes the 6- to 7-year outcomes of 190 of the 208 infants enrolled in a landmark study of TH: the Eunice Kennedy Shriver National Institutes of Child Health and Human Development (NICHD) Neonatal Research Network (NRN) Randomized Clinical Trial of Whole Body Therapeutic Hypothermia. Analyses of outcomes at age 6 to 7 found significantly reduced risk of the composite outcome death or intelligence quotient (IQ) less than 70 among infants who were randomly assigned to the TH group. There was a significant, TH-associated reduction in death (28% among TH-treated and 44% among controls [relative risk], 0.66 [0.45–0.97]) and a trend in the direction of reduced risk of the primary outcome, death, or an IQ less than 70 (47% in the TH group and 62% among control subjects [relative risk, 0.78 (0.61–1.01; $P = .06$)]). Although the study was not powered for long-term outcomes, trends also were observed for TH-associated reductions in other specific morbidities, including cerebral palsy, blindness, and seizures. These findings provide additional evidence in support of TH. On the other hand, nearly half of TH-treated babies either died or exhibited an IQ score less than 70 at age 6 by rigorous standardized testing. Thus, TH represents an effective but insufficient treatment for HIE. Further work is needed to determine optimal use of TH (eg, mode, depth, and duration of hypothermia) and to identify complimentary therapies, such as erythropoietin or xenon, which might offer synergistic benefit when used in conjunction with TH. In a related report,[2] NICHD NRN classifications of magnetic resonance imaging (MRI) patterns of brain injury at 44 weeks PMA also were found to correlate with later outcomes. Additional TH/HIE research efforts must be directed at developing improved diagnostic methods (eg, aEEG, NIRS, early MRI findings) that more promptly and accurately identify babies most likely to benefit from TH and provide a window on expected outcomes with TH.

L. J. Van Marter, MD, MPH

References

1. Shankaran S, Laptook AR, Ehrenkranz RA, et al. Whole-body hypothermia for neonates with hypoxic-ischemic encephalopathy. *N Engl J Med.* 2005;353: 1574-1584.
2. Shankaran S, Barnes PD, Hintz SR, et al. Brain injury following trial of hypothermia for neonatal hypoxic-ischaemic encephalopathy. *Arch Dis Child Fetal Neonatal Ed.* 2012;97:F398-F404.

Neurodevelopmental Outcomes Following Two Different Treatment Approaches (Early Ligation and Selective Ligation) for Patent Ductus Arteriosus
Wickremasinghe AC, Rogers EE, Piecuch RE, et al (Univ of California San Francisco)
J Pediatr 161:1065-1072, 2012

Objective.—To examine whether a change in the approach to managing persistent patent ductus arteriosus (PDA) from early ligation to selective ligation is associated with an increased risk of abnormal neurodevelopmental outcomes.

Study Design.—In 2005, we changed our PDA treatment protocol for infants born at ≤27 6/7 weeks' gestation from an early ligation approach, with prompt PDA ligation if the ductus failed to close after indomethacin therapy (period 1: January 1999 to December 2004), to a selective ligation approach, with PDA ligation performed only if specific criteria were met (period 2: January 2005 to May 2009). All infants in both periods received prophylactic indomethacin. Multivariate analysis was used to compare the odds of a composite abnormal neurodevelopmental outcome (Bayley Mental Developmental Index or Cognitive Score <70, cerebral palsy, blindness, and/or deafness) associated with each treatment approach at age 18-36 months (n = 224).

Results.—During period 1, 23% of the infants in follow-up failed indomethacin treatment, and all underwent surgical ligation. During period 2, 30% of infants failed indomethacin, and 66% underwent ligation after meeting prespecified criteria. Infants treated with the selective ligation strategy demonstrated fewer abnormal outcomes than those treated with the early ligation approach (OR, 0.07; $P = .046$). Infants who underwent ligation before 10 days of age had an increased incidence of abnormal neurodevelopmental outcome. The significant difference in outcomes between the 2 PDA treatment strategies could be accounted for in part by the earlier age of ligation during period 1.

Conclusion.—A selective ligation approach for PDAs that fail to close with indomethacin therapy is not associated with worse neurodevelopmental outcomes at age 18-36 months.

▶ Despite decades worth of clinical studies, the optimal management of a patent ductus arteriosus (PDA) in the extremely preterm infant remains unclear. In a recent survey, the majority of US neonatologists reported that they initially would treat a symptomatic PDA with indomethacin.[1] However, there are few data to inform clinical management when indomethacin fails to close a PDA.

In this observational, retrospective single-center study, the authors took advantage of a change in their neonatal intensive care unit's approach to managing a persistent PDA to determine if prolonged exposure to a persistent PDA increases the risk for poor neurodevelopmental outcome in early childhood. In the first epoch (1999 to 2004), a persistent PDA was surgically ligated as soon as possible (early ligation), while in the second epoch (2005 to 2009), a persistent PDA was surgically ligated only if there were specific clinical signs indicating an increase in the left-to-right shunt through the PDA (selective ligation). In both epochs, each infant was treated with a course of prophylactic indomethacin initiated within 15 hours of birth. The decision of whether to administer a second course of indomethacin if the PDA did not close was made by the attending neonatologist.

In a previous publication, it was noted that the cohort of infants treated with the selective ligation approach had decreased PDA ligation and necrotizing enterocolitis, but the incidence of bronchopulmonary dysplasia, sepsis, retinopathy of prematurity, or death was unchanged.[2]

The authors' conclusion in this article that selective ligation is not associated with worse neurodevelopmental outcomes needs to be interpreted cautiously for several reasons. Although the follow-up rate for infants who had their PDAs surgically ligated is not stated, the overall follow-up rate was only 67%. In addition, the number of infants in the early and late PDA ligation cohorts who were evaluated was only 30 and 29, respectively. Caution is also needed regarding the authors' speculation that young postnatal age at the time of surgical ligation is a significant predictor of abnormal neurodevelopmental outcome. Ligation before 10 days of age occurred in a total of 12 infants (9 in the first epoch and 3 in the second epoch), and although the odds ratio is 11.44, the 95% confidence interval is 1.85 to 70.72.

L. A. Papile, MD

References

1. Kiefer AS, Wickremasinghe AC, Johnson JN, et al. Medical management of extremely low-birth-weight infants in the first week of life: a survey of practices in the United States. *Am J Perinatol.* 2009;26:407-418.
2. Jhaveri N, Moon-Grady A, Clyman RI. Early surgical ligation versus a conservative approach for management of patent ductus arteriosus that fails to close after indomethacin treatment. *J Pediatr.* 2010;157:381-387.

Perinatal Origins of First-Grade Academic Failure: Role of Prematurity and Maternal Factors

Williams BL, Dunlop AL, Kramer M, et al (Emory Univ, Atlanta, GA; et al)
Pediatrics 131:693-700, 2013

Objective.—We examined the relationships among gestational age at birth, maternal characteristics, and standardized test performance in Georgia first-grade students.

Methods.—Live births to Georgia resident mothers aged 11 to 53 years from 1998 through 2003 were deterministically linked with standardized test results for first-grade attendees of Georgia public schools from 2005 through 2009. Logistic models were used to estimate the odds of failure of the 3 components of the first-grade Criterion-Referenced Competency Test (CRCT).

Results.—The strongest risk factor for failure of each of the 3 components of the first-grade CRCT was level of maternal education. Child race/ethnicity and maternal age at birth were also associated with first-grade CRCT failure irrespective of the severity of preterm birth, but these factors were more important among children born moderately preterm than for those born on the margins of the prematurity distribution. Adjusting for maternal and child characteristics, there was an increased odds of failure of each component of the CRCT for children born late preterm versus term, including for math (adjusted odds ratio [aOR]: 1.17, 95% confidence interval [CI]: 1.13—1.22), reading (aOR: 1.13, 95% CI: 1.08—1.18), and English/language arts, for which there was an important interaction with being born small for gestational age (aOR: 1.17, 95% CI: 1.07—1.29).

Conclusions.—Preterm birth and low maternal education increase children's risk of failure of first-grade standardized tests. Promoting women's academic achievement and reduce rates of preterm birth may be important to achieving gains in elementary school performance.

▶ Most developed countries in the West have a variety of national databases that contain vital information regarding their citizens. Because the United States lacks such systems, epidemiologic studies in the US rely on data from several sources. In this study, the authors extracted data from birth records in Georgia and linked them to standardized testing data obtained from the Georgia State Department of Education. There were 628 115 births to Georgia-resident mothers from 1998 through 2003. Of this cohort, 314 328 (53%) were successfully linked to their first-grade standardized test scores. Possible sources of loss to follow-up, including interstate migration and enrollment in private school or home schooling, accounted for approximately 29%. The remaining 18% loss most likely related to changes or errors in the recording of identifying variables used in the linkage.

Children were categorized as either passing or failing each of the 3 components of the standardized test (math, reading, and English/language arts). The child's gestational age at birth was considered to be extremely preterm (20—27 weeks), moderately preterm (28—33 weeks), late preterm (34—36 weeks), term (38—42 weeks) or postterm (42—43 weeks). Race/ethnic categories were non-Hispanic white, non-Hispanic African-American, or Hispanic of any race. Maternal age at the time of delivery was divided into 8 categories (from 10 to 14 years to > 40 years) with 25 to 29 years used as the reference age. Maternal education at the time of delivery was divided into 4 categories, with a college degree or greater considered the reference category.

In both the crude and logistic models, the strongest risk factor for failure of each of the 3 components of the standardized test was maternal education. Maternal age and the child's race/ethnicity also were significantly associated with failure of each component of the standardized educational test, irrespective of the degree of prematurity. The relative influence of these factors on the probability of test failure varied considerably across the gestational age categories, with the greatest effect noted among the moderately preterm cohort. As the authors note, because the test failure rate at the first-grade level is inherently low, it is reasonable to expect that the synergism among maternal education and socioeconomic status, preterm birth, and subsequent academic performance may become more apparent as a child progresses through the grade levels.

L. A. Papile, MD

Neonatal seizures and post-neonatal epilepsy: a seven-year follow-up study
Pisani F, Piccolo B, Cantalupo G, et al (Univ-Hosp of Parma, Italy)
Pediatr Res 2012 [Epub ahead of print]

Background.—Seizures are one of the most common symptoms of acute neurological disorders in newborns. This study aims at evaluating predictors of epilepsy in newborns with neonatal seizures.

Methods.—We recruited consecutively eighty-five neonates with repeated neonatal video-EEG-confirmed seizures between Jan 1999 and Dec 2004. The relationship between clinical, EEG and ultrasound data in neonatal period and the development of post-neonatal epilepsy was investigated at 7 years of age.

Results.—Fifteen patients (17.6%) developed post-neonatal epilepsy. Partial or no response to anticonvulsant therapy (OR 16.7, 95% CI: 1.8-155.8, $p = .01$; OR 47, 95% CI: 5.2-418.1, $p < .01$ respectively), severely abnormal cerebral ultrasound scan findings (OR: 5.4; 95% CI: 1.1-27.4; $p < .04$), severely abnormal EEG background activity (OR: 9.5; 95% CI: 1.6-54.2; $p = .01$) and the presence of status epilepticus (OR: 6.1; 95% CI: 1.8-20.3; $p < .01$) were found to be predictors of epilepsy. However, only the response to therapy seemed to be an independent predictor of post-neonatal epilepsy.

Conclusion.—Neonatal seizures seem to be related to post-neonatal epilepsy. Recurrent and prolonged neonatal seizures may act on an epileptogenic substrate, causing further damage, which is responsible for the subsequent clinical expression of epilepsy.

▶ The wide variability in the reported risk for developing childhood epilepsy in patients with a history of neonatal seizures most probably relates to differences in patient selection and the definition of seizures. In this observational report, the authors restricted their patient population to newborns with seizures confirmed by video electroencephalogram (video-EEG) that was performed before starting antiepileptic therapy. Infants were considered as having epilepsy when unprovoked, recurring epileptic seizures either occurred in the neonatal period and persisted beyond the third month of corrected age or had an onset after the neonatal period.

Overall, 15 of the 85 newborn infants with video-EEG evidence of seizures developed epilepsy. The frequency of epilepsy was similar in term and preterm newborns (18.1% vs 17.1%). The diagnosis of epilepsy was made in the neonatal period for 60%, between 3 and 12 months of age for 13%, and after the first year in 27%. Twelve of the 15 patients with epilepsy had evidence of moderate/severe brain injury on neonatal head sonograms (HUS) and subsequent evidence of cerebral palsy and developmental delay at 7 years of age. The predominant neuromotor impairment was spastic quadriplegia (11/13).

The authors suggest that the response to antiepileptic drug therapy, status epilepticus (SE), severe abnormal EEG background activity, and moderate/severe brain injury as seen on HUS are independent variables predictive of subsequent epilepsy. Because only 42% of infants with SE, 27% of infants who had abnormal EEG background activity, and 34% of those with moderate/severe brain injury noted on HUS developed epilepsy, the usefulness of these parameters in predicting which encephalopathic infants need ongoing surveillance for the occurrence of epilepsy is uncertain.

L. A. Papile, MD

Outcomes at 7 years for babies who developed neonatal necrotising enterocolitis: the ORACLE Children Study

Pike K, Brocklehurst P, Jones D, et al (Univ of Bristol, UK; Univ College London, UK; Univ of Leicester, UK; et al)
Arch Dis Child Fetal Neonatal Ed 97:F318-F322, 2012

Background.—Within the ORACLE Children Study Cohort, the authors have evaluated long-term consequences of the diagnosis of confirmed or suspected neonatal necrotising enterocolitis (NEC) at age of 7 years.

Methods.—Outcomes were assessed using a parental questionnaire, including the Health Utilities Index (HUI-3) to assess functional impairment, and specific medical and behavioural outcomes. Educational outcomes for children in England were explored using national standardised tests. Multiple logistic regression was used to explore independent associates of NEC within the cohort.

Results.—The authors obtained data for 119 (77%) of 157 children following proven or suspected NEC and compared their outcomes with those of the remaining 6496 children. NEC was associated with an increase in risk of neonatal death (OR 14.6 (95% CI 10.4 to 20.6)). At 7 years, NEC conferred an increased risk of all grades of impairment. Adjusting for confounders, risks persisted for any HUI-3 defined functional impairment (adjusted OR 1.55 (1.05, 2.29)), particularly mild impairment (adjusted OR 1.61 (1.03, 2.53)) both in all NEC children and in those with proven NEC, which appeared to be independent. No behavioural or educational associations were confirmed. Following NEC, children were more likely to suffer bowel problems than non-NEC children (adjusted OR 3.96 (2.06, 7.61)).

Conclusions.—The ORACLE Children Study provided opportunity for the largest evaluation of school age outcome following neonatal NEC and demonstrates significant long-term consequences of both gut function (presence of stoma, admission for bowel problems and continuing medical care for gut-related problems) and motor, sensory and cognitive outcomes as measured using HUI-3.

▶ Neonatologists are intimately familiar with the devastating effects of necrotizing enterocolitis (NEC) in neonatal mortality and short-term morbidity; however, information regarding NEC-associated long-term outcomes remains sparse. This follow-up investigation of more than 6000 infants born to mothers enrolled in the ORACLE study of perinatal antibiotic treatment for preterm labor or premature rupture of fetal membranes, conducted in the United Kingdom between 1994 and 2000, attempts to breach this knowledge gap. The study of NEC embedded within ORACLE confirmed higher rates of neonatal mortality among infants with NEC and evaluated the long-term effects of NEC among survivors. A total of 119 of 157 ORACLE-enrolled infants who later had proven or suspected NEC were evaluated at age 7 via parent questionnaire (the Multi-Attribute Health Status classification system) as well as by National Curriculum test results at Key Stage 1. In both unadjusted analyses and analyses adjusted for antenatal and neonatal factors, the odds of functional impairment at any level and ongoing bowel problems were greater among children who had experienced suspected or proven NEC than among those who experienced neither. Unadjusted analyses also revealed increased risks of educational attainment less than level 2 at Key Stage 1 (reading, writing, and math), cerebral palsy, and attention deficit hyperactivity disorder—associations that were no longer significant after adjustment for antenatal and neonatal factors. A caveat regarding the latter finding is that some of the potential confounding factors included in the multivariate model might constitute the intermediates through which NEC leads to adverse long-term outcomes. Hopefully, one or more of the promising research avenues focused on NEC now being pursued will lead to accurate prediction and effective prevention of this terrible disorder.

L. J. Van Marter, MD, MPH

Self-Reported Adolescent Health Status of Extremely Low Birth Weight Children Born 1992–1995

Hack M, Schluchter M, Forrest CB, et al (Case Western Reserve Univ, Cleveland, OH; Univ of Pennsylvania School of Medicine, Philadelphia; et al)
Pediatrics 130:46-53, 2012

Objectives.—To compare the self-reported health of extremely low birth weight (ELBW, <1 kg) adolescents with that of normal birth weight (NBW) controls and the children's assessments of their general health at ages 8 versus 14 years.

Methods.—One hundred sixty-eight ELBW children and 115 NBW controls of similar gender and sociodemographic status completed the Child Health and Illness Profile—Adolescent Edition at age 14 years. It includes 6 domains: Satisfaction, Comfort, Resilience, Risk Avoidance, Achievement, and Disorders. At age 8 years, the children had completed the Child Health and Illness Profile—Child Edition. Results were compared between ELBW and NBW subjects adjusting for gender and sociodemographic status.

Results.—ELBW adolescents rated their health similar to that of NBW adolescents in the domains of Satisfaction, Comfort, Resilience, Achievement and Disorders but reported more Risk Avoidance (effect size [ES] 0.6, $P < .001$). In the subdomain of Resilience, they also noted less physical activity (ES -0.58, $P < .001$), and in the subdomain of Disorders, more long-term surgical (ES -0.49) and psychosocial disorders (ES -0.49; both $P < .01$). Both ELBW and NBW children reported a decrease in general health between ages 8 and 14 years, which did not differ significantly between groups.

Conclusions.—ELBW adolescents report similar health and well-being compared with NBW controls but greater risk avoidance. Both ELBW and NBW children rate their general health to be poorer at age 14 than at age 8 years, possibly due to age-related developmental changes.

▶ As survival rates for extremely-low-birth-weight (ELBW) infants have dramatically increased over the past decade, there has been increasing interest in their long-term outcomes over and above neurosensory and cognitive sequelae. Previous reports of ELBW adolescents and young adults born before the 1990s indicated that they considered their health and well-being to be similar to that of their normal-birth-weight (NBW) peers, despite higher rates of chronic medical and neurodevelopmental problems.[1] In contrast, risk-taking behavior was reported to be less among ELBW young adults.[2-4] In this report, the health and well-being of ELBW 14-year-olds who were born in the 1990s was compared with that of a NBW-matched cohort.

The primary outcome measure was the Child Health and Illness Profile-Adolescent Edition, a self-administered questionnaire that includes 150 items related to perceived health, functioning, and well-being and 46 disease- or injury-specific questions. The questions are organized into 20 subdomains and 6 conceptually based domains: 1) satisfaction, which includes items concerning self-worth and satisfaction with one's health; 2) comfort, which includes physically and emotionally experienced feelings and limitations in activity; 3) resilience, which includes states and behaviors that promote health, including social problem-solving, physical activity, home safety, and health and family involvement; 4) risk avoidance, which includes avoidance of individuals risks, behaviors that may disrupt social development and subsequent health, and influences of peers who are involved in risky behaviors; 5) achievement, which includes both academic achievement in school and work performance; and 6) disorders, which include biomedically defined states of ill health, injuries, and impairments.

ELBW children differed significantly from NBW children only in the domain of risk avoidance. The findings were similar after excluding children with neurosensory disorders. The greater risk avoidance among ELBW children pertained to 3 activities: drinking alcohol, marijuana use, and engaging in sexual intercourse either individually or by their friends. Although the overall scores for the domains of achievement, resilience, and disorders did not differ between ELBW and LBW children, there were significant differences in several areas; fewer ELBW children reported ever driving a car, doing something risky or dangerous on a dare, breaking parental rules, or having trouble getting along with teachers. They also reported less physical activity, more long-term surgical disorders, such as vision and hearing problems, and more long-term psychosocial disorders compared with NBW peers.

Comparison of the 8- with the 14-year-old assessment questionnaires showed no difference between the ELBW and NBW children in the mean score for the question rating general health. Both groups rated their health significantly poorer at 14 years than 8 years.

The results of the current study are in agreement with previous reports of ELBW adolescents and young adults born before the 1990s, both with regard to perceptions of their health and well-being and their engagement in less risk-taking behavior. The reasons for less risk-taking behavior are not fully understood, but may include emotional problems, relative social isolation because of disabilities, or an increase in parental protection and supervision.

L. A. Papile, MD

References

1. Zwicker JG, Harris SR. Quality of life of formerly preterm and very low birth weight infants from preschool to adulthood: a systemic review. *Pediatrics.* 2008; 121:e366-e376, www.pediatrics.org/cgi/content/full/121/2/e366.
2. Hack M, Flnnery DJ, Schluchter M, Cartar L, Borawaaki E, Klein N. Outcomes in young adulthood for very-low-birth-weight infants. *N Engl J Med.* 2002;346: 149-157.
3. Cooke RW. Health, lifestyle and quality of life for young adults born very preterm. *Arch Dis Child.* 2004;89:201-206.
4. Hille ET, Dorrepaal C, Perenboom R, Gravenhorst JB, Brand R, Verloove-Vanhorick SP; Dutch POPS-19 Collaborative Study Group. Socail lifestyle, risk-taking behavior, and psychopathology in young adults born very preterm or with a very low birthweight. *J Pediatr.* 2008;152:793-800.

Clinical and psychosocial functioning in adolescents and young adults with anorectal malformations and chronic idiopathic constipation

Athanasakos EP, Kemal KI, Malliwal RS, et al (The Royal London Hosp, UK; Queen Mary Univ of London, UK)

Br J Surg 100:832-839, 2013

Background.—Faecal incontinence (FI) and constipation occur following corrective surgery for anorectal malformations (ARMs) and in children or adults with chronic constipation without a structural birth anomaly (chronic idiopathic constipation, CIC). Such symptoms may have profound effects on quality of life (QoL). This study systematically determined the burden of FI and constipation in these patients in adolescence and early adulthood, and their effect on QoL and psychosocial functioning in comparison with controls.

Methods.—Patients with ARMs or CIC were compared with age- and sex-matched controls who had undergone appendicectomy more than 1 year previously and had no ongoing gastrointestinal symptoms. Constipation and FI were evaluated using validated Knowles—Eccersley—Scott Symptom (KESS) and Vaizey scores respectively. Standardized QoL and psychometric tests were performed in all groups.

Results.—The study included 49 patients with ARMs (30 male, aged 11—28 years), 45 with CIC (32 male, aged 11—30 years) and 39 controls (21 male, aged 11—30 years). The frequency of severe constipation among patients with ARMs was approximately half that seen in the CIC group (19 of 49 *versus* 31 of 45); however, frequencies of incontinence were similar (22 of 49 *versus* 21 of 45) ($P < 0.001$ *versus* controls for both symptoms). Physical and mental well-being were significantly reduced in both ARM and CIC groups compared with controls ($P = 0.001$ and $P = 0.015$ respectively), with generally worse scores among patients with CIC. Both were predicted by gastrointestinal symptom burden ($P < 0.001$). There were no statistically significant differences in state or trait psychiatric morbidity between groups.

Conclusion.—FI and constipation are major determinants of poor QoL in adolescents and young adults with ARMs and in those with CIC.

▶ Neonatologists and pediatric surgeons caring for children in tertiary and quaternary centers will frequently care for babies who have anorectal malformations (ARMs), either isolated as imperforate anus or with vertebral, anorectal, cardiac, trachea–oesophageal, renal, and limb association. Parents often ask what the prognosis of these children is as they grow.

This study from London partially addressed this question by comparing adolescents who have had a previous appendectomy as a control group with those who had previous surgery for ARMs and a third group with chronic idiopathic constipation (CIC) (with absence of a well-defined cause). The patients with ARMs and CIC exhibited signs of increased constipation, incontinence, and gastrointestinal quality of life index, as would be expected. Overall, the physical and mental well-being scores were also slightly but statistically lower in the CIC and ARM groups when compared with the controls. A large overlap was found in the results of the 3 groups in all of these outcomes, signifying that many of these individuals would be within a normal range despite their incontinence or constipation. Of major interest was that several important psychological assessments, such as anxiety, depression, hopefulness, honesty, and coping mechanisms, showed no significant differences among the groups. The authors cite 1 limitation of the study, which is that it was probably skewed toward worse outcomes because the patients were primarily attenders to tertiary pediatric and adolescent surgical practices with a high intervention requirement. Overall, this study provides data for cautious optimism for those infants with ARMs, especially in the emotional responses that influence how the individual copes with the stressors involved with fecal incontinence and chronic constipation.

J. Neu, MD

Default options and neonatal resuscitation decisions

Haward MF, Murphy RO, Lorenz JM (Children's Hosp at Montefiore, Bronx, NY; Decision Theory and Behavioral Game Theory, Zurich, Switzerland; Columbia Univ College of Physicians and Surgeons, NY)
J Med Ethics 38:713-718, 2012

Objective.—To determine whether presenting delivery room management options as defaults influences decisions to resuscitate extremely premature infants.

Materials and Methods.—Adult volunteers recruited from the world wide web were randomised to receive either resuscitation or comfort care as the delivery room management default option for a hypothetical delivery of a 23-week gestation infant. Participants were required to check a box to opt out of the default. The primary outcome measure was the proportion of respondents electing resuscitation. Data were analysed using χ^2 tests and multivariate logistic regression.

Results.—Participants who were told the delivery room management default option was resuscitation were more likely to opt for resuscitation (OR 6.54 95% CI 3.85 to 11.11, $p < 0.001$). This effect persisted on multivariate regression analysis (OR 7.00, 95% CI 3.97 to 12.36, $p < 0.001$). Female gender, being married or in a committed relationship, being highly religious, experiences with prematurity, and favouring sanctity of life were significantly associated with decisions to resuscitate.

Discussion.—Presenting delivery room options for extremely premature infants as defaults exert a significant effect on decision makers. The information structure of the choice task may act as a subtle form of manipulation. Further, this effect may operate in ways that a decision maker is not aware of and this raises questions of patient autonomy.

Conclusion.—Presenting delivery room options for extremely premature infants as defaults may compromise autonomous decision-making.

▶ Many bioethical discussions regarding how to manage the problem of extremely premature birth when viability is highly uncertain tend to concentrate on traditional analyses of ideas like "best interests" or "nonmaleficence". Providers, especially, tend to have rather set ideas about what the available data on mortality and morbidity ought to mean when a neonate is born between 22 and 24 weeks of gestation. That is, we move rather seamlessly from fact to value and impute this to our daily clinical practice.

In this interesting study, the authors remind us that ethics is not just about getting the analysis right but also mastering the art of communication. Regardless of our informed opinions, as medical professionals who sit in positions of authority, what we say and how we say it have tremendous effects on what parents understand and what they decide. The science behind the psychology of decision making and framing effects is robust and perhaps even stronger in evidence base than much of standard neonatal practice. Yet, few physicians, in the course of their training, and even fewer neonatologists, have ever been required to study or learn how to speak carefully and reflectively in moments of high-stakes decision making with families. This is not only regrettable, it is shameful. It is also predictable. Unless and until those of us responsible for setting the agenda for our clinical practice, research, and training for the next generation begin to prioritize understanding these phenomena as much as we do the neat biological problems we face, things are destined to stay the same.

S. Sayeed, MD, JD

16 Ethics

Parents' experiences of information and communication in the neonatal unit about brain imaging and neurological prognosis: a qualitative study

Harvey ME, Nongena P, Gonzalez-Cinca N, et al (Imperial College London and Hammersmith Hosp, UK; et al)
Acta Paediatr 102:360-365, 2013

Aim.—To explore parental information and communication needs during their baby's care in the neonatal unit with a focus on brain imaging and neurological prognosis.

Methods.—Eighteen parents recruited from one neonatal unit in the United Kingdom participated in semi-structured qualitative interviews using a grounded theory approach. The topic guide focused on information received about neonatal brain imaging, diagnosis and prognosis, emotional impact and support.

Results.—Parents expressed different information needs influenced by their history, expectations, coping strategies and experiences. Most felt they initially were passive recipients of information and attempted to gain control of the information flow. Nurses were the main providers of information; doctors and other parents were also valuable. Attending ward rounds was important. Some parents felt accessing specific information such as the results of brain imaging could be difficult. Concerns about long-term developmental outcomes and the need for information did not diminish over time. The emotional impact of having a preterm baby had a negative effect on parents' ability to retain information, and all had an ongoing need for reassurance.

Conclusion.—The findings provide insights about the needs and experiences of parents who have a continuing requirement for information about their infant's care, development and prognosis.

▶ In their qualitative study of parents in a UK neonatal intensive care unit (NICU), Harvey et al have provided a concise, accessible, and illuminating view of the experience of parenting a hospitalized preterm infant. Although those of us who provide care in newborn intensive care units have frequent and diverse interactions with our patients' parents, rarely are we afforded these rich and candid insights. The study is small and limited to a single center, but this was a well-designed and conducted investigation into the parental experience of receiving and processing information about infants' brain imaging and neurologic prognosis. The report brings home a message that is easy to forget—parents want to hear from us, to know what we know, and to understand what it all means for their baby. This report also emphasizes the importance of context, using vivid descriptions of the first weeks in the NICU. It is in these early days that physicians probably spend the most time with parents, but, as we learn here, this time is turbulent and hazy, and information-sharing meetings early in NICU admission may have a much lower yield than those we could be having later on the hospital course.

This report would make an excellent addition to an educational syllabus for residents and fellows as well as for nurses and other NICU staff. I would have liked to know a bit more about the patient group represented here to help me understand how much the experiences of these parents might resemble those of the families I care for and to elucidate whether there would be value in expanding this study to a more geographically and culturally diverse group. But this critique should not detract from the lessons—that qualitative research is an excellent approach to empirical bioethics research, that empirical bioethics research in neonatology is a valuable tool to learn about our patients and their families (and improve the care we provide to them), and that we have work to do when it comes to supporting parents of premature infants.

N. Laventhal, MD, MA

The politics of probiotics: probiotics, necrotizing enterocolitis and the ethics of neonatal research

Janvier A, Lantos J, Barrington K (Sainte Justine Univ Health Ctr, Montreal, Quebec, Canada; Univ of Missouri, Kansas City, OR)
Acta Paediatr 102:116-118, 2013

There have been over twenty prospective, randomized trials of the use of probiotics to prevent necrotizing enterocolitis (NEC) in premature babies. A Cochrane meta-analysis of 16 of the studies by Khalid Al Faleh and colleagues, enrolling 2842 preterm infants, reported that "enteral probiotics supplementation significantly reduced the incidence of severe NEC (stage II or more) (typical RR 0.35, 95% CI 0.24 to 0.52) and mortality (typical RR 0.40, 95% CI 0.27 to 0.60) with no evidence of harm. They concluded, "Enteral supplementation of probiotics prevents severe NEC and all-cause mortality in preterm infants."

▶ The use of probiotics to prevent necrotizing enterocolitis (NEC) is not routine in the United States, yet it is routine in many other parts of the world. Evidence exists to support their use, yet most of the evidence is not homegrown, which complicates matters, as the authors point out in this brief, insightful commentary.

Provincial though it sounds, it might be ethically defensible to argue that we need local studies using locally, readily available probiotics to try and prevent locally generated NEC before adopting widespread use locally. However, we should all lament (and not confuse as providing a sound ethical argument) the current commercialized US regulatory and research environment that makes it difficult to conduct such studies.

If the authors are correct, and we never get to the point at which we can systematically evaluate the utility of probiotics to prevent one of the major causes of morbidity and mortality in our premature population—primarily because of free market considerations—we might need to reconsider our claim that our primary allegiance in academic medicine is to our neonatal patients. It is one thing to call for more contextually relevant evidence and quite another to collectively fail to advocate for a less-encumbered process that would permit us to carry out the necessary studies.

In the meantime, the authors are correct to highlight practical problems that we might anticipate facing—as our patients' families bring more Internet evidence to the clinical neonatal intensive care unit (NICU) encounter. One thing seems predictable: parents who are inquisitive enough to learn that there is a treatment that may reduce the incidence of NEC that is used in European and Asian NICUs are not likely to be satisfied with an excuse that sounds like regulatory red tape.

S. A. Sayeed, MD, JD

Which newborn infants are too expensive to treat? Camosy and rationing in intensive care
Wilkinson D (Univ of Adelaide, North Adelaide, South Australia, Australia)
J Med Ethics 2013 [Epub ahead of print]

Are there some newborn infants whose short- and long-term care costs are so great that treatment should not be provided and they should be allowed to die? Public discourse and academic debate about the ethics of newborn intensive care has often shied away from this question. There has been enough ink spilt over whether or when for the infant's sake it might be better not to provide life-saving treatment. The further question of not saving infants because of inadequate resources has seemed too difficult, too controversial, or perhaps too outrageous to even consider. However, Roman Catholic ethicist Charles Camosy has recently challenged this, arguing that costs should be a primary consideration in decision-making in neonatal intensive care.

In the first part of this paper I will outline and critique Camosy's central argument, which he calls the 'social quality of life (sQOL)' model. Although there are some conceptual problems with the way the argument is presented, even those who do not share Camosy's Catholic background have good reason to accept his key point that resources should be considered in intensive care treatment decisions for all patients. In the second part of the paper, I explore the ways in which we might identify which infants are too expensive to treat. I argue that both traditional personal 'quality of life' and Camosy's 'sQOL' should factor into these decisions, and I outline two practical proposals.

▶ The "R" word remains dirty in the United States, despite the fact that we ration health care goods and services every minute of every day in this country.

Rationing is best understood as "the allocation of health care resources in the face of limited availability, which necessarily means beneficial interventions are withheld from some individuals."[1] We cannot deny that we already ration in the neonatal intensive care unit (NICU). Not every neonate who might benefit from both small and large interventions receives them. We make clinical decisions that most often reflect our expert judgment about what kinds of treatments and interventions to offer our patients or potential patients. But, we also have a nagging tendency to disguise all sorts of considerations ripe with subjective value judgment (eg, quality of life) into our purportedly objective clinical judgment calculus. That such decisions are understood and conveyed as reflective of our considered clinical judgment does not deny that they are still rationing decisions. Our clinical judgments incorporate implicit risk-benefit and cost-benefit analyses that are systematically biased toward one particular—but not the only plausible—view of benefit.

Wilkinson's commentary on rationing in the NICU is worth a close read because it forces us to acknowledge and address some unspoken and uncomfortable truths. As a profession, many of us want to openly talk with society about the cost of intensive care and the efficient use of resources—both within the NICU and at the other end of the age spectrum. However, we feel prohibited from doing so because of the primacy of individual autonomy in our modern bioethical and legal discourse. The notion of denying a potential benefit to a few for the sake of many remains public anathema, so we carry on in private, continuing to do a disservice not only to our patient families but also ourselves in the process. There are no easy solutions and no single one will satisfy all stakeholders. However, as a society, we need to get over pretending that we live in a world of infinite health care goods and services.

S. Sayeed, MD, JD

Reference

1. Brock DW. Health care resource prioritization and rationing—why is it so difficult? *Soc Res.* 2007;74:125-148.

The Experience of Families With Children With Trisomy 13 and 18 in Social Networks

Janvier A, Farlow B, Wilfond BS (Univ of Montreal, Quebec, Canada; Patients for Patient Safety Canada, Mississauga, Ontario; Univ of Washington School of Medicine, Seattle)

Pediatrics 130:293-298, 2012

Background.—Children with trisomy 13 and trisomy 18 (T13-18) have low survival rates and survivors have significant disabilities. For these reasons, interventions are generally not recommended by providers. After a diagnosis, parents may turn to support groups for additional information.

Methods.—We surveyed parents of children with T13-18 who belong to support groups to describe their experiences and perspectives.

Results.—A total of 503 invitations to participate were sent and 332 questionnaires were completed (87% response rate based on site visits, 67% on invitations sent) by parents about 272 children. Parents reported being told that their child was incompatible with life (87%), would live a life of suffering (57%), would be a vegetable (50%), or would ruin their family (23%). They were also told by some providers that their child might have a short meaningful life (60%), however. Thirty percent of parents requested "full" intervention as a plan of treatment. Seventy-nine of these children with full T13-18 are still living, with a median age of 4 years. Half reported that taking care of a disabled child is/was harder than they expected. Despite their severe disabilities, 97% of parents described their child as a happy child. Parents reported these children enriched their family and their couple irrespective of the length of their lives.

Conclusions.—Parents who engage with parental support groups may discover an alternative positive description about children with T13-18. Disagreements about interventions may be the result of different interpretations between families and providers about the experiences of disabled children and their quality of life.

▶ Children afflicted with trisomy 13 or 18 (T13-18) do not flourish by most sensible renditions of the term and their lives are invariably shortened. These are the statistical facts. The truth is there is very little we can do as doctors to change these probabilities and this, no doubt, frustrates us.

In the pursuit of an ever-better evidence base, our conventional professional values often embed inside what appear to be robust empirical probabilities. Health care providers, trained in curing or minimizing disease, are inclined to understand and interpret the evidence in a predictably normative manner. The probabilities are so overwhelmingly suggestive of some outcome, that the only reasonable conclusion about what to do must be this or that. However, it is precisely when we fail to make transparent not only our values, but also what drives our prioritization of these values over others, that the potential for ethical conflict arises. The authors of this provocative article remind us of this by drawing our attention back to the families who have little choice in who they get to deal when facing these profound dilemmas.

(T13-18) are genetic descriptions of clinical diagnoses that affect real children and their families. These family narratives challenge us to reconsider—to what the fact of severe life diminishment morally equates. No one could plausibly have an interest in being afflicted with (T13-18), but it is a distinct and different question to ask whether living with that affliction is worse than death. The fact is we cannot know. The facts are also that some children do survive for some period, are nurtured by informed parents who shower them with affection, and appear to have lives filled with meaningful joys rather than constant suffering.

The question we must ask ourselves is: What makes it unreasonable for a parent who is informed of the predicted outcomes to nevertheless believe that such a compromised human life is better than immediate death? Critically, we should accept with a measure of humility that even really thoughtful physicians possess no unique or superior moral insight into this hard question.

Finally, it deserves mention that although it may be an imprudent use of resources to provide life-sustaining treatment to those who have no chance for a flourishing human life in the fullest sense, this is not an argument that is grounded in best interests analysis, tempting though it is to disguise it as such. If we want to have a debate about distributive justice, about who among us should get medical therapy when we face scarcity, we should do it transparently and with honesty about why and when devaluing some human lives over others might make ethical sense.

S. A. Sayeed, MD, JD

Medical practice and legal background of decisions for severely ill newborn infants: viewpoints from seven European countries
Sauer PJJ, On behalf of the European Neonatal EoL Study group 2010 (Univ Med Ctr Groningen, the Netherlands; et al)
Acta Paediatr 102:e57-e63, 2013

Aim.—To comparing attitudes towards end-of-life (EOL) decisions in newborn infants between seven European countries.

Methods.—One paediatrician and one lawyer from seven European countries were invited to attend a conference to discuss the practice of EOL decisions in newborn infants and the legal aspects involved.

Results.—All paediatricians/neonatologists indicated that the best interest of the child should be the leading principle in all decisions. However, especially when discussing cases, important differences in attitude became apparent, although there are no significant differences between the involved countries with regard to national legal frameworks.

Conclusion.—Important differences in attitude towards neonatal EOL decisions between European countries exist, but they cannot be explained solely by medical or legal reasons.

▶ "Not on one strand are all life's jewels strung."—William Morris

The combination of an emphasis on evidence-based medicine and improving the quality of care along with better data collection has led to an increased recognition of the variability of care that is provided. In some situations, there is clear cause for concern and need for improvement. For example, pneumococcal vaccination rates for unvaccinated adult patients with pneumonia ranged from less than 45% of patients in one region of the United States to more than 95% in another. In other situations, such as end-of-life (EOL) decisions for neonates, there also appears to be variability, likely caused by cultural, ethical, and legal factors.

In this study, the authors look at the factors involved in decision making for EOL care for neonates in 7 European countries (Belgium, France, Germany, Italy, Portugal, Sweden, and the Netherlands). They do so through a 2-day invitational conference with a pediatrician representative and health lawyer representative from each country. At the meeting, medical participants presented the national opinion of their country on neonatal EOL care. Although all the pediatricians agreed that the best interests of the neonate "should be the leading principle in all decisions regarding continuation or forgoing of treatment," there was major variation in clinical practice. In the Netherlands, neonatal euthanasia is condoned under certain circumstances, whereas in Italy, treatment is continued in all cases until the infant dies. The topic was explored further on the second day of the conference when 4 relevant cases were discussed. Once again, there was variation in care. An infant with severe epidermolysis bullosa whose parents wish for active euthanasia might have their wishes respected in the Netherlands, France, Belgium, and Germany. It would never happen in Sweden, Italy, and Portugal.

As the authors note, the main issue is whether "differences in attitude regarding EOL decisions in newborn infants in Europe [is] a problem that needs to be solved?" It is highly unlikely that there is complete consensus on these controversial issues even within the countries. One of the cases presented involved resuscitation of a 23-week-old infant, with different countries having different responses. Studies in the US have similarly shown a variation in opinion among neonatologists on what to do in this situation.[1-3] Variation in these situations may be appropriate as long as there is a continued dialogue and always a compassionate, humanistic approach toward the baby and family.

J. Fanaroff, MD, JD

References

1. Wennberg JE. Time to tackle unwarranted variations in practice. *BMJ.* 2011;342: d1513.
2. Sauer P, Dorscheidt J, Verhagen A, Hubben JH. Medical practice and legal background of decisions for severely ill newborn infants: viewpoints from seven European countries. *Acta Paediatr.* 2013;102:e57-e63.
3. Singh J, Fanaroff J, Andrews B, et al. Resuscitation in the "grey zone" of viability: determining physician preferences and predicting infant outcomes. *Pediatrics.* 2007;120:519-526.

Maternal autonomy and low birth weight in India
Chakraborty P, Anderson AK (Univ of Georgia, Athens)
J Womens Health (Larchmt) 20:1373-1382, 2011

Background.—The prevalence of low birth weight (LBW) is a major public health issue in India (30.0%) and is the highest among South-Asian countries. Maternal autonomy or the mother's status in the household indicates her decision-making power with respect to movement, finance, healthcare use, and other household activities. Evidence suggests that autonomy of the mother is significantly associated with the child's nutritional status. Although previous studies in India reported the determinants of LBW, literature on the association between mother's autonomy and birth weight are lacking. This study, therefore, aims to examine the influence of maternal autonomy on birth weight of the newborn.

Methods.—The study, a secondary data analysis, examined data from the 2005-2006 National Health and Family Survey (NFHS 3) of India. A maternal autonomy score was created through proximal component factor analysis and categorized as high, medium, and low autonomy levels. The main outcome variable included birth weight of the index child obtained from health cards and mother's recall. Descriptive and logistic regression analyses were performed.

Results.—Results from the study indicate that 20.0% of the index children included in the analysis were born at LBW. Low maternal autonomy was an independent predictor of LBW (odds ratio [OR] 1.28, 95% confidence interval [CI] 1.07-1.53, $p = 0.007$) after adjusting for other factors, and medium autonomy level was not significant.

Conclusions.—These findings clearly indicate the importance of empowering women in India to combat the high incidence of LBW.

▶ The low birth weight (LBW) incidence of nearly 27% in South Asia is a major health issue. This innovative study is an important reminder that the social determinants of health must be addressed if any headway is to be made in combating such health issues.

A secondary analysis of India's National Family Health Survey data examined 14 407 mothers and their infants' measured birth weight and interviewed 33 881 mothers for their perception of their infants' birth size. (Half of the deliveries in India are outside health care institutions and infants are therefore not weighed, yet a consistent relationship between the infant's birth weight and the mother's assessment of birth size has been shown.)

For this study, a composite maternal autonomy score was derived from four dimensions regarding participants' responses to who had the final say on their own health care, on making large household purchases, on making purchases for daily needs, and on visits to family and relatives.

It is certainly not a surprising finding that low maternal autonomy is an independent predictor of LBW and unfavorable birth outcomes, after adjusting for many other coexisting factors. This study is a powerful reminder that programs aimed at combating LBW infants need to consider women's status and decision-making autonomy as an independent determinant to be addressed. A similar study from Nepal is further emphasis that a mother's literacy and involvement in health care decision making are the most powerful means of reducing infant mortality.[1]

J. Hellmann, MBBCh, FCP(SA), FRCPC, MHSc

Reference

1. Adhikari R, Sawangdee Y. Influence of women's autonomy on infant mortality in Nepal. *Reprod Health.* 2011;8:7-14.

Article Index

Chapter 1: The Fetus

Chapter 2: Epidemiology and Pregnancy Complications

Chapter 3: Genetics and Teratology

Chapter 4: Labor and Delivery

Chapter 5: Infectious Disease and Immunology

Chapter 8: Central Nervous System and Special Senses

Chapter 9: Behavior and Pain

Chapter 10: Gastrointestinal Health and Nutrition

Chapter 11: Hematology and Bilirubin

Chapter 12: Renal, Metabolism, and Endocrine Disorders

Chapter 13: Miscellaneous

Chapter 14: Pharmacology

Chapter 15: Postnatal Growth and Development/Follow-up

Chapter 16: Ethics

Author Index

A

Abele J, 40, 41
Aby J, 206
Ades A, 51
Agakidis C, 177
Ah Mew N, 244
Al-Hosni M, 17
Allegro D, 224
Amon E, 17
Anderson AK, 295
Anderson D, 195
Andrade C, 265
Ang JY, 143
Argyri I, 235
Athanasakos EP, 285
Audibert F, 13
Ayers K, 178
Azad MB, 158

B

Badger GJ, 247, 249
Baird R, 252
Ballard RA, 259
Bancalari E, 99
Barrington K, 290
Bartholoma NM, 70
Bartz BH, 153
Bassareo PP, 86
Bauer LA, 259
Bauserman MS, 63
Beal J, 171
Bear KA, 29
Bebbington MW, 7
Becker KC, 58
Been JV, 172
Bellant J, 171
Benjamin DK, 58
Benkoe T, 170
Bennett NJ, 70
Bhatia J, 195
Bhutani VK, 222
Bin-Nun A, 231
Bingham P, 46
Binkhorst M, 106
Boivin A, 13
Bonifacio SL, 238, 239
Bora S, 129
Bos AF, 216
Bosschaart N, 225
Bouman K, 11

Boylan GB, 123
Braga LH, 236
Bresnahan M, 193
Brocklehurst P, 282
Bromiker R, 231
Brouwers HAA, 180
Browning KR, 43
Brunskill G, 241
Brynjarsson H, 103
Buiter HD, 11
Burgos AE, 206

C

Cabrera-Rubio R, 164, 204
Caeymaex L, 150
Caldwell DM, 16
Campbell DM, 219
Canpolat FE, 97
Cantalupo G, 281
Carletti A, 8
Carpenter JH, 247, 249
Castellano A, 254
Chakraborty P, 295
Chang T, 118, 119
Chen Y, 178
Cheong JL, 273
Chor CM, 14
Chu TC, 262
Claesson R, 207
Clark CAC, 129
Claure N, 84, 99
Cogo PE, 98
Collado MC, 164, 204
Contro E, 8
Corkins MR, 196
Cowan FM, 132
Cui S, 33
Czaba C, 113

D

Däbritz J, 169
Danhaive O, 98
Danzer E, 7
Dassler A-M, 148
Davies MJ, 25
Davis JS, 108
Davis MM, 67
D'Costa W, 109

De Buyst J, 78
de Melo Bezerra CT, 233
de Zegher F, 185
Dedhia K, 140
Dempsey EM, 123
DePass K, 31
Derikx JPM, 168
Di Fiore JM, 136
Diaz M, 185
Domar AD, 4
Donovan EF, 64
Doyle LW, 272
Dunlop AL, 279
Duty SM, 250
Dyer JA, 255

E

Edwards EM, 46
Edwards WH, 65
Erdeve O, 97
Espinosa-Martos I, 190

F

Fajardo MF, 84
Fallon EM, 175
Farlow B, 292
Farrokhyar F, 236
Feng Y, 20
Fergusson DA, 212, 215
Flaherman VJ, 206
Flidel-Rimon O, 57
Flore G, 86
Forrest CB, 283
Friedberg I, 161

G

Galstyan S, 57
Gandolfi Colleoni G, 8
Ganguli K, 166
Gibbins KJ, 43
Gleiss A, 170
Gomez P, 9
Gómez de Segura A, 190
Gonzalez-Cinca N, 289
Gothwal S, 37

Printed and bound by CPI Group (UK) Ltd, Croydon, CR0 4YY

08/05/2025

01864755-0010